THE ERA OF GLOBAL RISK

The Era of Global Risk

An Introduction to Existential Risk Studies

Edited by
SJ Beard, Martin Rees, Catherine Richards, and
Clarissa Rios Rojas

OpenBook
Publishers

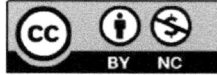

ISBN Paperback: 978-1-80064-786-2
ISBN Hardback: 978-1-80064-787-9
ISBN Digital (PDF): 978-1-80064-788-6
ISBN Digital ebook (epub): 978-1-80064-789-3
ISBN XML: 978-1-80064-791-6
ISBN HTML: 978-1-80064-792-3
DOI: 10.11647/OBP.0336

Cover image: Anirudh, *Our Planet* (October 14, 2021), https://unsplash.com/photos/Xu4Pz7GI9JY. Cover design by Jeevanjot Kaur Nagpal.

Table of Contents

Preface

Martin Rees

This book is about our entire planet's future. The stakes have never been higher. The Earth has existed for 45 million centuries, but this is the first century in which one dominant species—ours—can determine, for good or ill, the future of the entire biosphere. Over most of history, the benefits we garner from the natural world have seemed an inexhaustible resource; the worst terrors humans confronted—floods, earthquakes, and diseases—came from nature too. But we are now deep in the 'Anthropocene' era. The human population, now exceeding eight billion, makes collective demands on energy and resources that are not sustainable without new technology and threaten irreversible changes to the climate. Novel technologies—especially bio and cyber—are socially transformative, but open up the possibility of severe threats if misapplied. The worst threats to humanity are no longer 'natural' ones; they are caused (or at least aggravated) by us.

Moreover, the world is far more interconnected by travel, the internet and supply chains; a disaster in one region will cascade globally.

Despite the concerns, there are some countervailing grounds for optimism. For most people in most nations, there has never been a better time to be alive, thanks to advances in health, agriculture, and communication, which have boosted the Global South as well as the northern world. Everyday life has been transformed in less than two decades by mobile phones, social media, and the internet; we would have been far less able to cope with recent shutdowns without these facilities. Computers double their power every two years. Gene-sequencing is a million times cheaper than it was 20 years ago: spin-offs

    https://doi.org/10.11647/OBP.0336.12

from genetics could soon be as pervasive as those we've already seen from the microchip.

And this optimism about science need not be eroded by COVID-19. Indeed, in dealing with this globe-spanning plague, science has been our salvation. The response has shown the scientific community's strengths—a colossal worldwide effort to develop and deploy vaccines, combined with honest efforts to keep the public informed. The crucial role of the underlying science—and the 'scenario planning' needed to minimise the likelihood of bio- and cyber- catastrophes—are key themes of the present book.

The challenges to governance posed by COVID-19 were unprecedented (at least in peacetime) in their urgency, impact, and global scope; 'experts' had to engage with politicians and the wider public in order to overcome them. But the world would have coped far better had there been more planning and preparedness at international levels. And there are conjectural threats—engineered pandemics and massive cyber attacks, for instance—that could create at least equal devastation at any time. Indeed, their probability and potential severity is increasing. COVID-19 must act as a wake-up call, reminding us—and our governments—of our vulnerabilities.

Looming over the world in this century is the threat of climate change. This is potentially a 'global fever', in some ways resembling a slow-motion version of COVID-19. For instance, both crises aggravate the level of inequality within and between nations. Those in megacities in the majority of the world can't isolate from rogue viruses; medical care is minimal, and they are less likely to have access to vaccines. Likewise, it is those countries, and the poorest people in them, that will suffer most from global warming and the subsequent effects on food production and water supplies. Climate change and environmental degradation may well, later this century, have global consequences that are even graver than pandemics and could last longer (or, indeed, be irreversible). So too could the loss of biodiversity, leading to mass extinctions. Many, from Pope Francis downward, believe that the natural world's diversity has value in its own right, quite apart from its crucial importance for us humans.

But a potential slow-motion catastrophe doesn't engage our public and politicians: our predicament resembles that of the proverbial boiling frog, content in a warming tank until it's too late to save itself. We fail to prioritise prevention and countermeasures, because their worst impact stretches beyond the time-horizon of political and investment decisions. Politicians recognise a duty to prepare for floods, terrorist acts, and other risks that are likely to materialise in the short term—and are localised within their own domain. But unless there is a clamour from voters, they have minimal incentive to address longer-term threats that aren't likely to occur while they're still in office—and which are global rather than local.

And of course most of the challenges are global. Coping with COVID-19 is plainly a global challenge. Similarly, the threats of potential shortages of food, water, and natural resources—and the challenge of transitioning to low carbon energy—can't be overcome by each nation separately. Nor can the regulation of potentially threatening innovations, especially those spearheaded by globe-spanning conglomerates. Indeed, a key issue is to what extent, in a 'new world order', nations will need to yield more sovereignty to new organisations along the lines of the IAEA, WHO, etc. And how do we manage the tension between privacy, security, and freedom in a world where small groups (or even a malign individual) empowered by bio or cyber technology could cause global devastation?

Scientists have an obligation to promote beneficial applications of their work in meeting these global challenges. Their input is crucial in helping governments decide wisely which scary scenarios—ecothreats or risks from misapplied technology—can be dismissed as science fiction, and how best to avoid the serious ones. We also need the insights of social scientists to help us envisage how human society can flourish in a networked and AI-dominated world.

The case for intense study of these extreme threats is compelling. But, until recently, they received minimal attention—far less than has been devoted to 'routine' accidents. Unless voters speak up, governments won't properly prioritise the study of mega-threats that could jeopardise the very survival of future generations. So scientists must enhance their leverage by involvement with NGOs, via blogging and journalism, and by enlisting charismatic individuals and the media to amplify their voices and change the public mindset. It is encouraging to witness the number of activists increasing, especially the young—who can hope to live into the 22nd century. Their campaigning is welcome. Their commitment gives grounds for hope.

These areas of study, crucial to the world's future, are still underprioritised in the world of academia and policy studies. I am glad that my university, Cambridge, is one of a still-small number that has created a Centre for the Study of Existential Risks (CSER). Staffed by idealistic young researchers, with expertise spanning natural and social sciences, the CSER has helped to deepen and solidify our understanding of this crucial agenda, and has thereby gained traction with policymakers.

This book, marking the 10th anniversary of CSER's foundation— and written in collaboration with experts from other centres—offers a perspective on the key topics, in a clear format and style which we hope will spread an informed awareness of the epochal issues that it addresses.

I am an astronomer, and would like to close with a cosmic perspective. Our Earth—this tiny 'pale blue dot' in the cosmos—is a special, maybe even unique, place. We are its stewards during an especially crucial era. That is an important message for us all.

We need to think globally, we need to think rationally, we need to think long-term—we need to be 'good ancestors', empowered by 21st-century technology but guided by values that science alone cannot provide. This book should provide some grounding for these aspirations.

Introduction

SJ Beard, Martin Rees, Catherine Richards, and
Clarissa Rios Rojas

We are living in an era of global risk. While policymakers were once able to focus exclusively on the risks facing their particular constituency—be that a country, corporation, community, or institution—now, everybody must take account of the threats that endanger humanity as a whole. These come in many forms, from global-scale natural disasters (like volcanic super-eruptions) to anthropogenic environmental destabilisation (like climate change and loss of biosphere integrity), and from calamities that spread rapidly around our highly networked planet (like viruses and cyber threats) to the development of novel technologies with high destructive potential (such as artificial intelligence and biotechnologies). Reflecting this trend, the recent sixth edition of the United Nations Global Assessment Report on Disaster Risk Reduction, *Our World at Risk*, calls on member states for transformative governance that will lead to a resilient future, particularly given the increased occurrence and intensity of disasters. Similarly, the UN Secretary General's report, '*Our Common Agenda*', seeks to centralise the initiatives needed for better management to major global risks within discussions of global policy and governance.

One of the most prominent advocates for the importance of global risk has been the World Economic Forum, who defines a global risk as "the possibility of the occurrence of an event or condition that, if it occurs, could cause significant negative impact for several countries or industries". Since 2006, the Forum's annual *Global Risk Report*, based on a comprehensive risk perception survey of its members and stakeholders,

 https://doi.org/10.11647/OBP.0336.13

has provided something of a barometer showing which risks are of greatest concern. For instance, their inaugural report found that:

> The 2006 risk landscape is dominated by high impact headline risks, such as terrorism and an influenza pandemic, which top the global risk mitigation agenda and are increasingly well understood. Other risks, like climate change, whose cumulative impact will only be felt over the longer term, have begun to move to the centre of the policy debate and may offer the greatest challenges for global risk mitigation in the future.[1]

However, by the time of its most recent 2022 edition, the focus of the report has shifted markedly, now finding that over the next five years, leaders are most concerned about societal risks (such as social cohesion, livelihood, and mental health) and environmental risks, but that "over a 10-year horizon, the health of the planet dominates concerns: environmental risks are perceived to be the five most critical long-term threats to the world as well as the most potentially damaging to people and planet".[2] One trend that can be observed in this shift in risk perception is a long-term move away from concern about external threats we need to secure ourselves against (such as specific viruses or terrorism) and towards systemic risks that we, as human beings, are creating for ourselves, through poor governance, short-termism, and a too narrow focus on economic productivity.

Such a shift is very much in line with the developing understanding of global risk at the Centre for the Study of Existential Risk, located at the University of Cambridge. However, our concern is not simply to understand what risks decision-makers are most concerned by, but which ones they should be more concerned about, and what they need to do to mitigate those risks. There is an increasingly rich vocabulary for understanding global risks,[3] and with this, it has become clear that not all risks are the same. Some are also 'extreme', both in the sense that they involve extreme amounts of harm and that they could push global systems outside of their 'normal operating space'.[4] Within this class, two further subcategories have received particular attention. Global catastrophic risks (GCRs) involve events with one or more of the following characteristics: (a) "sudden, extraordinary, widespread disaster beyond the collective capability of national and international governments and the private sector to control";[5] (b) significant harm at the global scale, such as a large and sudden reduction in the global population,[6] and/or (c) a failure of critical global systems,[7] including the cluster of sociotechnological systems we sometimes call 'human civilisation'. Finally, existential risks are those with the very worst potentialities, usually understood to involve either the extinction of humanity[8] or "the permanent and drastic destruction of its potential for desirable future development" (according to some assumptions about what desirable futures might be).[9] While these two are often conflated, it might be best to separate them into extinction risk and existential risk.[10]

There are many reasons why we should be especially concerned about extreme global risks, global catastrophic risks, and existential risks. Moral philosophers have argued that we have the strongest possible moral duty to mitigate these risks, whether on utilitarian,[11] idealist,[12] agent-centred,[13] or social-contract-based[14] grounds. Psychologists have also shown how people are systemically biased towards downplaying and ignoring these risks, and thus we need to work hard if we are to overcome these biases and give the risks the attention they deserve.[15] However, increasingly, we can also see that paying attention to risks such as these has tremendous practical importance. It seems likely that the current level of these risks is such that they could significantly impact the lives and futures of many people who are alive today, as well as being a significant threat to the long-term goals of many kinds of institution, from governments and charities to investors and corporations. In this book, we will not pay much attention to the reasons why one should focus on extreme global risks. Instead, we simply note that, if given the choice, most people would unquestionably want to protect themselves and others from such risks, and thus focus on the dual questions of how to understand these risks and manage them effectively.

The following ten chapters set out a number of different approaches to thinking about global, extreme, global catastrophic, and existential risks. The first five focus on the emerging science of global risk itself and build the case for an open and creative approach to studying these risks, drawing on lessons from the past—from the rich interdisciplinary literature on social and ecological collapse, from the experiences of people working on the governance of science and technology, from discussions about global injustice, and from the diversity of human beings with an interest in safeguarding our collective future. The second set of chapters then go on to provide more detailed assessments of different risk drivers (including natural disasters, environmental breakdown, biotechnology, the potential of transformative future artificial intelligence (AI) in general, and the military application of AI in particular); the peculiar challenges to studying and mitigating each of these; and how they compare. Most, but not all, of these chapters were written by researchers affiliated to, or associated with, the Centre for the Study of Existential Risk at the University of Cambridge, and the chapters aim to provide those researchers' personal accounts of how best to think about this aspect of global risk while also engaging with, and surveying, a far broader range of literature and perspectives on the subject.

Our first chapter, 'A Brief History of Existential Risk and the People Who Worked to Mitigate It' by SJ Beard and Rachel Bronson, provides a historical account of our growing understanding of global risks and how scientists and others have worked to mitigate them. Looking back over the past 75 years, the chapter shows us how humanity has had to grapple with threats from nuclear weapons, environmental breakdown, and novel technologies to the political and technological forces that created them. However, it also surveys the many active scientific and political movements that have worked to avert disaster, as curious, compassionate, and courageous people have sought to understand these terrifying forces, bring them to wider public attention, and work to prevent human extinction and the collapse of civilisation. Using the iconic Doomsday Clock of the Bulletin of Atomic Scientists as a guide, it briefly tells the story of some of these people and organisations who sought to guide us safely through the 20th century and beyond. Understanding this history both helps us to understand the risks that continue to threaten humanity and offers opportunities to learn from the successes and failures of the past, rather than focusing only on whatever catastrophe is most immediate in our collective attention. In particular, the chapter highlights the importance of reinforcing key messages about risks, modelling extreme scenarios, managing the pace of scientific research, and placing its findings in the public domain— messages which are echoed in subsequent chapters.

The second chapter, 'Theories and Models: Understanding and Predicting Societal Collapse' by Sabin Roman, looks at what those who study global risks can learn from efforts to understand and model the process of societal and ecological collapse, which is a significant global risk in itself and also an example of the kind of extreme, non-linear, and potentially dangerous transition that is associated with extreme global risks more generally. Surveying the extensive and interdisciplinary literature on this subject, in some cases extending back several centuries, the chapter illustrates the ways in which many qualitative and quantitative modelling approaches can be applied to shed insight on the causes and nature of such collapses. Some of these approaches are primarily concerned with the exogenous causes of collapse, such as conflict or environmental catastrophes. However, other approaches view collapse as endogenous to societies themselves, originating in economic inequality or shifting societal dynamics, and it is argued that even in the presence of external causes we cannot fully understand collapse unless we take account of these endogenous effects that ultimately make societies vulnerable in the first place. Perhaps most promisingly, the chapter indicates how we can create constructive new approaches based around modelling a variety of feedback loops between different elements, and how these can be adapted to generate and test new hypotheses about social and ecological collapse (either past or future).

Chapter 3, 'Existential Risk and Science Governance' by Lalitha S. Sundaram, looks at how the governance of science might matter for the production and prevention of existential risk, and whether there are options for making science and technology less risky that are being ignored. In particular, it focuses on the ways in which scientific governance is conventionally framed within the global risk community— as something extrinsic to be regulated, with either greater top-down control to promote safety, or greater libertarian freedom to promote innovation—and highlights the potential shortcomings of this approach. As an alternative, it proposes considering scientific governance more broadly as a constellation of socio-technical processes that shape and steer technology, and argues that research culture and self-governance within science need to be seen as central to how science and technology developments play out. This alternative framing highlights many new levers at our disposal for ensuring the safe and beneficial development of technologies; overlooking such possibilities could mean robbing humanity of some of our most effective tools for mitigating global risk. The chapter ends by proposing some areas where scientists and the global risk community might together hope to influence those existing modalities, such as via education, professional bodies, two-way policy engagement, collective action, and public outreach.

Chapter 4, 'Beyond "Error and Terror": Global Justice and Global Catastrophic Risk' by Natalie Jones, serves as an invitation to consider global political, economic, social, and legal systems (particularly in relation to global justice and inequality) when studying and addressing global catastrophic risks. While the previous chapter showed how our understanding of risk was hampered by too great a focus on top-down approaches to mitigation and governance, this chapter highlights a no less important blind spot in much of the thinking about global risk: the tendency to focus more on individuals and institutions as agents of risk, and neglect the importance of systems of extraction, oppression, marginalisation, and corruption. While individuals and institutions are undoubtedly important drivers of global risk, studying global risk while ignoring global injustice can distort our understanding of risk. In contrast, adding a global justice lens onto our existing strategies helps us see the nature of risks more clearly. Furthermore, as the case of climate change shows, strategies to reduce global catastrophic risk will be more effective if they take account of global justice considerations. It follows that policies to reduce global catastrophic risk can—and should—be designed to simultaneously mitigate risk and achieve justice.

Chapter 5, 'We Have to Include Everyone: Enabling Humanity to Reduce Existential Risk' by Sheri Wells-Jensen and SJ Beard, argues for the importance of considering diversity and inclusion as integral both to a flourishing science of global risk and to efforts to mitigate such risks. Given the scale and importance of global risk, it can be tempting to believe that only the most able would be able to understand and mitigate it effectively. However, the chapter argues that such thinking is clearly mistaken. Far from being merely vulnerable and unable to help, disabled people and others who are marginalised or excluded are the real experts in vulnerability, adaptation, and resilience, and have a lot to contribute to studying and managing risks, even on the global scale. Moreover, diversity and inclusion are vital sources of creativity and insight. This chapter explores the limitations and costs of standard narratives around diversity and inclusion in global risk, and shows how the global risk community would benefit from championing inclusive futures and paying more attention to disabled people and other marginalised groups. It focuses on the benefits of diversity and inclusion across three case studies (foresight and horizon scanning, space colonisation, and bioethics) to highlight this point, while also considering the wider costs of marginalisation and exclusion to society as a whole.

Moving onto specific drivers of risk, Chapter 6, 'Natural Global Catastrophic Risks' by Lara Mani, Doug Erwin, and Lindley Johnson, considers risks from 'natural' disasters. It explores the dichotomies that are often neglected and left on the peripheries of discussions about such risks falling somewhere between hazard and vulnerability. The chapter shares a similar perspective to Chapter 2, that while the historical and geological record of such disasters can be used to study their impact, we need to consider more than just the rate of disasters as exogenous events and also take account of the factors that make societies and species more or less vulnerable to them if we are to understand the evolving nature of this risk. The chapter argues that, while humanity has lived with global-scale natural threats (such as large magnitude volcanic eruptions and Near-Earth Object impacts) throughout history, the risk of such events is currently growing due to the increasing scale and complexity of human society. Thus, while the probability of potentially catastrophic natural hazards of this kind may be relatively low, it is certainly not negligible, and the societal and economic impacts are potentially vast; however, this type of hazard is frequently underestimated in the literature. The chapter surveys the state of current thinking around extreme natural risks and asks what can be learned from efforts to reduce some of these risks (such as Planetary Defense against near-Earth objects) for improving our resilience to natural global-scale catastrophes more generally.

Chapter 7, 'Ecological Breakdown and Human Extinction' by Luke Kemp, explores the catastrophic potential of anthropogenic environmental risks, and (in particular) climate change. The chapter considers both the scale and nature of global risk from climate change and the arguments for prioritising climate mitigation as a way of reducing global risk. Reviewing the available evidence, it notes the weaknesses of certain arguments that climate change is and is not a risk with global catastrophic and existential potential. However, while there are many plausible reasons to be concerned about the catastrophic potential of climate change, it finds that attempts to argue that we should not consider climate change as being of the same severity as technological global risks often depend upon spurious notions of what a climate-induced catastrophe might involve. It then considers the appropriateness of using existing discourse around existential and global catastrophic risk to talk about climate change in the first place, given that this often frames risks in terms of their potential impact on long-term economic and technological growth, which is a questionable goal and one that (in many ways) assumes that possible ecological limits to human growth should be disregarded out of hand. Finally, however, in considering the case for climate mitigation as a global risk reduction strategy, the chapter makes the case that there is compelling evidence in favour of this, not only due to the direct impacts of climate mitigation but also the substantial co-benefits to human health and flourishing that many policies aimed at climate mitigation might provide. However, it also argues that many of the strategies proposed for climate mitigation at the global scale are problematic because they misidentify the root causes of the problem in identifying climate change as a 'tragedy of the commons' when it is actually a 'tragedy of the elite' where, as previously discussed in Chapter 4, systems of global injustice are empowering a small number of agents with the capacity to do large amounts of harm and also incentivising them to do so.

Chapter 8, 'Biosecurity, Biosafety, and Dual Use: Will Humanity Minimise Potential Harms in the Age of Biotechnology?' by Kelsey Lane Warmbrod, Kobi Leins, and Nancy Connell, discusses a number of recent advances in the life sciences that may serve to contribute to the current level of global risk (both positively and negatively), their convergence with developments in many other fields (such as AI and nanotech), and the harms that might be caused by their misuse. The chapter surveys recent developments across genomics, gain of function experiments, gene drives, synthetic biology, and AI-enabled biological research. It contrasts the rapid development and interdisciplinarity of these fields with the slow-moving pace of efforts to govern their use, often relying on the now decades-old Biological Weapons Convention. It thus emphasises the need for new approaches that fully embrace the power and flexibility of bottom-up science governance, as described in Chapter 3, and also the empowerment of communities who are often disproportionately affected by the quest for new technologies, as advocated for in Chapters 4 and 5. Grappling with the multiple potentialities of new technologies requires careful thought, but it also requires researchers and practitioners to work collectively to address the challenges we currently face as biology marches towards a global bioeconomy. This is an achievable goal but will require action to be taken soon. Urgent actions include creating and conducting a robust risk assessment methodology and implementing appropriate biosafety measures; strengthening frameworks for obtaining and enforcing consent for research, including at the community level; and requiring higher standards of interpretability for algorithms and big datasets used in biological research and the development of biotechnologies (a problem also discussed in the next chapter).

Chapter 9, 'From Turing's Speculations to an Academic Discipline: A History of AI Existential Safety' by John Burden, Sam Clarke, and Jess Whittlestone describes the development of thought related to artificial intelligence (AI) and existential risk. These risks are more likely to be realised by future AI systems with greater capabilities and generality than current systems; however, the field of AI is moving extremely swiftly and AI systems are becoming more ubiquitous in the daily lives of people around the world. Great care must, therefore, be taken to ensure these systems are safe. The chapter describes how the field of existential AI safety has matured from pure speculative concerns in the 20th century into a rigorous academic discipline of technical expertise. In particular, it focuses on the problem of *alignment*. An AI system is considered aligned if it behaves according to the values of a particular entity, such as a person, an institution, or humanity as a whole. There are many ways in which AI systems may become misaligned, or in which the need for different alignments may pull it in conflicting directions, and the problem could thus arise in a wide variety of contexts, with different but no less serious existential consequences in each of these. Just as important as our evolving understanding of the problems of AI safety, however, have been the development of new approaches to achieving AI safety and ensuring meaningful—and beneficial—human control over AI systems. Furthermore, despite the significant progress that has been made, the field remains surprisingly small, and its recent history only serves to highlight the many prospects for further development in the near future.

Finally, Chapter 10, 'Military Artificial Intelligence as a Contributor to Global Catastrophic Risk' by Matthijs M. Maas, Kayla Lucero-Matteucci, and Di Cooke, focuses specifically on the uses of AI to increase humanity's destructive capabilities within the military context. After reviewing past military GCR research and recent pertinent advancements in military AI, the chapter focuses on lethal autonomous weapons systems (LAWS) and the intersection between AI and nuclear weapons, both of which have received the most attention thus far. Regarding LAWS, it argues that, while the destructive capabilities of this technology are increasing, it is unlikely these will constitute a global catastrophic or existential risk in the near future, based primarily on current and anticipated costs and production trajectories. On the other hand, it argues that the application of AI to nuclear weapons has a significantly higher GCR potential. The chapter cites the danger of this within existing debates over when, where, and why nuclear weapons could lead to a GCR, as well as the recent geopolitical context, by identifying relevant converging global trends that may be raising the risks of nuclear warfare. The chapter turns its focus to the existing research on specific risks arising at the intersection of nuclear weapons and AI, and outlines six hypothetical areas where the use of AI systems in, around, or against nuclear weapons could increase the likelihood of nuclear escalation and result in global catastrophes. These systems include the automation of nuclear decision-making, the pressurisation of human decision-making, AI deployment in systems peripheral to nuclear weapons, AI as a threat to information security, AI as a threat to nuclear integrity, and broader impacts on strategic stability. The chapter concludes with suggestions for future directions of study, and sets the stage for a research agenda that can gain a more comprehensive and multidisciplinary understanding of the potential risks from military AI, both today and in the future.

While nowhere near fully comprehensive in scope, these chapters provide a snapshot of a rapidly evolving field: the scientific study of global risk as a phenomenon of urgent but tractable problems with global importance.[16] It is a field that, although undergoing significant growth in recent years, still remains surprisingly small and neglected. Unfortunately, it is also a field that is already showing signs of disciplinary fracture (for instance, between researchers working primarily on environmental risks and those working primarily on technological risks) that desperately needs to be understood and addressed. This book represents the first interdisciplinary survey of the topic to come out since Nick Bostrom and Milan Cirkovic's *Global Catastrophic Risks* in 2008,[17] and its intention is precisely to provide both a survey and prospectus for this science as a vibrant, open, and rigorous field of academic research. Each of these chapters presents a clear call for action and has been specially written with an educated lay audience in mind, although we submit that, given the range and nature of material being presented, they may not always be for the faint of heart. Nevertheless, we believe that, in this era where no one can ignore the threats that endanger all humanity, it is imperative that this science should be available to all, and that everyone should ask themselves: what is my role and how can I contribute to bringing the era of global risk to a close and move towards an era of global safety?

Acknowledgements

The editors of this volume would like to thank Clare Arnstein, Esmé Booth, Laura Elmer, Alice Jondorf, Jess Bland, Seán Ó hÉigeartaigh, and the staff at Open Book Publishing for invaluable assistance in preparing this volume. Many of the chapters here grew out of panel discussions from the 2020 Cambridge Conference on Catastrophic Risk at the Centre for the Study of Existential Risk and we would also like to thank Lara Mani, Catherine Rhodes, and Annie Bacon for helping to organise this as well as the other panellists and participants for their contributions. This publication was made possible through the support of a grant from Templeton World Charity Foundation, Inc. The opinions expressed in this publication are those of the author(s) and do not necessarily reflect the views of Templeton World Charity Foundation, Inc.

Notes and References

1   World Economic Forum, *Global Risks 2006* (2006).

2   World Economic Forum, *The Global Risks Report 2022: 17th Edition* (2022).

3   Cremer, Carla Zoe and Luke Kemp, 'Democratising risk: In search of a methodology to study existential risk', *arXiv preprint arXiv:2201.11214* (2021); Sundaram, Lalitha S., Matthijs M. Maas and S.J. Beard, 'From Evaluation to Action: Ethics, Epistemology and Extreme Technological Risk' in Catherine Rhodes (ed), *Managing Extreme Technological Risk. World Scientific Publishing* (forthcoming).

4   Broska, Lisa Hanna, Witold-Roger Poganietz, and Stefan Vögele, 'Extreme events defined—A conceptual discussion applying a complex systems approach', *Futures, 115* (2020), p.102490.

5   Schoch-Spana, Monica, Anita Cicero, Amesh Adalja, Gigi Gronvall, Tara Kirk Sell, Diane Meyer, Jennifer B. Nuzzo, et al. 'Global catastrophic biological risks: Toward a working definition', *Health Security, 15*(4) (2017), pp.323-328.

6   For instance: Cotton-Barratt Owen, Sebastian Farquhar, John Halstead, Stefan Schubert, and Andrew Snyder-Beattie, *Global Catastrophic Risks 2016. Global Challenges Foundation* (2016) use a 10% reduction; Kemp, Luke, Chi Xu, Joanna Depledge, Kristie L. Ebi, Goodwin Gibbins, Timothy A. Kohler, Johan Rockström et al. 'Climate Endgame: Exploring catastrophic climate change scenarios', *Proceedings of the National Academy of Sciences, 119*(34) (2022): e218146119 use a 25% reduction (while referring to risks involving a 10% reduction as 'Decimation Risks'), and Maas, Lucero-Matteucci, and Cooke (this volume) use a threshold of 1 million fatalities.

7   Avin, Shahar, Bonnie C. Wintle, Julius Weitzdörfer, Seán S. Ó hÉigeartaigh, William J. Sutherland, and Martin J. Rees, 'Classifying global catastrophic risk', *Futures, 102* (2018), pp.20-26.

8   Kemp et al. (2022).

9   Bostrom, Nick. 'Existential risks: Analyzing human extinction scenarios and related hazards,' *Journal of Evolution and Technology, 9* (2002).

10   Cremer and Kemp (2021).

11   Bostrom, Nick, 'Existential risk prevention as global priority,', *Global Policy, 4*(1) (2013), pp.15–31.

12   Parfit, Derek, *Reasons and Persons*. Oxford University Press (1984); Beard, S.J. and Patrick Kaczmarek, 'On Theory X and what matters most', *Ethics and Existence: The Legacy of Derek Parfit* (2021), p.358.

13 Scheffler, Samuel, *Why Worry About Future Generations?* Oxford University Press (2018).

14 Finneron-Burns, Elizabeth, 'What's wrong with human extinction?', *Canadian Journal of Philosophy, 47*(2–3) (2017), pp.327–43; Beard, S.J. and Patrick Kaczmarek, 'On the wrongness of human extinction', *Argumenta, 5* (2019), pp.85–97.

15 Yudkowsky, Eliezer, 'Cognitive biases potentially affecting judgement of global risks', *Global Catastrophic Risks, 1*(86) (2008), p.13.

16 One work that is foundational for both this science in general and this volume in particular was published by Martin Rees in 2003. It was originally intended that this work should be titled *Our Final Century?*; however, its publishers sought to outdo one another in making this sound more alarmist, first removing the question mark for the UK edition and then substituting 'Hour' for 'Century' for the American market. For this reason, the international group of authors behind these chapters cite this important work as both Rees, M., *Our Final Century: Will Civilisation Survive the Twenty-First Century?* Random House (2003) and Rees, M., *Our Final Hour: A Scientist's Warning.* Basic Books (2003).

17 Bostrom, Nick and Milan M. Ćirković (eds), *Global Catastrophic Risks.* OUP (2008).

1. A Brief History of Existential Risk and the People Who Worked to Mitigate It

SJ Beard and Rachel Bronson

Despite garnering significant academic, political, and public attention, the existential risks posed by nuclear weapons, environmental breakdown, and disruptive technologies continue to threaten human survival, and we may now be in a more perilous position than at any other time in history. For over 75 years we have been dragooned into unacceptable gambles by political and technological forces, and were lucky to survive thus far. However, this story has not just been about luck. Since the emergence of such risks, curious, compassionate, and courageous people (including many scientists) have sought to understand these terrifying forces, bring them to wider public attention, and work with every tool at their disposal to prevent human extinction and the collapse of civilisation. In this chapter, we seek to revisit the ups and downs of this perilous journey, using as our guide the shifting time of the Doomsday Clock, and to briefly tell the story of some of the people and organisations who sought to guide us safely through it. Understanding this history is vital, not only because these risks remain pressing, but also because it offers an opportunity for those currently working to reduce existential risk (and especially those in the nascent academic field of Existential Risk Studies) to learn from the successes and failures of the past. In particular, we show the importance of reinforcing key messages about risks and how to manage them, modelling extreme scenarios to understand them better, managing the pace of scientific

  https://doi.org/10.11647/OBP.0336.01

research, and placing its findings in the public domain. If we can learn these lessons and apply them rigorously, then history shows we can turn back the hands of the Doomsday Clock, and ensure that our future is no longer a hostage to our fortune.

The origins of our understanding of Existential Risk

People have speculated about the 'the end of the world' since the dawn of history—indeed, the oldest story that has been passed down may well be the Mesopotamian deluge myth, which tells of a flood that wiped out all but a few humans, and is familiar to most in the west through the biblical story of Noah.[1] However, such eschatological speculation has largely been bound up with religious beliefs and invariably ends with humanity continuing on Earth, in the afterlife, or via an eternal cosmic cycle of rebirth. Furthermore, as Martin Rees argued in his book *Our Final Century*:

> Throughout most of human history the worst disasters have been inflicted by environmental forces—floods, earthquakes, volcanos, and hurricanes—and by pestilence. But the greatest catastrophes of the twentieth century were directly induced by human agency.

Virtually everyone alive today is familiar (to some degree) with the anthropogenic risks that threaten global disaster, like nuclear war, climate change, and risks from disruptive technologies such as artificial intelligence (AI) and biotech. These risks are both naturalistic—in the sense that we understand how they could happen within the laws of nature—and absolute, in the sense that there may be no reprieve for humanity and no afterlife.

In fact, the very idea that humanity was vulnerable to going extinct in this way may be a relatively recent invention. It arose from the scientific discovery of prehistoric fossils and its implication of a 'deep past' during which evidence of extinctions was incontrovertible, our growing awareness that there is no great difference in kind between humans and other species, the spread of secular atheism, and the acceleration of social, scientific, and technological change.[2]

Perhaps the first group to fully express this change in thinking were authors of speculative fiction. For instance, Mary Shelley, one of the founders of science fiction, wrote *The Last Man* in 1826,[3] which tells the story of Lionel, who witnesses the death of all other humans in the last few decades of the 21st century from a series of apocalyptic events, most notably a worldwide plague. The first mention of human extinction being caused by self-improving machines comes from Samuel Butler's 1863 *Darwin Among the Machines*, later reprinted as part of his novel *Erewhon*.[4, 5] Similarly, the first discussion of the existential risk posed by atomic weaponry is arguably found in H.G. Wells's *The World Set Free*,[6] while more recently, sci-fi authors have been among the first to explore how humanity may bring about its own demise through our harmful influence on planet Earth.[7]

Such writers not only captured the popular imagination but also directly influenced academic research. H.G. Wells's 1901 book *Anticipations of the Reaction of Mechanical and Scientific Progress Upon Human Life and Thought*,[8] for instance, is a foundational text for the academic discipline of Futures Studies, a subject of vital importance to our understanding of existential risk.[9] Wells also wrote at least two non-fiction, if not entirely serious, essays on the risk of human extinction, 'On Extinction' and 'The Extinction of Man',[10] while the first book-length non-fiction work to classify and explore the entire range of possible existential catastrophes was Isaac Asimov's *A Choice of Catastrophes*.[11]

Yet, while they have a vital role in raising awareness and exploring different futures, science-fiction authors are often the first to argue for the importance of the hard science on which they draw. Thus, the true foundation of the study of existential risk belongs to a group of pioneering scientists and philosophers working during and shortly after World War II, who became concerned about several overlapping trends and developments with the potential to significantly threaten humanity's future.

The threat of nuclear weapons

Worries about the risk of a global catastrophe first gained major scientific attention after World War II, with widespread concern about nuclear weapons and their potential to wipe humanity off the face of the Earth. The speed and violence with which nuclear technology evolved was breathtaking, even to those closely involved in its development.

As early as 1939, world-renowned scientists Albert Einstein and Leo Szilard penned a letter to US President Franklin D. Roosevelt about a breakthrough in nuclear technology that was so powerful, and could have such tremendous battlefield consequences, that a single nuclear bomb, "carried by boat and exploded in a port, might very well destroy the whole port", a possibility seen as too significant for the President to ignore. A mere six years later, one such bomb was used to destroy an entire city and its population, followed by another one. A few years after that, nuclear arsenals were capable of destroying civilisation as we know it.

The first scientific concern that nuclear weapons might have the potential to end humanity as a whole appears to have come from scientists involved in the first nuclear tests, and related to whether they might accidentally ignite the Earth's atmosphere, although these concerns were quickly dismissed.[12]

However, many who worked on the Manhattan Project continued to have severe reservations about the power of the weapons they helped to produce. After successfully performing the first controlled nuclear chain reaction at the University of Chicago in 1942, confirming its potential to release energy, the team of scientists working on the Manhattan Project dispersed, with some going off to Los Alamos and other research laboratories to develop nuclear weapons, while others stayed in Chicago to undertake their own research. Many of those who stayed were themselves immigrants to the United States and were keenly aware of the intertwining of science and politics. They, with the help of colleagues, began actively organising and engaging on how to keep the future of nuclear technology safe. For instance, they helped advance the Franck report in June 1945 that foreshadowed a dangerous and costly nuclear arms race, and argued against a surprise nuclear attack on Japan. This group went on to establish the *Bulletin of the Atomic Scientists of Chicago (The Bulletin)*, whose first issue was published a mere four months after the atomic bombs were dropped on Hiroshima and Nagasaki. With support from the University of Chicago's President, Robert Hutchins, and colleagues in international law, political science, and other related fields, they helped kick off and support a global citizen-scientist movement that had a powerful effect on the creation of the global nuclear order.[13] Many of these same individuals were also instrumental in establishing the Federation of Atomic (now American) Scientists, which was located in Washington DC to ensure proximity to key decision-makers whose views they hoped to sway. In contrast, *The Bulletin*'s headquarters in Chicago focused more on engaging and educating the public about the political and ethical challenges presented by the advancement of science, which they anticipated would only accelerate in the years to come. The founders believed that public pressure was key to political responsibility, and education was the best channel to ensure it.[14]

Two years after its founding, *The Bulletin* published Martyl Langsdorf's now iconic 'Doomsday Clock' to serve as the first cover of its new magazine. Over time, the Clock became globally recognised, in part because of its simplicity and bluntness. Married to a Manhattan Project scientist, Martyl was an artist who understood the urgency and desperation her husband and colleagues felt about managing nuclear technology. She created the Clock to convey their deep concern, as well as to draw attention to their belief that responsible citizens could prevent catastrophe by mobilising and engaging. The message of the Clock is clear: humans can prevent this clock from striking midnight. In that, it provides both a challenge and some hope.

In 1949 the USSR tested its first nuclear weapons, and in reaction to this, *The Bulletin*'s editor moved the hands of the Clock from seven to three minutes to midnight. In doing so, he activated the Clock, turning it from a static to a dynamic metaphor. The clock would evolve into a symbol that, according to Kennette Benedict, former Executive Director of *The Bulletin*:

> [warns] the public about how close we are to destroying our world with dangerous technologies of our own making. It is a metaphor, a reminder of the perils we must address if we are to survive on the planet.[15]

In 1953 the clock moved to two minutes to midnight, after the United States and USSR detonated the first thermonuclear weapons (H-bombs). This was the latest the clock was ever set in the 20th century (the furthest away it has been to midnight was 17 minutes in 1991, following the end of the Cold War). The Doomsday Clock, and its now annual setting, remains perhaps the most widely recognised and oft-cited symbol of our existential predicament, as well as the most easily understood representation of our attempts to come to terms with it.

Another factor that increased both public and scientific concern about nuclear weapons was growing awareness of the risk that radioactive particles could contaminate the environment, with catastrophic effects. This theory was promoted by Hermann Muller, who discovered that radiation can induce genetic mutations and received the first post-war Nobel Prize in physiology for this work. Muller—along with Einstein, Bertrand Russell, and other prominent scientists of the day—later wrote the *Russell-Einstein Manifesto* in 1955, according to which:

> No one knows how widely such lethal radioactive particles might be diffused, but the best authorities are unanimous in saying that a war with H-bombs might possibly put an end to the human race... sudden only for a minority, but for the majority a slow torture of disease and disintegration.[16]

An important consequence of this manifesto was the establishment of the Pugwash Conferences on Science and World Affairs, which were initiated in 1957 by Russell and Joseph Rotblat, a physicist who also worked on the Manhattan Project. The Pugwash Conferences were vital for establishing communication channels at a time when Cold War tensions were at their highest, and the Conferences undertook vital background work to establish key non-proliferation treaties such as the 1963 Partial Test Ban Treaty, the 1968 Non-Proliferation Treaty, and the 1972 Biological Weapons Convention. Joseph Rotblat and the Pugwash Conferences were awarded the 1995 Nobel Peace Prize for their "efforts to diminish the part played by nuclear arms in international politics and, in the longer run, to eliminate such arms".[17] To this day, Pugwash remains the existential risk organisation with the widest global reach.[18]

Alongside these efforts of scientists, popular protest and resistance to the development, creation, and use of nuclear weapons was also vitally important. This resistance has taken many forms. For instance, in the UK, Bertrand Russell helped to establish both the Campaign for Nuclear Disarmament, a large and conventional pressure group, and the Committee of 100, a group set up specifically to perform acts of civil disobedience. He explained the need for both groups as follows:

> The Campaign for Nuclear Disarmament has done and is doing valuable and very successful work to make known the facts, but the press is becoming used to its doings and beginning to doubt their news value. It has therefore seemed to some of us necessary to supplement its campaign by such actions as the press is sure to report. There is another, and perhaps more important reason for the practice of civil disobedience in this time of utmost peril. There is a very widespread feeling that however bad their policies may be, there is nothing that private people can do about it. This is a complete mistake. If all those who disapprove of government policy were to join massive demonstrations of civil disobedience they could render government folly impossible and compel the so-called statesmen to acquiesce in measures that would make human survival possible.[19]

In founding this group, Russell established a justification for civil disobedience in the face of existential risk that remains to this day, most prominently in the Extinction Rebellion protests.

Russell was far from the only person to lead such a movement. Martin Luther King Jr and other civil rights leaders saw nuclear disarmament as essential and inextricably linked to the quest for social justice and racial equality. Many shared the view of Langston Hughes that American racism had played an important role in Harry Truman's decision to use nuclear weapons aggressively against Japanese people, and feared that they would be used selectively against non-whites in future.[20] There was also the argument that nuclear weapons were simply the latest, and most dangerous, manifestation of oppressive and destructive attitudes that marginalised groups had struggled against for centuries. As Dr King put it in his very final speech delivered at the Bishop Charles Mason Temple in Memphis on April 3rd 1968:

> Another reason that I'm happy to live in this period is that we have been forced to a point where we're going to have to grapple with the problems that men have been trying to grapple with through history, but the demands didn't force them to do it. Survival demands that we grapple with them. Men, for years now, have been talking about war and peace. But now, no longer can they just talk about it. It is no longer a choice between violence and nonviolence in this world; it's nonviolence or nonexistence.[21]

Also of great significance, but often overlooked, has been the resistance of indigenous peoples to nuclear colonialism. Indigenous lands and lives were often the first to be co-opted for the production of nuclear weapons, from being displaced to make way for nuclear test sites to being hired at low wages to work in the mining and refining of uranium and other materials at significant costs to their own health.[22]

While concerned scientists and others did much to expose the risks from nuclear weapons as they developed, the nature of these risks meant that many people, including some of those who were responsible for creating these risks, were not aware of their immediacy. For instance, the 1963 Arkhipov incident, in which a Russian submarine commander wished to use nuclear weapons in retaliation for a perceived attack during the Cuban Missile Crisis before his junior officer overruled him, remained largely unknown until 2002.[23]

Policies can—and have—made a difference in reducing risk. For instance, Robert McNamara sent a memo to President John F. Kennedy in 1963 arguing that falling production costs made it realistic to expect at least eight new nuclear powers to emerge in the next ten years, while Kennedy himself predicted that perhaps 25 nuclear weapon states would emerge by the end of the 1970s.[24] Yet nuclear powers have emerged at a far slower pace. By some estimates, up to 56 states may have, at one time or another, possessed the capability to develop a nuclear weapons programme, yet the vast majority of these either chose not to engage in nuclear weapons activity or voluntarily terminated their programmes, with only ten states ever having developed nuclear weapons of their own—one of which (South Africa) has since disarmed.[25] In this, and other ways, the various initiatives we describe here have helped to make our world safer, though it remains far from safe. One 2013 study estimated the odds of a nuclear war having occurred between 1945 and 2011 as 61%;[26] however, in truth it is likely still too early to say what our chances really were and, indeed, we may never know.

Environmental breakdown and climate change

Concerns about risks to humanity from our own environmental impacts are nothing new. In *The Epochs of Nature* (1778), Georges-Louis Leclerc, the Comte de Buffon, wrote contemptuously of those who have "ravaged the land, starve it without making it fertile, destroy without building, use everything up without renewing anything".[27] In 1821, Charles Fourier wrote *The Material Deterioration of the Planet*, concerning humanity's negative impacts on our environment and the harmful consequences for ourselves. While his theories do not match with our modern understanding of the planetary system, his concern that "we bring the axe and destruction, and the result is landslides, the denuding of mountain-sides, and the deterioration of the climate" still rings true today.[28] Similarly, Fredrich Engels noted how:

> In relation to nature, as to society, the present mode of production is predominantly concerned only about the immediate, the most tangible result. Then surprise is expressed that the more remote effects of actions directed to this end turn out to be quite different, are mostly quite the opposite in character.[29]

In 1896 Svante Arrhenius was the first to uncover the basic principles of anthropogenic climate change. As he later explained his findings to a general audience: "any doubling of the percentage of carbon dioxide in the air would raise the temperature of the earth's surface by 4°", while "the slight percentage of carbonic acid in the atmosphere may, by the advances of industry, be changed to a noticeable degree in the course of a few centuries."[30]

Yet prior to the mid-20th century, and the post-war 'great acceleration' of population, economic productivity, and environmental destruction, such concerns remained marginal. Some of the earliest general studies of the possibility for human extinction and the collapse of civilisation, including William Vogt's *Road to Survival*[31] and Fairfield Osborne's *Our Plundered Planet*,[32] linked this threat specifically to environmental harms such as soil erosion and pollution. Another pivotal early work was Rachel Carson's *Silent Spring*,[33] which not only echoed these earlier concerns, but increased their scientific rigour and added a crucial policy edge by raising public awareness about the danger from chemical pesticides, such as DDT. Carson was a marine biologist, nature writer, and pioneering conservationist who became concerned about the ecological effects of indiscriminate overuse of pesticides, which she called "biocides". As she wrote in *Silent Spring*:

> Along with the possibility of the extinction of mankind by nuclear war, the central problem of our age has ... become the contamination of man's total environment with such substances of incredible potential for harm—substances that accumulate in the tissues of plants and animals

and even penetrate the germ cells to shatter or alter the very material of heredity upon which the shape of the future depends (Carson, 1962).

A further growth in public concern about environmental harms came in 1968, when two young biologists, Paul and Anne Ehrlich, were commissioned to write *The Population Bomb*,[34] which received widespread attention in both the academic and popular press. It warned about the catastrophic impacts of overpopulation, which the Ehrlichs claimed could lead to "hundreds of millions" of deaths from starvation. Early manifestations of this concern included the founding of organisations such as Friends of the Earth and Greenpeace (both in 1969) and the first Earth Day (April 22nd 1970), which saw 20 million Americans march in cities across the country. In 1972, the Club of Rome—an organisation of scientists, economists, diplomats, government officials, and other influencers from around the world—published *The Limits to Growth*,[35] which developed the first global systems models to investigate the long-run impacts of trends in population, consumption, environmental degradation, and technology.[36] Its conclusions were stark: "If the present growth trends in world population, industrialization, pollution, food production, and resource depletion continue unchanged, the limits to growth on this planet will be reached sometime within the next one hundred years". By 1978, *The Bulletin* weighed in with a cover story asking *Is Mankind Warming the Earth?*—to which its author answered, "Yes."[37]

One of the more optimistic pronouncements within the *Limits to Growth* report was that the advent of nuclear energy might mean that the atmospheric concentration of greenhouse gases may cease to rise, "one hopes before it has had any measurable ecological or climatological effect". History has not borne this prediction out. Nor did it take long for scientists to confirm that humanity's emission of greenhouse gases was already having deleterious climatic and ecological impacts, with grave implications for our future. Less than a decade later, James Hansen led a ground-breaking study in *Science*, showing that:

> the anthropogenic carbon dioxide warming should emerge from the noise level of natural climate variability by the end of the century, and there is a high probability of warming in the 1980s. Potential effects on climate in the 21st century include the creation of drought-prone regions in North America and central Asia as part of a shifting of climatic zones,

erosion of the West Antarctic ice sheet with a consequent worldwide rise in sea level, and opening of the fabled Northwest Passage.[38]

Hansen would go on to greatly increase public awareness of the reality of climate change when he testified before the US Senate Committee on Energy and Natural Resources, although the fame of this event was as much due to attempts by the Office for Budgetary Responsibility to censor Hansen's explanation of climate models and what they indicated.[39] However, while Hansen's climate research from this period is especially well-known, he was only one part of a vast array of scientists arriving at the modern consensus about anthropogenic climate change, a consensus that was well-established by the 1980s and has only strengthened since.[40]

This consensus has helped us to achieve some impressive feats of global governance and policy change, including the formation of the Advisory Group on Greenhouse Gases in 1985, and its development into the Intergovernmental Panel on Climate Change in 1988, as well as the signing of the United Nations Framework Convention on Climate Change at the Earth Summit in Rio de Janeiro in 1992, and its subsequent amendments (such as the 1997 Kyoto Protocol and 2015 Paris Agreement). However, equally important have been the consistent efforts of a small number of vested interests to undermine this consensus and spread misinformation about climate change and other risks, limiting the impact of what might otherwise have been possible.[41] As with nuclear weapons, however, this is not a gap that scientists can bridge on their own. Support for public efforts of advocacy and resistance is also needed if progress is to be made, especially those of the people who will be worst affected by climate change, such as poor, landlocked, small island nations and marginalised and indigenous communities around the world.[42]

As public awareness of, and concern about, environmental risks facing humanity has grown, people have increasingly come to talk about nuclear weapons and climate change in the same breath as equal threats to the future of humanity. For instance, in 2007 *The Bulletin* updated their framing of the Doomsday Clock to formally recognise climate change as a factor in setting it.[43] Of course, the timescale of these risks remains quite different: a nuclear exchange could happen within minutes, while climate risk is slowly accumulating year after year. Similarly, responsibility for the world's nuclear weapons lies in the hands, or at the fingers, of only a few global decision-makers, while we are all engaged in climate change and environmental destruction, even if to a very unequal extent.[44] However, the severity of these risks— both in terms of their potential to cause global catastrophes and their likelihood of doing so—are undoubtedly comparable, and we should also assess both risks in terms of whether or not the current level of global action being taken to combat them is proportional to this severity and the rising urgency of reducing it.

The convergence of nuclear and environmental risks in the nuclear winter hypothesis

Yet, in at least one instance, concerns about environmental and nuclear risks have intertwined, and it is an event that warrants special attention as it may have been the occasion when scientific concern about existential risk most directly influenced global policy—the publication of the 'nuclear winter' hypothesis. By the early 1980s, some scientists had become worried that the greatest threat posed by nuclear conflict was not radioactivity but the massive firestorms that could inject soot into the stratosphere, blocking incoming solar radiation and causing global agricultural failures, environmental catastrophes, and maybe even human extinction. The result would be what the atmospheric scientist Richard Turco called "the nuclear winter". This hypothesis arose at a time when nuclear tensions were increasing, with events such as stalled US-USSR nuclear negotiations, rising numbers of global conflicts, and the entry of India as a nuclear weapons state, causing the Doomsday Clock to tumble forward nine minutes in 12 years and reach three minutes to midnight by 1984.

This possibility was rendered more plausible because of a study published in 1980 by Luis and Walter Alvarez that hypothesised that the non-avian dinosaurs became extinct because an asteroid struck Earth.[45] This impact threw dust into the stratosphere, blocking out sunlight and compromising photosynthesis. This hypothesis threatened the then-dominant paradigm that there is a 'balance of nature' that enforces gradual changes on life and protects the Earth from catastrophes, which had reigned for more than a century.[46] When the hypothesis was subsequently corroborated by the discovery of the Chicxulub crater on the Yucatan Peninsula, it prompted the scientific community to acknowledge that events in the past had caused globally catastrophic effects, and this raised the possibility that it might happen again, this time due to anthropogenic causes.[47]

One of the most prominent scientists who warned about nuclear winter was the cosmologist, planetary physicist, and exobiologist Carl Sagan. Sagan had gained significant scientific prominence through his research, especially in the search for extra-terrestrial life, and had a pre-eminent reputation as a science communicator through his books and TV programmes such as *Dragons in Eden* and *Cosmos*.[48] Sagan and four other scientists published an influential study modelling the possibility of nuclear winter in the journal *Science*.[49] However, he also pre-empted this publication with more popular works and media appearances to increase the potential impact of the research on politicians and the public. For instance, Sagan wrote a cover story for the October 30th edition of the popular Sunday news supplement *Parade* magazine arguing that, should a nuclear conflict occur:

> Many species of plants and animals would become extinct. Vast numbers of surviving humans would starve to death. The delicate ecological relations that bind together organisms on Earth in a fabric of mutual dependency would be torn, perhaps irreparably. There is little question that our global civilization would be destroyed. The human population would be reduced to prehistoric levels, or less. Life for any survivors would be extremely hard. And there seems to be a real possibility of the extinction of the human species.[50]

To further develop this point, Sagan joined forces with Paul Ehrlich to co-organise a two-day conference and co-author the 1984 book on the "long-term biological consequences of nuclear war," *The Cold and the Dark*.[51]

Both the research behind the nuclear winter hypothesis and the strategy for its promotion were controversial. While the hypothesis itself was plausible in many respects, the modelling used to support it was seen as quite primitive, even at the time, and debate still rages about how significant a cooling effect a limited nuclear war might have. However, the greater controversy was about the scientists' decisions to go public before their paper had been published, and harness the power of the media to get their idea across quickly. This may have been inspired (in part) by Sagan's health issues; he is said to have dictated a letter opposing Ronald Reagan's Strategic Defense Initiative (popularly known as Star Wars) from his hospital bed while recovering from an operation. However, it may also have been influenced by the involvement of Ehrlich and his earlier popular successes.

The article, along with others, certainly had an impact.[52] The work of Sagan and his counterparts harnessed public attention and helped to spur opposition to the Strategic Defense Initiative, inspire a Soviet moratorium on nuclear weapons tests in 1985, and ensure both parties continued negotiating towards the Strategic Arms Reduction Treaty (START). Soviet Premier Mikhail Gorbachev told Ronald Reagan in 1988 that Sagan was "a major influence on ending [nuclear] proliferation".[53] This was brought about by a swathe of new arms control initiatives including the 1987 Intermediate-Range Nuclear Forces Treaty (which banned all Russian and US land-based ballistic missiles with ranges between 500 and 5,500 km and saw 2,692 nuclear missiles removed from service), the 1991 signing of START (which would eventually lead to the removal of around 80% of nuclear weapons), the 1991 Presidential Nuclear Directives (that removed the vast majority of nuclear weapons out of the European theatre), and the Nunn-Lugar Cooperative Threat Reduction program (which wound down and ended the USSR's secret, illegal biological weapons programme).

These developments, together with political changes around the world at the end of the Cold War, saw a rapid improvement in humanity's existential situation, as charted by a shift of the Doomsday Clock from three minutes to midnight in 1984 to 17 minutes to midnight in 1991, the safest we had been since the end of World War II. The work of so many people to understand and draw attention to existential risks over the 20th century had undoubtedly helped to bring about this favourable state. While political leaders may have driven these outcomes, scientists provided the technical foundation and helped support a global grassroots civic effort that improved the safety and security of what Sagan evocatively described as this "pale blue dot, the only home we've ever known".[54]

The road to 90 seconds to midnight: Growing risks, disruptive technologies, and the foundation of Existential Risk Studies

Yet this positive state of affairs was not to last. A mere 12 years later, in 2003, the Doomsday Clock was back to where it began in 1947, at seven minutes to midnight. That same year, in his book *Our Final Century*, the British Astronomer Royal Martin Rees predicted that: "The odds are no better than fifty-fifty that our present civilization on earth will survive to the end of the present century."[55] Sadly, subsequent events have very much borne out such pessimism and the Doomsday Clock has continued its slide and today stands at 90 seconds to midnight, closer than it was even at the height of the Cold War. How has this happened?

One factor that has undoubtedly contributed to this massive decline in fortune has been the continued emergence of new kinds of threats. The pages of *The Bulletin* have long considered the challenges posed by new disruptive technologies, and these have recently been adopted as a third contributing factor when setting the Doomsday Clock.[56] Scientists first identified technological threats to human survival decades ago, including those associated with AI,[57] biological weapons,[58] nanotechnology,[59] and high-energy physics experiments.[60, 61] As well as threats from specific technologies, many have also come to see that our future is increasingly imperilled by the convergence of disruptive technologies with existing nuclear and environmental threats. These discoveries in turn precipitated the gradual formation of a dedicated academic discipline for studying existential risk, such as the publication of *Our Final Century* and the establishment of new research institutes like the Future of Humanity Institute, the Future of Life Institute, the Global Catastrophic Risk Institute, and the Centre for the Study of Existential Risk.[62] Many of these centres originated out of a view that transformative technologies were necessary precisely because they were required to help humanity reach a more safe and beneficial future, by giving us greater control over our environment, our societies, and ourselves, but that we could only achieve this if we could find out how to develop them safely. However, this original vision has now been joined by many other ways of understanding existential risks and how to manage them, such as by applying lessons from disaster studies[63] and security studies,[64] viewing risks from a global systems perspective,[65] placing risk mitigation in a broader policy context,[66] and identifying opportunities to increase global resilience.[67]

As the number and variety of threats facing humanity has multiplied, so has the seriousness of the challenges posed by nuclear and environmental risks. By 2015 *The Bulletin* had moved its Doomsday Clock from five to three minutes to midnight. There were three key issues behind this move. Firstly, deteriorating relations between the US and Russia—who together possess 90% of the world's nuclear arsenal—and the actual and threatened dismantling of many of the Cold War instruments designed to keep those arsenals safe, such as the successor to the START treaty (New START).[68] Secondly, every major nuclear state was investing massively in its nuclear weapons systems, including replacement, expansion, and modernisation.[69] Finally, the global architecture needed to address climate threats was nowhere in sight.

In 2016 *The Bulletin*'s science and security board identified two possible bright spots, with the potential to reverse some of these negative trends: the Iran nuclear deal and the Paris climate agreement. However, they also noted that both agreements still had to be implemented, and in 2017 were forced to conclude that the situation had significantly worsened, with both of these bright spots being dimmed by changes in US domestic politics and growing evidence of a global disparagement of expertise and a recklessness about nuclear language and leadership. They thus moved the clock to two and a half minutes to midnight, and in 2018 moved it further to two minutes to midnight due to the continuing deterioration of international diplomacy.

In 2020, *The Bulletin* moved the clock closer to midnight than it has ever been before, a decision also endorsed by researchers at the Centre for the Study of Existential Risk.[70] Above all, the new time reflected the sheer instability of the current global situation, and the failure of international institutions to respond to the ticking clock of existential risk, including the collapse of the Intermediate Nuclear Forces Treaty that had marked the beginning of the end of the Cold War itself. We are back to a global political situation that is akin to what it was during the Cold War, and yet the risks we face now are so much more numerous and complex. If we are to turn back the Clock, we need a new wave of foresight, creativity, engagement, and education to study and manage these risks. Sadly, recent events such as the COVID-19 pandemic and Russian invasion of Ukraine indicate that the scale of this challenge may only be growing, and this was recognised when, just a few days before this chapter went to press, *The Bulletin* moved the clock further forward to 90 seconds to midnight.

Learning from the pioneers of existential risk

How can studying the history of existential risk help us succeed in mitigating it? For one thing, it helps those fighting for humanity to focus on our long-term goals and the need for lasting safety, rather than getting stuck passing from urgent crisis to urgent crisis with only transient respites (like the one experienced at the end of the Cold War).

There are also more specific things we can learn from this history. First, certain key messages require constant reinforcement, such as that global catastrophes are a real possibility against which we have no fundamental protection. There have been times in the past, such as during the Cuban Missile Crisis, when politicians took these messages to heart, such as by frequently reiterating that "a nuclear war can never be won and must never be fought", but evidence suggests that this does not last. Second, if we are to understand these catastrophes we will have to engage in some speculation and modelling, such as that which was used to develop the nuclear winter hypothesis, as it will be too costly to wait until we can observe disasters directly. Third, if we are to prevent these catastrophes then we need to place this science in the public domain and be willing to publicly advocate for it, even if that is (at times) difficult or controversial, and especially if it involves working across cultural, geographical, or political divides, as the Pugwash Conferences were able to. Fourth, scientists and their allies must be called on repeatedly to attest to the fact that our current pace of scientific and technological development carries risks as well as benefits. While we all sincerely wish for scientific advancement to be wholly beneficial, this rarely—if ever—is the case. And yet, it is not in the province of scientists alone to ensure the benefits outweigh the risks. It requires diplomacy, governance, and public engagement. Finally, we need to build closer links between scientists and the public, and recognise that grassroots efforts (and even civil disobedience) may be essential components for managing existential risk in the current geopolitical situation—what Nick Bostrom refers to as our "semi-anarchic default condition".[71]

We need, therefore, to be both realistic and respectful in our evaluation of this pioneering work. Many of the theoretical frameworks within which scientists work tend to be useful only for linking discrete exogenous shocks with catastrophic effects; for instance, by considering a simple causal chain from nuclear conflict, to firestorms, to stratospheric soot injection, to famine. Questions about the exact size of such risks, or the timeframes within which they might be expected to occur, are not amenable to precise answers and, while understandable, the public's demand for such answers has encouraged some to make claims that have not been borne out by the subsequent facts. How to handle such tensions responsibly is a challenge facing all who work on existential risk, and one we have heard few address with the directness it deserves. Furthermore, such studies are hard to reconcile with the need for a science of existential risk that can move beyond direct drivers of risk to embrace complexity and chaos in all its forms. This is one area where the integrated approaches to the study of existential risk that have emerged in the field of Existential Risk Studies may be especially valuable.[72] However, even here, approaches will undoubtedly continue to be indebted to systems thinkers and complexity scientists.

The founding objectives of *The Bulletin*, which echo the hopes of many who have sought to work on existential risks, were two-fold: to make scientists aware of "the relationship between their own world of science and the national and international politics", and to educate the public about the need to manage the "dangerous presents from Pandora's box of modern science".[73] Focusing attention on threats to human existence is not for the faint of heart, and the founders of *The Bulletin* were well aware that their aims would only be realised by a long, sustained effort. Political solutions can appear inconsequential against such extreme outcomes. Technological advancement will bring, and has brought, such grand benefits that it is disquieting to advocate for ethical and political roadblocks to reduce potential—and sometimes merely theoretical—risks. While the concerned scientists who have helped to keep humanity safe and flourishing are often labelled as pessimistic, history shows us that this charge is unfair. To assume that scientific, social, and technological change only carries risks would leave us unable to explain the indisputable benefits they have given to humanity, and their potential to do even more good in future. However, to focus only on these benefits could lead us to fatally ignore some of the very real challenges currently facing us.

For the last 75 years, the Doomsday Clock has served as one of the few popular images that is able both to break through the global public discourse and to define such difficult trade-offs. Still, knowing the risks is never enough; we must also figure out the space of safe and beneficial scientific development and create the restraints necessary to govern it. These are hard problems. However, we can see from the history of existential risk that when talented scientists work together with committed politicians and motivated activists, it is possible to do more than simply cross our fingers and hope for the best. We can weigh the dice in our favour; we can turn back the hands of the Clock.

Notes and References

1   There are many instances of this myth. Another prominent version can be found in Tablet XI of the Epic of Gilgamesh. Some have suggested that the prevalence of the deluge in Mesopotamian culture attests to folk memories of real catastrophic floods caused by prehistoric global warming at the end of the last glacial age.

2   For more on this history, see Moynihan, T., *X-risk: How Humanity Discovered Its Own Extinction*. MIT Press (2020); and Torres, E., *Human Extinction A History of the Science and Ethics of Annihilation*. Routledge (2023).

3   Shelley, M.W., *The Last Man*. Henry Colburn (1826).

4   Butler, S., 'Darwin among the machines', *The Press, June 13 1863* (1863); Butler, S., 'The book of the machines', *Erewhon: Or, Over the Range*. Trübner and Ballantyne (1872).

5   The first mention of autonomous machines causing human extinction due to 'value misalignment', the principle concern for many scholars of existential risk today, can be found in Jack Williamson's short story *With Folded Hands* (Williamson, J., 'With folded hands', *Astounding Science Fiction*. Street & Smith (1947)), implying that this facet of AI ethics predates even other canonical AI-related thought experiments, such as John Searle's *Chinese Room* (Searle, J.R., 'Minds, brains, and programs', *Behavioral and Brain Sciences*, 3(3) (1980), pp.417–57. https://

doi.org/10.1017/S0140525X00005756) or Alan Turing's *Imitation Game* (Turing, A.M., 'Computing machinery and intelligence', *Mind LIX* (236) (1950), pp.433–60. https://doi.org/10.1093/mind/LIX.236.433). A comprehensive record of when different kinds of AI-induced catastrophes were first described can be found at https://timelines.issarice.com/wiki/Timeline_of_AI_safety#Timeline.

6   Wells, H.G., *The World Set Free: A Story of Mankind*. E.P. Dutton (1914).

7   The earliest example of this genre (often known as 'cli-fi' or climate fiction) may be Ballard, J.G., *The Burning World*. Berkley Pub (1964).

8   Wells, H.G., *Anticipations of the Reaction of Mechanical and Scientific Progress Upon Human Life and Thought*. Chapman & Hall (1901).

9   Warren, W.W., 'H.G. Wells and the genesis of future studies', *World Future Society Bulletin, 17*(1) (1983), pp.25–29.

10   Wells, H.G., 'On extinction', *Chambers's Journal* (30 September 1893) and Wells, H.G., 'The extinction of man', *Certain Personal Matters: A Collection of Material, Mainly Autobiographical*. William Heinemann (1897).

11   Asimov, I., *A Choice of Catastrophes: The Disasters That Threaten Our World*. Simon & Schuster (1979).

12   Konopinski, E.J., C. Marvin, and E. Teller, *Ignition of the Atmosphere With Nuclear Bombs*. Los Alamos National Laboratory (1946). https://fas.org/sgp/othergov/doe/lanl/docs1/00329010.pdf

13   Kimball Smith, A., *A Peril and a Hope: The Scientists' Movement in America: 1945–47*. University of Chicago Press (1965).

14   One early success of these citizen-scientists was contributing to the establishment of the 'nuclear taboo' against use that has lasted to this day. In private conversations, Eisenhower's Secretary of State complained that the "stigma of immorality" prevented the US from using nuclear weapons. The next generation of citizen-scientists in the 60s and 70s built on this by taking the ideas of arms control into government and helping to achieve the first agreements with the Soviets. See Adler, Emanuel, 'The emergence of cooperation: National epistemic communities and the international evolution of the idea of nuclear arms control', *International Organization*, 46(1) (1992), pp.101–45; and Tannenwald, Nina, *The Nuclear Taboo: The United States and the Non-Use of Nuclear Weapons Since 1945*. Cambridge University Press (2007).

15   Benedict, J., 'Doomsday Clock', *Bulletin of the Atomic Scientists* (January 2018). https://thebulletin.org/2018/01/doomsday-clockwork/

16 The full text of this manifesto can be read at https://pugwash. org/1955/07/09/statement-manifesto/

17 Norwegian Nobel Committee, 'The Nobel Peace Prize 1995' [Press Release] (1995) https://www.nobelprize.org/prizes/peace/1995/press-release/

18 Many of the founders of Pugwash, including Einstein and Russell, had initially believed that establishing a world government might be necessary to prevent humanity eradicating itself as a result of the advent of nuclear weapons, by eradicating the divisions that were seen as the causes of conflict. However, the organisation itself stands as a lasting testament to the ability of individual scientists to work across ideological and geographical divides to make the world safer, in spite of its divisions. For more on this distinction between 'top-down' and 'bottom-up' approaches to tackling existential risk and the history of Pugwash and similar initiatives, see the chapter by Lalitha S. Sundaram: 'Existential Risk and Science Governance'.

19 Russell, B., 'Civil disobedience', *New Statesman*, 17 February 1961 (1961).

20 Williams, P., 'Physics made simple: The image of nuclear weapons in the writing of Langston Hughes', *Journal of Transatlantic Studies*, 6(2) (2008), pp.131–41.

21 King Jr, M.L., 'I see the promised land', in J.M. Washington (ed.), *A Testament of Hope: The Essential Writings and Speeches of Martin Luther King, Jr.* HarperOne (1986), pp.279–86.

22 For further resources on nuclear colonialism and indigenous people's resistance to it, see https://www.nirs.org/resisting-nuclear-colonialism-on-indigenous-peoples-day/ and http://www.environmentandsociety. org/exhibitions/risk-and-militarization/nuclear-colonialism

23 Savranskaya, S.V., 'New sources on the role of Soviet submarines in the Cuban Missile Crisis', *Journal of Strategic Studies*, 28(2) (2005), pp.233–59.

24 Yusuf, M., *Predicting Proliferation: The History of the Future of Nuclear Weapons.* Brookings Institution (2009).

25 van der Meer, S., 'Forgoing the nuclear option: States that could build nuclear weapons but chose not to do so', *Medicine, Conflict and Survival*, 30(supplement 1) (2014), pp.27–34.

26 Lundgren, C., 'What are the odds? Assessing the probability of a nuclear war', *The Nonproliferation Review*, 20(2) (2013), pp.361–74.

27 Leclerc, G.L., *The Epochs of Nature.* University of Chicago Press (2018).

28 Fourier, C., *Selections From the Works of Fourier.* Sonnenschein & Company (1901).

29   Engels, F., 'The part played by labour in the transition from ape to man', first published in *Die Neue Zeit 1895–06*. Published in English by Progress Publishers (1934), translated by Clemens Dutt.

30   Arrhenius, S., *Worlds in the Making: The Evolution of the Universe*. Harper (1908). Note, however, that both Fourier and Arrhenius were actually more concerned about the possibility of global cooling than global warming, and that such (now widely discredited) anxieties continued to receive significant scientific interest well into the 20th century. For further discussion of this history see Locher, F. and Fressoz, J.B. 'Modernity's frail climate: A climate history of environmental reflexivity', *Critical Inquiry*, 38(3) (2012), pp.579–98.

31   Vogt, W., *Road to Survival*. William Sloan Associates (1948).

32   Osborn, F., *Our Plundered Planet*. Little, Brown and Company (1948).

33   Carson, R., *Silent Spring*. Houghton Mifflin Company (1962).

34   Ehrlich, P.R., *The Population Bomb*. Ballantine Books (1968).

35   Meadows, D.H., D.L. Meadows, J. Randers, and W.W. Behrens, *The Limits to Growth*. Universe Books (1972).

36   While this was the earliest (and, to date, most prominent) research by the Club of Rome, it is far from the only attempt to model the risks and causes of societal collapse. For more on the techniques employed by the Club of Rome and other researchers, see the chapter by Sabin Roman: 'Understanding and Predicting Societal Collapse'.

37   Kellogg, W.K., "Is mankind warming the earth?" *Bulletin of the Atomic Scientists*, 34(2) (1978), pp.10–19 (1978), https://doi.org/10.1080/009634 02.1978.11458464

38   Hansen, J., D. Johnson, A. Lacis, S. Lebedeff, P. Lee, D. Rind, and G. Russell. 'Climate impact of increasing atmospheric carbon dioxide', *Science*, 213(4511), pp.957–66 (1981). Similar concerns were raised the following year in an internal report for ExxonMobil that predicted a one-degree average global temperature rise by 2022—a prediction that, regrettably, has now been shown to have been highly accurate. See Supran, G. and N. Oreskes, 'Assessing ExxonMobil's climate change communications (1977–2014)', *Environmental Research Letters*, 12(8) (2017), p.084019.

39   Rich, N., *Losing Earth: The Decade We Could Have Stopped Climate Change*. Pan Macmillan (2019).

40   However, note that, while this consensus has existed since the 1980s, the topic of climate change as a global catastrophic risk has received

surprisingly little attention from the scientific community, even as it has become a hot topic of public and political debate. A full assessment of the research currently existing in this space—most of which has only been conducted within the last decade—can be found in Luke Kemp's chapter 'Ecological Breakdown and Human Extinction'.

41   Oreskes, N. and E.M. Conway, *Merchants of Doubt: How a Handful of Scientists Obscured the Truth on Issues From Tobacco Smoke to Global Warming*. Bloomsbury (2011).

42   However, the importance of working with groups seeking racial, indigenous, and other forms of justice in reducing existential threats like nuclear weapons and climate change is not merely that they have (in fact) been important agents of change. As Natalie Jones sets out in her chapter 'Beyond "Error and Terror": Global Justice and Global Catastrophic Risk', a failure to understand issues of global injustice, inequality, corruption, and oppression can give us a flawed understanding of the risks facing humanity; however, privileged academics in elite universities are often poorly situated to fully understand this.

43   Not that this was an especially new departure for the magazine. *The Bulletin*'s first article to mention anthropogenic climate change came out in 1954 (albeit in a satire of different public attitudes towards fossil fuels and nuclear power) while in 1961 it published further articles on climate change as part of a three-volume special on *Man and His Habitat*. See Frisch, O.R., 'On the feasibility of coal-driven power stations', *Bulletin of the Atomic Scientists, 10*(6) (1954), p.224. https://doi.org/10.1080/0096340 2.1954.11453480 and Suess, H.E., 'Fuel residuals and climate', *Bulletin of the Atomic Scientists, 17*(9) (1961), pp.374–75.

44   Hickel, J., 'Quantifying national responsibility for climate breakdown: An equality-based attribution approach for carbon dioxide emissions in excess of the planetary boundary', *The Lancet Planetary Health, 4*(9), pp.e399-e404 (2020).

45   Alvarez, L.W., W. Alvarez, F. Asaro, and H.V. Michel, 'Extraterrestrial cause for the cretaceous-tertiary extinction', *Science 208*(4448), pp.1095–108 (1980), https://doi.org/10.1126/science.208.4448.1095.

46   Palmer, T., *Controversy Catastrophism and Evolution: The Ongoing Debate*. Springer Science & Business Media (2012).

47   Of course, it also drew scientific attention to the possibility of similar catastrophes occurring due to asteroid impacts or volcanic eruptions in the future, as discussed by Lara Mani, Doug Erwin, and Lindley Johnson in their chapter 'Natural Global Catastrophic Risks'.

48   Sagan, C., *The Dragons of Eden: Speculations on the Evolution of Human Intelligence*. Penguin Random House (1977); Sagan, C., A. Druyan, and S. Soter, *Cosmos: A Personal Voyage*. PBS (1980).

49   Turco, R.P., O.B. Toon, T.P. Ackerman, J.B. Pollack, and C. Sagan, 'Nuclear winter: Global consequences of multiple nuclear explosions', *Science*   222(4630),   pp.1283–92   (1983),   https://doi.org/10.1126/science.222.4630.1283.

50   Sagan, C., 'Would nuclear war be the end of the world?' *Parade* (October 30th 1983).

51   Ehrlich, P.R., C. Sagan, D. Kennedy, and W.O. Roberts, *The Cold and the Dark: The World After Nuclear War*. W.W. Norton & Company (1984). While Ehrlich was initially sceptical that a nuclear conflict could cause human extinction, his view eventually changed. In his words: "it was the consensus of our group that, under those conditions, we could not exclude the possibility that the scattered survivors simply would not be able to rebuild their populations, that they would, over a period of decades or even centuries, fade away. In other words, we could not exclude the possibility of a full-scale nuclear war entraining the extinction of Homo sapiens." Badash, L., *A Nuclear Winter's Tale: Science and Politics in the 1980s*. MIT Press (2009).

52   Although it is worth noting that other important work on nuclear war and human extinction of the time did not depend on the nuclear winter hypothesis, such as Jonathan Schell's highly influential article series and book *The Fate of the Earth* (Schell, J., 'The fate of the Earth', *The New Yorker* (February 1982).

53   Frances, R.M., 'When Carl Sagan warned the world about nuclear winter', *Smithsonian Magazine* (2017).

54   Sagan, C., *Pale Blue Dot: A Vision of the Human Future in Space*. Random House (1994).

55   Rees, M., *Our Final Century: Will Civilisation Survive the Twenty-First Century?* Random House (2003).

56   For instance, *The Bulletin* has been raising awareness of the risks from biotechnology since the 1940s, geoengineering since the 1960s, AI since the 1970s, and nanotech since the 2000s. See Thimann, K.V., 'The role of biologists in warfare', *Bulletin of the Atomic Scientists*, 3(8), pp.211–12 (1947), https://doi.org/10.1080/00963402.1947.11459090; Landsberg, H.E., 'Climate made to order', *Bulletin of the Atomic Scientists*, 17(9), pp.370–74 (1961), https://doi.org/10.1080/00963402.1961.11454271; Weizenbaum, J., 'Once more—A computer revolution', *Bulletin of the Atomic Scientists*, 34(7) (1978), pp.12–19. https://doi.org/10.1080/00963402.1978.11458531;

and Kosal, Margaret E., 'Nanotech: Is small scary?' *Bulletin of the Atomic Scientists, 60*(5) (2004), pp.38–47., https://doi.org/10.1080/00963402.2004.11460819.

57 Good, I.J., 'Speculations concerning the first ultraintelligent machine', *Advances in Computers 6* (1966), pp. 31-88, https://doi.org/10.1016/S0065-2458(08)60418-0.

58 Lederberg, J., 'Biological warfare and the extinction of man', in a statement before the Subcommittee on National Security Policy and Scientific Developments, House Committee on Foreign Affairs (1969).

59 Drexler, K.E., *Engines of Creation: The Coming Era of Nanotechnology*. Anchor Press/Doubleday (1986).

60 Dar, A., A. De Rújula, and U. Heinz. 'Will relativistic heavy-ion colliders destroy our planet?', *Physics Letters B, 470*(1–4), pp.142–48 (1999).

61 The history of thinking about AI as an existential risk is discussed in John Burden, Sam Clarke, and Jess Whittlestone's chapter: 'A History of AI Existential Safety', while the growing threat from biotechnology and developments in the life sciences is discussed in Kelsey Lane Warmbrod, Kobi Leins, and Nancy Connell's chapter: 'Biosecurity, Biosafety and Dual Use: Will Humanity Minimise Potential Harms in the Age of Biotechnology?'

62 And these have also been joined by a growing range of think tanks and policy bodies such as the Centre for Security and Emerging Technology, the Centre for Health Security, and the Nuclear Threat Initiative.

63 Liu, H.Y., K.C. Lauta, and M.M. Maas, 'Governing boring apocalypses: A new typology of existential vulnerabilities and exposures for existential risk research', *Futures, 102* (2018), pp.6–19.

64 Sears, N.A., 'Existential security: Towards a security framework for the survival of humanity', *Global Policy, 11*(2) (2020), pp.255–66.

65 Avin, S., B.C. Wintle, J. Weitzdörfer, S.S. Ó hÉigeartaigh, W.J. Sutherland, and M.J. Rees, 'Classifying global catastrophic risks', *Futures, 102* (2018), pp.20–26.

66 Cotton-Barratt, O., M. Daniel, and A. Sandberg, 'Defence in depth against human extinction: Prevention, response, resilience, and why they all matter', *Global Policy, 11*(3) (2020), pp.271–82.

67 Baum, S., 'Resilience to global catastrophe', in Benjamin D. Trump, Marie-Valentine Florin, and Igor Linkov (eds), *IRGC Resource Guide on Resilience (Vol. 2): Domains of Resilience for Complex Interconnected Systems*. EPFL International Risk Governance Center (2018).

68   New START was eventually renewed by the Biden Administration in 2021 before being suspended by Russia in 2023.

69   A particular concern within nuclear modernisation has been the combination of AI and nuclear weapons, as discussed by Matthijs Maas, Kayla Lucero-Matteucci, and Di Cooke's chapter: 'Military Artificial Intelligence as Contributor to Global Catastrophic Risk'.

70   See https://www.cser.ac.uk/news/doomsday-clock-2020/

71   Bostrom, N., 'The vulnerable world hypothesis', *Global Policy*, 10(4) (2019), pp.455–76.

72   For some introductory works on these approaches, see Leslie, J.A., *The End of the World: The Science and Ethics of Human Extinction*. Routledge (1996); Bostrom, N., 'Existential risks: Analyzing human extinction scenarios and related hazards', *Journal of Evolution and Technology*, 9(1) (2002). https://www.nickbostrom.com/existential/risks.pdf; Bostrom, N., 'The vulnerable world hypothesis', *Global Policy*, 10(4) (2019), pp.455–76; Walsh, Bryan, *End Times: A Brief Guide to the End of the World*. Hachette (2019); Ord, T., *The Precipice: Existential Risk and the Future of Humanity*. Hachette (2020); as well as the other chapters in this volume.

73   Rabinowitch, E. and M. Grodzins, 'Bulletin', *Bulletin of the Atomic Scientists*, 1(1), p. 1(1945), https://doi.org/10.1080/00963402.1945.11454590.

2. Theories and Models: Understanding and Predicting Societal Collapse

Sabin Roman

There have been numerous arguments put forth to explain why societies collapse. In this chapter we consider different approaches to understanding the risk of societal collapse. According to Joseph Tainter, collapse is a rapid and significant loss of an established level of socio-political complexity of a society.[1] A complex society usually exhibits a degree of social stratification and differentiation; specialisation of economic functions and occupations at the individual, group, and territorial level; centralised control, i.e. elites that regulate and integrate economic and political activity; regimentation and behavioural control (e.g. rule of law); investment in cultural property (e.g. monumental architecture, literary, and artistic creation etc.); information flow between individuals (e.g. education), between economic and political groups, and between centralised structures and the periphery; trading and redistribution of resources; the general coordination and organisation of individuals and groups; and a single political unit which integrates an extended territory. Practically, collapse is signalled by (or has been associated with) the disappearance or significant decline in these indicators of complexity.

A simple example of quantitative reasoning that gives some insight into the long-term future of our society is the doomsday argument. In 1964 the American cultural theorist Albert Goldman proposed 'Lindy's Law' after spending time in Lindy's delicatessen in New York listening

    https://doi.org/10.11647/OBP.0336.02

to comedians try to predict how long each other's shows would run for. According to this law, "the life expectancy of a television comedian is proportional to the total amount of his exposure on the medium", based on the observation that many comedians would overexpose themselves in ways that would ultimately prove unsustainable in the long run. This principle was later formalised by the mathematician Bernard Mandelbrot[2] and then generalised by Nassim Taleb into the idea that non-perishable things (like human projects and ventures, up to and including human civilisations, but not people or artefacts) 'age' in reverse so that "every year that passes without extinction doubles the additional life expectancy" and "the robustness of an item is proportional to its life".[3] Of course, this does not mean we can predict when any given society will collapse, but it does allow us to gain some indication of how long societies in general can be expected to survive, and also potentially which aspects of any given society will outlast which others.

A similar kind of argument was developed by J. R. Gott to consider future prospects for our species.[4] This is not based on assumptions about the way that things do or don't age, but rather on a Bayesian argument about what we can infer from the fact that we ourselves have observed something existing. The idea is that, if an item can only be observed for a finite length of time (e.g. the period of time during which it exists) then, unless we have some prior belief that we are observing it at a special time in its life (e.g. we are actually observing its creation or demise) we should expect our observation of that thing to be located randomly within this period. Thus, we might reason that there is a 95% probability that we will not be observing it at either the first or last 2.5% of its life, and an equal chance that we are observing it in the second half of its lifespan as in the first. Gott goes on to evaluate this argument against his observations of different aspects of civilisation, including Stonehenge, the Berlin Wall, the USSR, and the journal *Nature* (in which he was publishing). He also applied this argument to our observation of the existence of humanity itself, concluding that we should have 95% confidence that our species will survive between 5,100 years and 7,800,000 years into the future.

Gott, and most other theorists of the subject, were actually more interested in further development of the doomsday argument, which depends not on the temporal location of our observation of the existence of humanity, but rather on our own demographic location within the species itself. The argument is as follows: from a total of N humans that will be born, any one person is equally likely to find themselves at any position n of the total population N. So, the distribution of n/N is uniform over $[0; 1]$. There is a 95% chance that n/N is within $[0.05; 1]$, so $n/N > 0.05$, which implies that $N < 20n$. This places an upper limit on the total expected number of people that will ever be born. With different assumptions on birth rates, we can then determine the total time that humanity has to exist. If 60 billion people have been born by now, then a total of 1.2 trillion people is to be expected overall. This argument has been analysed from various perspectives. However, it has too many moving parts to give a robust time horizon for the end of humanity. The total number of humans up to the present day needs to be estimated, as well as the fraction this constitutes of the total N, and the likely population levels and birth rates over time. For example, population levels for humanity have varied from a few million (for most of our history) to billions (after 1800). Hence, depending on these estimates, the time our species has left can vary from thousands to millions of years so that, irrespective of its validity, the argument is simply not that informative.

While Lindy's Law and the temporal version of the doomsday argument have fewer moving parts, allowing timescales to be estimated with less uncertainty, the arguments still do not prove to be that informative, with the estimates for the future lifespan of our civilisation or species ranging over at least three orders of magnitude (similar to the demographic case). Nevertheless, the argument is not necessarily void, as the upper bound of its predictions are comparable with estimates of mammal species' lifetimes.

What makes the doomsday argument informative is its use of the 95% confidence interval, but this is not necessarily justified. Assuming that all the humans born up to the present moment (or the amount of time our species has existed for) amounts to 5% of the total is rather arbitrary. Nevertheless, since Sir Ronald Fisher introduced the 95% confidence interval, there has been a tyranny of the 5% in statistical testing.[5] The 5% feels like a 'safe', modest quantity to reference and changing the doomsday argument to use more than 10% (which crosses a psychological boundary for a civilisation with a decimal system) would likely be viewed with suspicion and unease.

Regardless of their potential value, however, Lindy's Law and the doomsday argument offer us only one way to assess the likely future of our species, and their axioms are limited by being almost entirely neutral regarding evidence that might shed light on this question (apart from the date at which our species/civilisation first emerged and the total size of previous populations, both of which are highly contestable and hard to determine with any precision). At its core, the doomsday argument relies on the assumption that there is some natural regularity that governs the past and future lifespan of humanity and our projects, arguing that we have no reason to consider our current observations of them to be special in history. Given the rapid changes that have been experienced in recent decades—in everything from the global population to the pace of technological development—both of these assumptions appear highly questionable.

However, we do not, in fact, need to adopt such an evidence-neutral approach. There have been numerous studies that address societal collapse within the field of archaeology (see the work of Tainter's *The Collapse of Complex Societies* and references therein)[6] and from an ecological perspective.[7] In the next sections, we review the main categories of theories put forward to explain societal collapse.

Exogenous factors and one-shot explanations

A popular reason that is proposed for the collapse of complex societies is the depletion of natural resources, which can take various forms, such as deforestation (as Jared Diamond has argued in the case of Easter Island)[8] or degradation of soil quality for the Maya.[9] This is a recurrent topic of concern for modern society, with emphasis ranging from water scarcity[10] to phosphorus shortages,[11] or, quite frequently, energy production.[12] The problem is often phrased in terms of reaching peak production of a certain resource, such as metals[13] or fossil fuels.[14]

The loss of resources can be gradual or rapid (such as in the case of a fast onset of environmental changes, with historic examples being the floods of the Nile river that favoured crop parasites in the Middle Kingdom of Egypt[15] or droughts for the Maya).[16] A contemporary example is climate change, which can lead to reduction in glacial cover and threaten freshwater supplies[17] or loss of arable land due to changes in temperature and precipitation.[18] Disruption via the loss of resources can also take the form of a shift to a new resource base that can destabilise prior social order and contribute to collapse.[19] A notable example for the modern world is the change to renewable energy resources and the move away from fossil fuels. A genuine transition to renewables is likely to be tumultuous.[20]

The general difficulty with natural resource arguments for the collapse of societies is that administrative structures, the allocation of labour, and numerous innovations are often developed and geared towards dealing with possible resource shortages and deteriorating environmental conditions.[21] Thus, the scarcity of resources first leads to an increase of the complexity of a society, rather than its collapse. While this can be a contributing mechanism to collapse, by itself it is not enough to adequately explain collapse. Overall, theories of collapse that rest on the depletion or scarcity of natural resources propose an almost paradoxical hypothesis that societies collapse in conditions they have been adapting to and dealing with since their inception.

Another broad category of explanations for collapse is focused on competition between societies, which can also take multiple forms. Historical cases that have been included in this category are the demise of the Huari and Tiahuanaco.[22] A common instance of competition is invasion from outsiders, which includes the Germanic invasion of the Roman Empire,[23] or the invasion of the Hittite Empire by seafaring nomads,[24] or contact with Europeans (in the case of Easter Island).[25] In recent history, the possibility of collapse via this competitive route has notable examples, such as the collapse of the Soviet Union in competition with the US.[26]

While appealing in its simplicity and the identification of a 'smoking gun' for collapse, this class of arguments misses an important point. Throughout its history, any given society has likely encountered many external threats, such as competition with several other societies on economic terms or, more directly, as conflict and warfare. None of these instances led to its collapse, but rather to a further increase in its complexity. Thus, blaming collapse on a certain instance of competition with another society is a type of cherry-picking.

Catastrophes are also a frequently quoted cause of collapse, with examples including the volcanic eruptions and earthquakes for the

Minoan Civilisation,[27] major epidemics for the Maya,[28] or rat infestation for Easter Island.[29] Catastrophes can be classified as extreme cases of contingent events, which form another class of explanations, where a sequence of detrimental events led to the collapse. The events need not be causally related, but represent a string of losses experienced by the society that weaken it and lead to its breakdown or collapse. Again, these types of arguments neglect the adaptive capacity a society has in managing shocks to its function. While a sizable catastrophe can effectively destroy an entire social system, such as with Pompeii,[30] they rarely have the geographical reach to lead to widespread collapse.

A related theory of collapse considers societies to be vulnerable and incapable of adaptation, so they cannot provide adequate and sufficient responses to their challenges and circumstances, e.g. the Aztec and Inca Empires.[31] If a society could not find and implement effective solutions to its problems, what prevented it from doing so? While these types of theories postulate the natural implication that if a society is not able to respond adequately to problems it will collapse, they do not account for the state of fragility.

For modern society, there are several examples of catastrophes that are threatening: the case of a solar flare, or asteroid impact, or a series of volcanic eruptions. While these can prove damaging worldwide in various regards (demographically, economically) it is questionable if they would pass the necessary threshold to lead to global collapse. The critical features lie in social organisation and how we are using the environment that gets impacted. In the case of the dinosaurs, the asteroid hitting the planet led to the destruction of their ecological niches and thus to their extinction,[32] but some species of mammals did survive. Thus, for the systems our society uses, our concern for their collapse does not necessarily stem from the gravity of any given catastrophe, but rather the high level of fragility we see they have. As with the ancient historical cases, to understand the vulnerability of the modern world in facing external threats, we need to account for its internal dynamics, which is of much higher complexity, and thus a greater challenge than any historical example. This is well exemplified by climate change, where the main driver of the phenomenon has been human activity since the start of the industrial revolution.

Overall, arguments based on competition with other societies, intruders, or catastrophes neglect the fact that these types of events have previously been encountered by a given society but no collapse occurred, e.g. earthquakes in the Minoan civilisation, barbarian attacks on the Roman front, or competition between the Mayan centres. In addition, these theories have the added difficulty of placing the drivers of the collapse outside of the society in question, which is incomplete from an epistemological perspective without accounting for changes in social structure and dynamics.

Social structure and class conflict

Some of the earliest proposed causes for the collapse of civilisations have been the conflict between social classes and the mismanagement by elites. Compared to the arguments above, one of the strengths of this class of explanations lies in placing the mechanism of collapse within the society in question. However, these explanations are accompanied by some mystical (vague, unmeasurable) factors underlying the collapse, e.g. a loss of social unity or of civic virtue.

One early theory of societal decline and collapse was put forward by Ibn Khaldun in 1377, who proposed a cyclical model for the rise and fall of civilisations.[33] Khaldun introduces the notion of 'asabiyyah', which roughly translates to social cohesion and unity. The theory can be summarised as follows: asabiyyah is strongly felt in the early stages of a society, but diminishes as the society grows and the leadership becomes too removed from the concerns of the majority of people. If a group at the periphery of the society enjoys a greater degree of social solidarity, it can grow in dominance and eventually lead to a change in the leadership. Then, a new cycle can start. One notable application of the theory has been to the Ottoman Empire to understand its development, which started at the periphery of the Byzantine Empire and grew to prominence.[34]

In the 18th century Edward Gibbon, in *Decline and Fall of the Roman Empire*, argued that the "virtue" of the citizens degraded, as they were less willing to protect their borders and outsourced their military defences to barbarian mercenaries.[35] In addition, he stated that Christianity diminished the martial spirit of the Romans, and belief in the afterlife made them reluctant to sacrifice themselves for the empire. We can observe that both Khaldun and Gibbon give explanations that rely on the loss of social cohesion—either due to the leadership or amongst the masses—and the subsequent invasion/replacement by an outside force.

As archaeology developed as a scientific field, the explanations based on class conflicts gained new popularity. A major systematic study, with a comprehensive review and integration of historical knowledge on societal development and collapse, was Arnold Toynbee's *A Study of History*, published in 1961, with volumes IV-VI covering the 'breakdown' and 'disintegration' of civilisations.[36] Toynbee does not consider environmental degradation or external invading forces as a root cause of the breakdown of a society. Rather, he argues that the mechanism behind the collapse is internal to the society and develops a theory of how this unfolds (as follows).

A "creative minority" is responsible for problem-solving within a society that leads to its growth and development, but eventually it ceases to be innovative, at which point it turns into a "dominant minority" which simply imposes rules and forces the majority into obedience. The majority is called the "proletariat" and is further divided into internal and external categories. The internal proletariat is under direct subjugation of the dominant minority, whereas the external one is left in poverty and disorganised. This state of affairs creates a tension that eventually leads to the disintegration of the social order. Toynbee applies the above theory to an extensive set of examples, including the Roman Empire, the Mayan civilisation, and the Old Egyptian Kingdom.

Recent applications of the class conflict hypothesis include Easter Island[37] and the Maya.[38] In the case of the modern world, we see a significant degree of social upheaval in the 18th and 19th century based on class conflict,[39] which (in part) likely inspired this category of theories for societal collapse. The main difficulty with theories of internal conflict and elite mismanagement is that these types of tensions and inefficiencies always exist in societies.[40] It is questionable that only at a certain point in a society's history did these recurrent themes cause the social structure to break down completely.

Prior to collapse, a high degree of social conflict can be present, as was the case with certain Chinese dynasties,[41] but direct causation cannot be inferred from this temporal succession. Similar to theories of resource depletion, the class conflict arguments encounter the difficulty that these types of challenges are characteristic to the structuring and functioning of a society since its inception. Similar to arguments based on external threats, the occurrence of internal conflicts is so common that explaining collapse based on the social upheaval happening just before collapse amounts to cherry-picking of events. Arguably, there is a long chain of events, with both internal and external factors, which occur throughout a society's history that are causally connected and can amount to its collapse. While the class conflict hypothesis highlights an important category of such contributing events, the causal structure is still short-sighted and the connection with other factors is neglected.

As seen above, most common theories of societal collapse either focus on factors that are not internal to the society in question or, in cases where the causes are intrinsic to the society, they refer to social conditions that have been characteristic to the society since its formation. The main difficulty in the explanations above is that they force the cause to be considered a single factor and posit the causal mechanism as a direct, linear process. Given the complexity of the systems involved, collapse is often a multi-faceted process that requires accounting for multiple interrelated factors. Simply listing the different contributing phenomena is insufficient to give us additional insight, but what can bridge the epistemological gaps is establishing the connection and causation between the different aspects affecting the operation of a society, such as its resource usage, its social organisation, main paradigms, norms, and institutions, and how it adapts to external threats. A consistent way to map these factors into one conceptual scheme is the identification of feedback mechanisms and the use of causal loop diagrams to illustrate the relationships that form and manifest over time.

The case of feedback mechanisms

A feedback mechanism is a multi-causal relationship between two or more variables. It can be represented by a causal loop diagram (CLD), where the different variables are listed and connections are illustrated with arrows. The variables are called stocks and represent quantities that change over time.

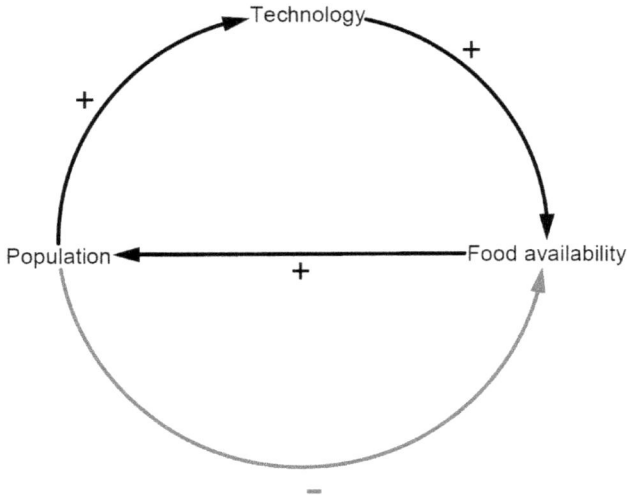

Fig. 1. A causal loop diagram (CLD) illustrating the relationship between population and food availability posited by Malthusian theory (lower half). An increase in population leads to a decrease in availability of food due to larger consumption. An increase in available food spurs an increase in population due to the higher amount of resources. The feedback tends to stabilise: any increase in population comes with a decrease in available food, which leads to a lower population. Boserup considers technology as adding a positive feedback loop (upper half), wherein a greater population leads to more technological innovation which allows more food production.[42]

The influence of one stock on another is shown through an arrow with a + (plus) or - (minus) depending on the growth of the starting stock, which leads to increase (+) or decrease (-) in the target stock. A CLD of a process can highlight its non-linear nature, represent how multiple factors influence each other, clarify the conceptual model of the dynamics, and be a stepping stone to a quantitative description.[43] Numerous physical, biological, social, and technological processes can be described through CLDs,[44] and they represent a natural explanatory framework for a process as complex as societal collapse.

An early example of a feedback mechanism applied to the sustainability of human society can be found in the 1798 work of Thomas Malthus, whose main argument can be summarised in the CLD of Fig. 1 (lower half).[45] The CLD can be understood as follows: an increase in population leads to a decrease in available food, while an increase in available food leads to an increase in population. The feedback mechanism is balancing, meaning that an increase in population leads to a decrease in available food, which would imply a decrease in the population. Thus, the variables tend to stabilise to certain values, because significant growth in one then leads to a counter-acting response from the other. The CLD only illustrates the simplest instance of Malthusian ideas, but does convey the point that population overshoot implies a later, possibly sharp, population decline.

An additional aspect Malthus points out is that population grows in exponential fashion, whereas agricultural production can only grow linearly. As described above, the mismatch will cause population levels to return to sustainable levels. In addition to food scarcity, with increasing population density, the chance of war breaking out increases, diseases are more easily transmitted, and general livelihood become harsher, which makes the bearing and raising of children more difficult. From the economic viewpoint, we can interpret this as saying that the costs of sustaining the population are growing faster than the capacity to sustain them.

With the industrial revolution, it became increasingly clear that technology could help eliminate—or at least delay—the negative population pressure Malthus hypothesised. Eventually, an alternative theory appeared with E. Boserup's *The Conditions of Agricultural Growth: The Economics of Agrarian Change Under Population Pressure*, which argued that, under conditions of rapid population growth and low land productivity, new, more intensive, agricultural technology would be developed to provide sufficient food.[46] Behind Boserup's thesis is the old tenet that 'necessity is the mother of all invention'. For example, the Mayan civilisation employed intensive agricultural practices (field-raising, terrace-building, etc.) and better irrigation and water management systems (e.g. building reservoirs) to cope with rainfall variability (including droughts) and their growing population.[47]

In Fig. 1 (upper half) we can see the CLD associated with Boserup's idea: an increase in population leads to an increase in technological development, that leads to an increase in food production. Thus, the decrease in food availability due to a large population growth can be compensated for through technological means. When conventional farming methods prove insufficient, the short-term response is likely the diversification and intensification of agricultural practice to compensate for any likely shortfall in production. But, as the Mayan case illustrates, on much longer time scales, the (ultimately) finite carrying capacity of the environment would constrain population growth (assuming all other factors are unchanged).[48] Thus, the theories of Malthus and Boserup can operate at different timescales, with a Malthusian catastrophe not necessarily avoided in the long term.

The question is then if technological innovation can continue to overcome environmental and production problems associated with the availability of food (and other necessary resources). Despite challenging Malthus by arguing that productivity per unit of land increases under intensification, Boserup argues that productivity per unit of labour actually decreases. Through factors such as preparation, fertilisation, and irrigation, human labour per unit of agricultural output increases but continues to be undertaken due to the growing population size. The work of Boserup received quantitative support through the data compiled by Clark and Haswell[49] and Wilkinson,[50] who show that the average and marginal return on agriculture does indeed decline with increasing labour.

Tainter generalises Boserup's observation of declining productivity per unit of labour to all problem-solving endeavours, not just procurement of food.[51] Specifically, Tainter posits that there are diminishing returns to investments in complexity (all activity geared towards problem-solving). In particular, this trend holds for technical innovation, e.g. to reach the same number of patent applications in 1958 as in 1946, the US required twice as many scientists and engineers, and three times as much investment as 12 years before.[52] Similar trends continue up to the present,[53] with examples including the decreasing number of patents per inventor,[54] the reduction in energy return on investment in oil production,[55] Eroom's law in pharmaceutical discoveries showing a decrease in R&D efficiency by a factor of 100 from 1950 to 2010,[56] and the rising economic and environmental costs of deep learning.[57]

The theories of Malthus, Boserup, and Tainter are not only applicable to modern society but also to past societies, and can (in part) account for historical cases of collapse, at least in cases relating to resource-harvesting in a fragile environment, such as for Easter Island[58] and the Classic Lowland Maya.[59] The idea of diminishing returns to investments in problem-solving is well exemplified by the Roman Empire,[60] whose early conquests were very profitable and allowed for the elimination of taxes for the citizens. With the expanding territory, the military and administrative costs grew as well.

At a certain point, further conquests/conflicts proved less beneficial and even amounted to a loss of resources, like the wars with the Germanic tribes. Maintenance of the empire ended up having larger costs than revenue, and territory was gradually lost. The Roman currency, the denarius, was being debased to expand the money supply and cover the costs (at least temporarily).[61] Throughout a period of 400 years, these negative returns manifested as a collapse. Similar arguments have been forwarded regarding the Chinese dynastic cycle,[62] the Ottoman Empire,[63] and the Maya.[64]

More generally, as was the case with the Roman Empire, the maintenance of a complex socio-political system requires resources and energy in various forms. Each new problem leads to an increase in the system's complexity due to the new institutions, more people, and different specialisations required to implement a solution. The increased complexity carries additional energy costs. The previously existing structures are not radically reformed but are expanded to incorporate new functionality, or additional ones are created.

So, the complexity tends to add increase with time, and hence, so do the costs of its maintenance. Furthermore, the benefits incurred in this enterprise suffer from the law of diminishing returns.[65] As such, "investment in socio-political complexity as a problem-solving response reaches a point of declining marginal returns".[66] At an advanced stage of socio-political growth, a society uses up most of its energy to maintain all the previously implemented solutions, and has very low returns on solving new problems. Thus, it becomes increasingly sensitive to—and incapable of—tackling internal or external threats and perturbations. In these conditions, collapse is a likely outcome, irrespective of specific factors or circumstances.

Another theoretical framework that significantly extends Malthus' work is structural demographic theory.[67] Beyond the population, the theory considers the role played by state structures and elites in stabilising or destabilising social order and dynamics. Multiple feedback mechanisms are posited within the social hierarchy, and several causal pathways are found for the emergence of political and wider social instability. The theory was developed by Peter Turchin and others to explain the emergence of rebellions and revolutions within a state, and it has led to numerous quantitative models that capture these phenomena in mathematical form.[68]

A theory of collapse built on feedback mechanisms describing social dynamics is consistent with the nature of a complex system, wherein multiple interacting factors are present, the evolution is non-linear, and causality cannot be assigned to singular aspects of the system. The frameworks outlined above are examples of influential theories on long-term sustainability (and collapse) that can be formulated as feedback mechanisms. While bridging epistemological gaps found in prior types of arguments, we can ask if these theories can provide specific predictions or remain as explanatory frameworks with no clear time horizons for their insights.

Quantitative models

To achieve specific, reliable, and quantitative predictions, it is necessary to formulate mathematical models of societal dynamics and evolution, such as within structural demographic theory.[69] Qualitatively describing the structure and dynamics of societies through feedback mechanisms is an important stepping stone towards the developments of realistic mathematical models.[70] A mathematical model can encapsulate the non-linear features of the relationships and dynamics found within a social system, and quantify and predict the time evolution of relevant variables (such as population levels, resource usage, economic metrics, etc.).

There are several different modelling methodologies that are commonly employed, and they differ in their complexity and calibration. There are large-scale models that attempt to capture multiple socio-environmental factors in a fine-grained fashion. These models fall into two broad classes:

(a) agent-based models (ABMs), which represent individuals (or communities) as agents with set attributes and behavioural rules, such that a realistic rendering of relevant behaviour is desired with the aim of obtaining larger scale emergent phenomena. Often, they also explicitly model the spatially extended features, such as terrain; and

(b) integrated world models, which employ a wide variety of modelling techniques (system dynamics, econometrics, etc.) and aim for an accurate, detailed representation of the system under study. They are complex models that use a large number of variables and parameters.

Early agent-based models were formulated and implemented in the 1970s and 80s. One of these models which we will mention is Schelling's model of racial segregation,[71] the iterated prisoner's dilemma,[72] and Craig Reynolds' "Boids" computer programme.[73] In the 1990s, the method expanded significantly, and became widely applied to modelling social and economic phenomena. Of particular interest is the Sugarscape model that is built up gradually and grows increasingly complex, when more realistic phenomena start to emerge (like wealth inequality, trade relations, and conflict).[74] This example is an excellent illustration of the general, non-trivial, and useful insights ABMs can provide by building social structure from the bottom-up.

There are several notable examples of agent-based models that address the dynamics of past societies and human activity (trade, migration, etc).[75] Arguably, the first significant effort in this sense was by Dean et al.,[76] Axtell et al.,[77] and Gumerman et al.,[78] who modelled the Kayenta Anasazi that lived in the Long House Valley in the Black Mesa area of north-eastern Arizona (US) from about 1800 BCE to 1300 CE. Other agent-based models focus on the Mayan civilisation[79] and the Bronze Age collapse,[80] but beyond the cases listed, agent-based models that aim to reproduce the archaeological records of complex, past societies are scarce. Effort in this area is directed more towards understanding prehistoric social dynamics and organisation.[81]

Given the large number of parameters and the many specific modelling choices that have to be made when designing such a high-resolution model, the problem of validating it is quite difficult. How many other parameter values and design decisions are compatible with the output of the model? To what extent are these possible models equivalent and insightful about the actual historical behaviour, decisions, and events? These questions cannot be answered in general, and despite the significant effort put into developing a realistic ABM, the whole endeavour can be at risk of becoming a very sophisticated curve-fitting exercise that provides little historical insight. Still, a variety of empirical approaches have been applied to ABMs, and this has led to a continued debate regarding their validation.[82]

The first major examples of mathematical models developed to account for collapse have not been aimed at ancient societies, but rather at modern society. The first global integrated models were initiated after the sustainability movement of the 1960s, when the Club of Rome was established by a group of economists and scientists with the goal to pursue a holistic understanding of—and solutions to—the world's major social and environmental problems.[83] In the mid-1950s, Professor Jay Forrester at MIT developed system dynamics, a diagrammatic method to aid the development of large-scale models consisting of differential equations.[84]

At the request of the Club of Rome, Forrester developed the World1 and World2 models, which incorporate complex feedback that characterises modern industrial society.[85] Eventually, the World3 model was developed, which led to the 'Limits to Growth' (LTG) study, led by Donella Meadows, that attempted to understand the development of society by taking into account a wide range of phenomena, including food production, pollution, economic wellbeing, population growth, and industrial output.[86] 'Limits to Growth' is based on the World3 model, which consists of 16 state variables (e.g. population, pollution, arable land) and 80 fixed parameters. The timeframe of the model is 200 years, between 1900 and 2100. The study focused on three scenarios: a base case with parameters best fitted to historical data, an environmentally sustainable case, and a technologically driven, industry-intensive scenario.

The first and third scenarios led to a peak in industrial output in the 21st century and a subsequent decline in economic activity and demographic levels. The sustainable case manages to reach a steady state with little loss of life, but it requires parameter choices that, in the real world, would require drastic action to curtail pollution and population growth. Given its dire outlook, the LTG study has received harsh criticism from economists,[87] but in recent years the standard run of the model has been found to match well with historical trajectories.[88] Since LTG was published, several other models have been developed, which are aimed at integrating social, ecological, and technological factors into a coherent whole to provide policy recommendations.[89]

There is another category of models where low-dimensional dynamical systems are employed to represent the dynamics of the system in an aggregated way. The models generally fall into one of two methodological approaches:

(a) economic-based models, in which individuals of the society are modelled as rational, utility-maximising agents. Typically, a utility function is chosen dependent on labour and land, and maximised under certain constraints. The relations that are obtained later inform the choice of dynamical system and parameters that influence the societal dynamics; and

(b) ecologically inspired models, which employ functional forms used in ecology to build the dynamical system and do not rely on neo-classical assumptions of consumer behaviour. The choice of dynamical system in this case is made by attempting to match the model structure to a theoretical framework (sociological or archaeological), along with empirical observations and measurements.

A broader trend started in the late 1990s—developing simple dynamical systems to model societal evolution. Renewed interest in the mathematical modelling of societal development (and collapse) was sparked by the work of Brander and Taylor.[90] Several papers that appeared following Brander and Taylor's also employed the economic methodology and analysed how different factors—such as property rights, technology, or growth—could have impacted and possibly modified the outcome on Easter Island.

With regard to economic models of societal dynamics, we can identify three weaknesses: (i) the fundamental assumption of rational human behaviour is not justified empirically,[91] (ii) the literature did not aim to improve the archaeological fit of the initial model by Brander and Taylor, and (iii) the models have increased in complexity over time with no discernible, testable features—e.g. more parameters were added or more complicated objective functions were proposed. Models which were developed on ecological and archaeological grounds, which we detail next, do not share these difficulties.

Some models do not employ an economic approach to modelling societies, but rather develop the dynamical systems more heuristically, from either ecological considerations or society-specific features consistent with the archaeology. In mathematical ecology, similarly to economics, an adequate representation of a system by a model is achieved by following certain general modelling principles.[92] But with regard to historical processes, there has not yet been a consensus on the appropriate modelling techniques. A new field called 'cliodynamics'[93] seeks to provide such a common framework for modelling historical processes, but the field is still in its infancy.

Discussion

We have reviewed the main theories put forward to explain how societies collapse, starting with qualitative theories with a focus on single exogenous factors, such as resource depletion, competition and conflict with other societies, catastrophes, and contingent events. Then, we considered theories with an endogenous explanation of collapse, which focus predominantly on class structures and elite mismanagement. In this regard, the theories of Khaldun, Gibbon, and Toynbee were highlighted as notable examples throughout the history of the field. The theories considered up to this point posit that collapse occurs in conditions that have been recurrent throughout the history of societies. Hence, taking any one given event (e.g. resource shortage, war, rebellion, etc.) as being the cause of the collapse means ignoring similar historical precedents and not accounting for how the society became susceptible to collapse.

Then, we considered theories that can be formulated as feedback mechanisms operating within societies. Historically, Malthus' theory provides an early example, upon which several refinements were made, notably by Boserup and Tainter, and later in structural demographic theory. These later theories provide frameworks compatible with the nature of a complex system (such as a society) and do not have the epistemological problems of previously mentioned theories, as they provide a mechanism and causal pathway for increased vulnerability to collapse. Furthermore, they provide a stepping stone to mathematical modelling of collapse, which moves beyond qualitative considerations and gives quantitative insight into the phenomenon.

Quantitative models of societal dynamics and collapse broadly fall into the following categories: agent-based models, integrated world models, and low-dimensional dynamical models. Agent-based models offer a bottom-up approach to understanding a system's structure and behaviour. The insight these models can provide is how basic building blocks of the system in question behave. The difficulty lies in matching underlying agent behaviour with large-scale features with the data, and discriminating between alternative assumptions regarding the agent's characteristics. Integrated world models have a high degree of complexity (many variables, equations, mechanisms, and sub-models) that hinder understanding and communication. Nevertheless, due to their complexity and comprehensiveness they are also the most realistic models, and are used in policy-making.

Low-dimensional dynamical systems models have been widely used to capture societal mechanisms from a top-down perspective.[94] The different schools of thought on the methodology of developing these models can be divided into either economically or ecologically focused; each one has different emphases and strengths. The advantage of low-dimensional models is that they can capture a specific idea or theory on how societal evolution takes place. This, plus their smaller number of variables, allows for comparison with the archaeological record. The main shortcoming of these models is the potential over-simplifications they make in describing the systems under study. However, searching for models at a mesoscopic scale of intermediate complexity can be advantageous, as sufficient societal elements can be accounted for to reproduce known data, but the model can also be kept manageable, so that it can be understood analytically and communicated more easily.

Still, the topic of societal collapse has generally been approached from a mostly qualitative perspective, which presents arguments in a narrative form without a mathematical understanding of the underlying dynamics. In some cases, there even appears to be an aversion to quantitative models.[95] Tainter argues that quantitative models are inadequate to capture the full scope of societal complexity and the underlying drivers of its evolution.[96] Turchin disagrees, and argues that "a discipline usually matures only after it has developed mathematical theory" especially if the discipline deals with dynamical quantities.[97] Informal verbal models are appropriate if the underlying mechanisms are sufficiently simple (acting in a linear and additive manner), but generally misleading if the system exhibits non-linear feedback and time lags.[98]

Casting hypotheses into quantitative models can help in illuminating uncertainties regarding the system, expose prevailing wisdom as incompatible with available data, guide data collection, or uncover new questions.[99] Mathematical models can thus be "indispensable when we wish to rigorously connect the set of assumptions about the system to predictions about its dynamics behavior".[100] However, as with Lindy's Law and the doomsday argument, there remains the general difficulty (as with any mathematical model) of choosing and calibrating its parameters. In addition, given the overall complexity of any given society, any proposed qualitative or quantitative description (feedback mechanism, models, etc.) can only aim to provide a partial description of societal dynamics and collapse. Establishing cause-effect relationships requires both empirical support and validated modelling, and remains subject to much debate. Applying this methodology to modern society comes with additional difficulties due to the system's highly interconnected nature, but progress is being made with regard to threats such as climate change.[101]

The use of quantitative models to test the validity of hypotheses has not been common in social sciences historically, and a new field called 'cliodynamics' has emerged to tackle this issue[102], and provide historical and current insight into social processes and emerging instability.[103]

Cliodynamics has the potential to follow in the footsteps of theoretical physics and mathematical biology in providing a robust, reliable modelling framework. The framework would be applicable to societal dynamics for ancient and modern cases. While the validation of any given model is difficult and debatable, by building a significant number of models with diverse features, a mathematical dictionary can be constructed that allows diverse social phenomena to be translated into equations or computational models. While economics provides one possible framework for modelling human behaviour, the models can be overly limiting in their underlying assumptions, whereas cliodynamics is more open to a diversity of assumptions from either an ecological or historical perspective.

Each term in an equation or rule in an agent-based model can form a foundation and a set of building blocks to obtaining certain emergent behaviours. For example, the law of mass action is a common functional term employed to model predator-prey interactions in population biology or population interactions in epidemiology. Similarly, the relationships between state resource, population, and war;[104] the impact of wealth on birth rates;[105] population shifts between specialisations;[106] the territory conquered by an army;[107] or transitions between a unified or turbulent period in history can be modelled through specific terms and equations proposed in the literature.[108] If a common set of historical mechanisms can be found throughout multiple time periods and a modelling framework with a toolkit of different methodologies adaptive to different scenarios can be built, then the science-fiction discipline of psychodynamics that Asimov imagined would be within reach.

Notes and References

1   Tainter, J., *The Collapse of Complex Societies*. Cambridge University Press (1988).

2   Mandelbrot, B.B., *The Fractal Geometry of Nature*. W.H. Freeman (1982).

3   Taleb, N.N., *Antifragile: How to Live in a World We Don't Understand*. Allen Lane (2012).

4   Gott III, J.R., 'Implications of the Copernican Principle for Our Future Prospects', *Nature*, 363(6427) (1993), pp.315–19.

5   Stigler, S., 'Fisher and the 5% Level', *Chance*, 21(4) (2008), p12.

6   Tainter (1988).

7   Costanza, R., L. Graumlich, W. Steffen, C. Crumley, J. Dearing, K. Hibbard, R. Leemans, C. Redman, and D. Schimel, 'Sustainability or collapse: What can we learn from integrating the history of humans and the rest of nature?', *Ambio* (2007), pp.522–27.

8   Diamond, J., *Collapse: How Societies Choose to Fail or Succeed: Revised Edition*. Penguin (2011).

9   Webster, D., *The Fall of the Ancient Maya: Solving the Mystery of the Maya Collapse*. Thames & Hudson (2002).

10 Mekonnen, M.M. and A.Y. Hoekstra, 'Four billion people facing severe water scarcity', *Science Advances*, 2(2), (2016), e1500323.

11 Cordell, D. and S. White, 'Peak phosphorus: Clarifying the key issues of a vigorous debate about long-term phosphorus security', *Sustainability*, 3(10) (2011), pp.2027–49.

12   Dorian, J.P., H.T. Franssen, and D.R. Simbeck, 'Global challenges in energy', *Energy Policy, 34*(15) (2006), pp.1984–91.

13   Ambrose, H. and A. Kendall, 'Understanding the future of lithium: Part 1, resource model', *Journal of Industrial Ecology, 24*(1) (2020), pp.80–89.

14   Chapman, I., 'The end of peak oil? Why this topic is still relevant despite recent denials', *Energy Policy, 64,* (2014) pp.93–101.

15   Butzer, K.W. and G.H. Endfield, 'Critical perspectives on historical collapse', *Proceedings of the National Academy of Sciences, 109*(10) (2012), pp.3628–31.

16   Kennett, D.J., S.F. Breitenbach, V.V. Aquino, Y. Asmerom, J. Awe, J.U. Baldini, P. Bartlein, B.J. Culleton, C. Ebert, C. Jazwa, and M.J. Macri, 'Development and disintegration of Maya political systems in response to climate change', *Science, 338*(6108) (2012), pp.788–91.

17   McDonald, R.I., P. Green, D. Balk, B.M. Fekete, C. Revenga, M. Todd, and M. Montgomery, 'Urban growth, climate change, and freshwater availability', *Proceedings of the National Academy of Sciences, 108*(15) (2011), pp.6312–17.

18   Zhang, X. and X. Cai, 'Climate change impacts on global agricultural land availability', *Environmental Research Letters, 6*(1) (2011), p.014014.

19   Harner, M.J., 'Population pressure and the social evolution of agriculturalists', *Southwestern Journal of Anthropology, 26*(1) (1970), pp.67–86; Bennett, J.W., *The Ecological Transition: Cultural Anthropology and Human Adaptation.* Routledge (2017).

20   Huber, N., R. Hergert, B. Price, C. Zäch, A.M. Hersperger, M. Pütz, F. Kienast, and J. Bolliger, 'Renewable energy sources: Conflicts and opportunities in a changing landscape', *Regional Environmental Change, 17*(4) (2017), pp.1241–55.

21   Isbell, W.H., 'Environmental perturbations and the origin of the Andean state', in C.L. Redman, M.J. Berman, E.V. Curtin, W.T. Langhorne, N.M. Versaggi, and J.C. Wanser (eds), *Social Archeology: Beyond Subsistence and Dating.* Academic Press (1978), pp.303–13; Dillehay, T.D. and A.L. Kolata, 'Long-term human response to uncertain environmental conditions in the Andes', *Proceedings of the National Academy of Sciences, 101*(12) (2004), pp.4325–30.

22   Lanning, E.P., *Peru Before the Incas.* Prentice-Hall (1967).

23   Manning, P. and T. Trimmer, *Migration in World History.* Routledge (2013).

24   Carpenter, R., *Discontinuity in Greek Civilization.* Cambridge University Press (1966).

25 Stevenson, C.M., C.O. Puleston, P.M. Vitousek, O.A. Chadwick, S. Haoa, and T.N. Ladefoged, 'Variation in Rapa Nui (Easter Island) land use indicates production and population peaks prior to European contact', *Proceedings of the National Academy of Sciences of the United States of America, 112*(4) (2015): 1025–30.

26 Nijman, J., 'The limits of superpower: The United States and the Soviet Union since World War II', *Annals of the Association of American Geographers, 82*(4) (1992), pp.681–95.

27 Marinatos, S., 'The volcanic destruction of Minoan Crete', *Antiquity, 13*(52) (1939), pp.425–39; Driessen, J. and C.F. Macdonald, *The Troubled Island: Minoan Crete Before and After the Santorini Eruption.* Aegaeum (1997).

28 Acuna-Soto, R., D.W. Stahle, M.D. Therrell, S.G. Chavez, and M.K. Cleaveland, 'Drought, epidemic disease, and the fall of classic period cultures in Mesoamerica (AD 750–950). Hemorrhagic fevers as a cause of massive population loss', *Medical Hypotheses, 65*(2) (2005), pp.405–09.

29 Hunt, T.L., 'Rethinking Easter Island's ecological catastrophe', *Journal of Archaeological Science, 34*(3) (2007), pp.485–502.

30 Scandonea, R. and L. Giacomellia, 'Vesuvius, Pompei, Herculaneum: A lesson in natural history', *Journal of Research and Didactics in Geography, 2* (2015), p.33.

31 Conrad, G.W. and A.A. Demarest, *Religion and Empire: The Dynamics of Aztec and Inca Expansionism.* Cambridge University Press (1984); Sinopoli, C.M., 'The archaeology of empires', *Annual Review of Anthropology, 23*(1) (1994), pp.159–80; Chepstow-Lusty, A.J., M.R. Frogley, B.S. Bauer, M.J. Leng, K.P. Boessenkool, C. Carcaillet, A.A. Ali, and A. Gioda, 'Putting the rise of the Inca Empire within a climatic and land management context', *Climate of the Past, 5*(3) (2009), pp.375–88.

32 Chiarenza, A.A., A. Farnsworth, P.D. Mannion, D.J. Lunt, P.J. Valdes, J.V. Morgan, and P.A. Allison, 'Asteroid impact, not volcanism, caused the end-Cretaceous dinosaur extinction', *Proceedings of the National Academy of Sciences, 117*(29) (2020), pp.17084–93.

33 Khaldun, I., *Muqaddimah* (1377).

34 Lewis, B., 'Ibn khaldun in Turkey', *Ibn Khaldun: The Mediterranean in the 14th Century: Rise and Fall of Empires.* Foundation El Legado Andalus (2006), pp.376–80.

35 Gibbon, E., *The History of the Decline and Fall of the Roman Empire.* Strahan & Cadell (1776).

36 Toynbee, A.J., *A Study of History* (12 vols). Oxford University Press (1961).

37   Pakandam, B., *Why Easter Island Collapsed: An Answer for an Enduring Question*. London School of Economics, Economic History Working Papers (117/09) (2009).

38   Hamblin, R.L. and B.L. Pitcher, 'The Classic Maya collapse: Testing class conflict hypotheses', *American Antiquity*, 45(2) (1980), pp.246–67; Chase, A.F. and D.Z. Chase, 'Contextualizing the collapse: Hegemony and Terminal Classic ceramics from Caracol Belize', in S.L. Lopez Varela and A.E. Foias (eds), *Geographies of Power: Understanding the Nature of Terminal Classic Pottery in the Maya Lowlands*. British Archaeological Reports (2006), pp.73–92.

39   Goldstone, J.A., *Revolution and Rebellion in the Early Modern World: Population Change and State Breakdown in England, France, Turkey, and China, 1600–1850*. Routledge (2016).

40   Tuchman, B.W., *March of Folly from Troy to Vietnam*. Alfred A. Knopf (1984); Tainter, (1988).

41   Eberhard, W., *A History of China*. University of California Press (2020); Roman, S., 'Historical dynamics of the Chinese dynasties', *Heliyon*, 7(6) (2021), p.e07293.

42   Boserup, E., *The Conditions of Agricultural Growth: The Economics of Agrarian Change Under Population Pressure*. Allen and Unwin (1965).

43   Meadows, D.H., *Thinking in Systems: A Primer*. Chelsea Green Publishing (2008).

44   Sterman, J., *Business Dynamics*. McGraw-Hill, Inc. (2000).

45   Malthus, T. R., *An Essay on the Principle of Population as it Affects the Future Improvement of Society, with Remarks on the Speculations of Mr. Godwin, M. Condorcet, and Other Writers*. Johnson (1798).

46   Boserup (1965).

47   Turner, B.L., 'Prehistoric intensive agriculture in the Mayan Lowlands: Examination of relic terraces and raised fields indicates that the Ro Bec Maya were sophisticated cultivators', *Science*, 185(4146) (1974), pp.118–24; Turner, B.L. and J.A. Sabloff, 'Classic Period collapse of the Central Maya Lowlands: Insights about human–environment relationships for sustainability', *Proceedings of the National Academy of Sciences*, 109(35) (2012), pp.13908–3914; Webster (2002).

48   Diamond (2011).

49   Clark, C. and M.R. Haswell, *The Economics of Subsistence Agriculture*. Springer (1970).

50 Wilkinson, R.G., *Poverty and Progress: An Ecological Model of Economic Development*. Taylor & Francis (2022).

51 Tainter (1988).

52 Machlup, F., *The Production and Distribution of Knowledge in the United States*. Princeton University Press (1962).

53 Tainter, J.A., 'Energy, complexity, and sustainability: A historical perspective', *Environmental Innovation and Societal Transitions*, 1(1) (2011), pp.89–95.

54 Strumsky, D., J. Lobo, and J.A. Tainter, 'Complexity and the productivity of innovation', *Systems Research and Behavioral Science*, 27(5) (2010), pp.496–509.

55 Taylor, T.G. and J.A. Tainter, 'The nexus of population, energy, innovation, and complexity', *American Journal of Economics and Sociology*, 75(4) (2016), pp.1005–043.

56 Scannell, P., 'The question of technology', *Narrating Media History*. Routledge (2012), pp.223–35.

57 Thompson, N.C., K. Greenewald, K. Lee, and G.F. Manso, 'Deep learning's diminishing returns: The cost of improvement is becoming unsustainable', *IEEE Spectrum*, 58(10) (2021), pp.50–55.

58 Roman, S., S. Bullock, and M. Brede, 'Coupled societies are more robust against collapse: A hypothetical look at Easter Island', *Ecological Economics*, 132 (2017), pp.264–78.

59 Roman, S., E. Palmer, and M. Brede, 'The dynamics of human–environment interactions in the collapse of the classic Maya', *Ecological Economics*, 146 (2018), pp.312–24.

60 Roman, S. and E. Palmer, 'The growth and decline of the Western Roman Empire: quantifying the dynamics of army size, territory, and coinage', *Cliodynamics*, 10(2) (2019); Tainter (1988).

61 Tainter, J.A., 'Problem solving: Complexity, history, sustainability', *Population and Environment* (2018), pp.3–41.

62 Lattimore, O., *Inner Asian Frontiers of China*. Beacon Press (1940).

63 Lewis, B., 'Some reflections on the decline of the Ottoman Empire', *Studia Islamica*, (9) (1958), pp.111–27.

64 Culbert, T.P., 'The collapse of the classic Maya civilization', in N. Yoffee and G.L. Cowgill (eds), *The Collapse of Ancient Civilizations*. University of Arizona Press (1991), pp.69–101.

65   Tainter, J.A., 'Complexity, problem solving, and sustainable societies', *Getting Down to Earth: Practical Applications of Ecological Economics* (1996), pp.61–76.

66   Tainter (1988), p.118.

67   Goldstone (2016).

68   Turchin, P., *Historical Dynamics*. Princeton University Press (2018).

69   Turchin, P. and A. Korotayev, 'The 2010 structural-demographic forecast for the 2010–2020 decade: A retrospective assessment', *PloS One*, *15*(8) (2020), p.e0237458.

70   Sterman (2000).

71   Schelling, T.C., 'Dynamic models of segregation', *Journal of Mathematical Sociology*, *1*(2) (1971), pp.143–86.

72   Axelrod, R. and W.D. Hamilton, 'The evolution of cooperation', *Science*, *211*(4489) (1981), pp.1390–396.

73   Reynolds, C.W., 'August. Flocks, herds and schools: A distributed behavioral model', *Proceedings of the 14th Annual Conference on Computer Graphics and Interactive Techniques* (1987), pp.25–34.

74   Epstein, J.M. and R. Axtell, *Growing Artificial Societies: Social Science From the Bottom up*. Brookings Institution Press (1996).

75   Kohler, T.A. and S.E. van der Leeuw (eds), *The Model-Based Archaeology of Socionatural Systems*. School for Advanced Research Press (2007), p.312; Barceló, J.A. and F. Del Castillo (eds), *Simulating Prehistoric and Ancient Worlds*. Springer International Publishing (2016).

76   Dean, J.S., G.J. Gumerman, J.M. Epstein, R.L. Axtell, A.C. Swedlund, M.T. Parker, and S. McCarroll, 'Understanding Anasazi culture change through agent-based modeling', *Dynamics in Human and Primate Societies: Agent-Based Modeling of Social and Spatial Processes* (2000), pp.179–205.

77   Axtell, R.L., J.M. Epstein, J.S. Dean, G.J. Gumerman, A.C. Swedlund, J. Harburger, S. Chakravarty, R. Hammond, J. Parker, and M. Parker, 'Population growth and collapse in a multiagent model of the Kayenta Anasazi in Long House Valley', *Proceedings of the National Academy of Sciences*, *99*(suppl 3) (2002), pp.7275–79.

78   Gumerman, G.J., A.C. Swedlund, J.S. Dean, and J.M. Epstein, 'The evolution of social behavior in the prehistoric American Southwest', *Artificial Life*, *9*(4) (2003), pp.435–44.

79 Heckbert, S., 'MayaSim: An agent-based model of the ancient Maya social-ecological system', *Journal of Artificial Societies and Social Simulation*, 16(4) (2013), p.11.

80 Chliaoutakis, A. and G. Chalkiadakis, 'Agent-based modeling of ancient societies and their organization structure', *Autonomous agents and multi-agent systems*, 30 (2016), pp.1072–116.

81 Barceló, J.A. and F. Del Castillo (eds) (2016).

82 Windrum, P., G. Fagiolo, and A. Moneta, 'Empirical validation of agent-based models: Alternatives and prospects', *Journal of Artificial Societies and Social Simulation*, 10(2) (2007), p.8; Moss, S., 'Alternative approaches to the empirical validation of agent-based models', *Journal of Artificial Societies and Social Simulation*, 11(1) (2008), p.5.

83 Ozbekhan, H., 'La planification prospective', *Actualité* économique, (3) (1976).

84 Forrester, J.W., *Industrial Dynamics*. MIT Press (1961).

85 Forrester, J.W., *World Dynamics*. Wright-Allen Press (1971).

86 Meadows, D.H., D.L. Meadows, J. Randers, and W.W. Behrens, *The Limits to Growth*. Universe Books (1972).

87 Bardi, U., *The Limits to Growth Revisited*. Springer Science & Business Media (2011).

88 Turner, G.M., 'A comparison of the Limits to Growth with 30 years of reality', *Global Environmental Change*, 18(3) (2008), pp.397–411.; Turner, G., 'Is global collapse imminent? An updated comparison of the Limits to Growth with historical data', *MSSI Research Paper*, 4 (2014), p.21.

89 Costanza, R., L. Graumlich, W. Steffen, C. Crumley, J. Dearing, K. Hibbard, R. Leemans, C. Redman, and D. Schimel, 'Sustainability or collapse: what can we learn from integrating the history of humans and the rest of nature?', *Ambio* (2007), pp.522–27.

90 Brander, J.A. and M.S. Taylor, 'The simple economics of Easter Island: A Ricardo-Malthus model of renewable resource use', *American Economic Review* (1998) pp.119–38.

91 Janssen, M.A. and M. Scheffer, 'Overexploitation of renewable resources by ancient societies and the role of sunk-cost effects', *Ecology and Society*, 9(1) (2004); Nell, E.J. and K. Errouaki, *Rational Econometric Man: Transforming Structural Econometrics*. Edward Elgar Publishing (2013).

92 Turchin, P., *Complex Population Dynamics*. Princeton University Press (2013).

93   Turchin, P., 'Arise 'cliodynamics'', *Nature*, *454*(7200) (2008), pp.34–35.

94   Roman, S., *Dynamic and Game Theoretic Modelling of Societal Growth, Structure and Collapse*. Doctoral dissertation, University of Southampton (2018).

95   Tainter, J.A., 'Plotting the downfall of society', *Nature*, *427*(6974) (2004), pp.488–89.

96   Tainter (2004).

97   Turchin (2013), p.1.

98   Sterman (2000).

99   Epstein, J.M., 'Why model?', *Journal of Artificial Societies and Social Simulation*, *11*(4) (2008), p.12.

100 Turchin (2013), p.4.

101 Kemp, L., 'US-proofing the Paris climate agreement', *Climate Policy*, *17*(1) (2017), pp.86–101; Richards, C.E., R.C. Lupton, and J.M. Allwood, 'Re-framing the threat of global warming: An empirical causal loop diagram of climate change, food insecurity and societal collapse', *Climatic Change*, *164*(3) (2021), pp.1–19.

102 Turchin (2008).

103 Turchin, P., *Ages of Discord*. Beresta Books (2016).

104 Turchin, P., 'Long-term population cycles in human societies', *Annals of the New York Academy of Sciences*, *1162*(1) (2009), pp.1–17.

105 Roman et al. (2017).

106 Roman (2018).

107 Turchin (2008); Roman and Palmer (2019).

108 Roman, S., 'Historical dynamics of the Chinese dynasties', *Heliyon*, *7*(6) (2021), p.e07293.

3. Existential Risk and Science Governance

Lalitha S. Sundaram

The study of existential risk has, since its earliest days, been closely linked with scientists (both their work and their concerns).[1] This is easily seen in key moments like the establishment of Pugwash and the creation of the Doomsday Clock, or in publications from prominent scientists in more recent years, such as *Our Final Century*.[2] From nuclear weapons to AI arms races, environmental crises, and, yes, even pandemics, science and technology are deeply implicated in the scholarship of existential risk, whether they are viewed as causes, risk multipliers, or potential mitigating forces (or, indeed, as all three).

In this chapter, I look at how the governance of science might matter for the production and prevention of existential risk in the context of what levers we, as a community, might be ignoring. In particular, I look at the ways in which scientific governance is conventionally framed— seeing science as something extrinsic to be regulated stringently or to be left alone to proceed without interference—and point out some of the shortcomings of this view. Instead, I propose considering scientific governance more broadly as a constellation of socio-technical processes that shape and steer technology, and in doing so, argue that research culture and self-governance not only exist but are central to how science and technology developments play out. I then put forward that there are many more levers at our disposal for ensuring the safe development of potentially very beneficial technologies than narrow views of scientific governance might suggest, and that overlooking them could rob us of much of our arsenal against existential risk. Many of the levers involve self-governance in some way, and I explore how that manifests in

    https://doi.org/10.11647/OBP.0336.03

different disciplines and settings. I end the chapter by proposing some areas where scientists and the existential risk community might together hope to influence those existing modalities.

Is top-down governance the only way?

One prominent narrative that concerns the intertwining of science and technology with existential risk stems from a number of scientists themselves 'raising the alarm', particularly in the wake of the Manhattan Project and the development and proliferation of nuclear weapons technology following the Second World War. Well-known examples are, of course, Robert Oppenheimer, Leo Szilard, and Enrico Fermi, but other examples include thinkers who were less directly involved in the development of these weapons, but who raised the possibility of anthropogenic civilisational destruction as a subject for serious academic and policy discussion, like Albert Einstein and Bertrand Russell, or even Winston Churchill and H.G. Wells. For this cadre of intellectuals, naturally, given the historical moment through which they lived, the greatest risks emerged from the possibility of technologically enhanced war, with Russell noting in a letter to Einstein that: "although the H-bomb at the moment occupies the centre of attention, it does not exhaust the destructive possibilities of science, and it is probable that the dangers of bacteriological warfare may before long become just as great".[3]

One possible solution that was frequently discussed and advocated by such groups was the establishment of world government, both as a means of preventing future wars that might now prove fatal to humanity and as a way of accelerating the creation and adoption of solutions to pressing global problems. Bertrand Russell, for instance, argued that science was destabilising modern society in the same way that nuclear physicists had recently learnt to destabilise atoms. He argued that science was increasingly disturbing the physical, biological, and psychological basis for societies to the point where "we must accept vast upheavals and appalling suffering" unless four conditions could be established. These were: 1) a single world government with a monopoly on all military force, 2) enough economic equality to eradicate envy between people, 3) a universally low birth rate to ensure a stable world population, and 4) opportunities for everyone to develop individual initiative "in work and play" and to exercise the greatest level of power over themselves.[4]

It is worth noting, however, that Russell saw these conditions as built on one another (to some extent), such that world government is seen as the basis on which to establish equality, sustainability, and individual freedom—rather than the other way around.

It is important to note, however, that despite the strong leanings that Russell, Einstein, and others had towards strong top-down governance (at least on the global stage), the organisation that is (one of their) most significant legacies in the field of existential risk—Pugwash—decidedly does not operate under that model. The Pugwash Conferences that have been organised since the Russell-Einstein Manifesto (see this volume's chapter by Beard and Bronson) "eventually came to be hosted, almost all of them in places other than Pugwash, by national 'Pugwash groups' whose character, institutional affiliations (if any) and methods of work and fundraising varied from country to country",[5] with the Pugwash website itself noting its "rather decentralized organizational structure".[6] Moreover, as noted in the chapter by Beard and Bronson, Pugwash co-existed with several civil movements—such as the Campaign for Nuclear Disarmament and the Committee of 100, established by Russell himself—which justify civil disobedience as a means to give voice to popular fears about existential risks and dissatisfaction with government policy.

Nevertheless, the view of top-down, formal oversight as the only way to achieve governance persists, especially when it comes to governance of existential risks stemming from science. In 2019, Nick Bostrom introduced the "Vulnerable World Hypothesis",[7] whereby technological advances are viewed as balls drawn from a large urn of infinite possibilities (possible technological ideas or advances, that is). The majority of these balls have thus far been beneficial (white) or not catastrophically damaging (grey). However, Bostrom posits, it is only a matter of time before we (human society) draw a "black ball": a "technology that invariably or by default destroys the civilization that invents it".[8] Bostrom's contention is that the primary reason for us not having done so yet is luck, rather than any kind of safeguarding mechanism or policy. In order not to continue relying on such luck (which must, to Bostrom's mind, eventually run out), he describes one way out: that of exiting what he terms the "semi-anarchic default condition".[9] This condition—namely the world as it exists—is one to be overcome if we are to avoid drawing a black ball. The three main features that Bostrom ascribes to it are a lack of preventative policing, a lack of global governance (in an obvious echo to Russell), and the fact that the actors involved have diverse motivations. Potential mitigations for some types of vulnerability that Bostrom proposes are options for technological curtailment, including differential technological development[10] and preference modification. Here, technologies deemed to be potentially "black ball" can be delayed in their development, or the actors involved could be monitored and their efforts re-focused. Overall, therefore, for Bostrom, a key macro-strategy would involve the strengthening of surveillance, and a global governance super-structure capable of "decisive action".[11] To be clear, Bostrom's argument is not that such a system is a desirable one (indeed, he is at pains to describe many of the potential downsides and concedes it may not be "desirable all things considered"[12]). Nevertheless, within the (hypothetical) context of the semi-anarchical condition of a "Vulnerable World", it is one of the few solutions that Bostrom sees as workable.

All this suggests a dichotomy between models in which science is allowed to develop on its own within existing social institutions (which are viewed as insufficiently overseen, in which case science is presumed to be more dangerous), or else sustained centralised action needs to be taken to reshape these institutions in order to direct scientific research and technological development away from what is risky and make society fit for receiving the benefits of science without being harmed. One way to think about this trade-off is in economic terms: either science (and thus scientists) is left to its own devices participating in an unregulated, *laissez-faire* 'market of ideas' or governments and regulators need to establish beforehand which topics will be most beneficial and safe, and then direct scientists and technology developers to work on those and avoid everything else. This dichotomy "between dirigism and laissez-faire"[13] has been characterised in biotechnology policy in terms of which parts of the biotechnology landscape are likely to yield the most public good, and as the Nuffield Council on Bioethics puts it, we are relying on state intervention on the one hand and market forces on the other.[14] While these ends of the spectrum (and options in between) have usually been considered in terms of their impact on future biotechnologies as a matter of social value, it is not a stretch to see how this could be reframed as a question of risk and safety, and of preventing catastrophic (or even existential) harm. Thus: either risks are foreseen by an authority and regulated against, or some notion of a market (largely informal, though this could be formalised as insurance)[15] naturally self-adjusts to drive riskier areas of work and practice into abandonment. Plainly, this latter option cannot be of much use when it comes to existential risks, since even the most well-funded insurers could not hope to pay out after humanity has gone extinct, and we might say the same about many of the more severe forms of global catastrophe as well. Extreme risks may prove to be a market failure in every conceivable sense.

A broader take on governance

Thinking about governance in this polarised way is very restrictive and ignores a great many realities about science and technology. For a start, science and technology do not exist as separate entities from human activity and society more broadly. Moreover, as an object of governance, they are neither distinct nor static. Science and technology are not monolithic either; their developments do not exist in a vacuum. They are enterprises engaged in by *people*, and so it matters a great deal who those people are. Not only that, it matters how they have been trained, not just in their professions but in how they approach the world and what responsibility they feel they have towards it. And these scientists—these people—do not act in isolation from each other and their communities or from the institutions and wider systems within which they operate either.

So, when it comes to 'governing science' in order to understand, prevent, and mitigate existential risks, instead of reaching immediately for some hegemonic form of extra-community governance, we need to better understand and learn how to shape these wider systems. Indeed, governance is best seen as 'how technologies are shaped and steered' rather than simply, as is too often the case, 'how they are regulated'. We need to think about governance as the group of mechanisms, processes, and communities that structures, guides, and manages technology— and this must include a consideration of systems and networks, as well as norms and culture. This is part of the view taken by Voeneky, who, while considering the legitimacy and efficacy of international law to govern global risk, describes "a multi-layer governance that consists of rules of international law, supranational and national law, private norm setting, and hybrid forms that combine elements of international or national law and private norm setting".[16]

There are two main failures of considering governance too narrowly (as a single law, policy, or other coercive measure to ensure scientists 'behave responsibly'). The first one is, as noted above, that it draws an artificial boundary around what 'science and technology' is: a boundary that tends to exclude the social and the political, seeing these instead as distinct realms into which technologies are injected or deployed. Instead, we need to acknowledge—and need our governance to acknowledge— that what we are looking at are sociotechnical systems,[17] where cross-pollination exists at every stage. Understanding these different levels of scientific governance is of utmost importance when thinking about existential risks because addressing these types of risk will require a combination of rules, norms, scientific vision, and an appreciation of the ways in which 'the social' and 'the scientific' constantly influence each other. Second, a narrow framing of scientific governance—in part a result of a too-narrow framing of science and technology—positions it solely as a gatekeeper. Viewing governance instead as a mechanism for steering allows us to harness the best of scientific and technological advances, while remaining mindful of the potential risks. However, this is not an easy path to tread; in the remainder of this chapter, I explore some of the reasons why, and propose some ways forward.

Responsibility for understanding and tackling existential risks is dispersed among a great many actors: how much of it is the responsibility of 'the scientific community'? The way 'the scientific community' is organised and how it operates is obviously a vast subject of study in and of itself, and outside the remit of this volume. A simplified (but by no means simple) view is that it involves myriad actors and institutions: governments and funders, the academy, the various institutions that 'house' the research, companies, industries and sectors, professional bodies that set standards and award qualifications, non-governmental organisations, international partnerships and coalitions and, of course, individual scientists and technology developers themselves.

A canonical example of a community's scientific self-governance is the Asilomar Conference on Recombinant DNA, which was prompted by a series of genetics experiments in the early 1970s. Experiments done in the laboratory of Paul Berg at Stanford demonstrated that DNA molecules could be 'recombined' using restriction enzymes to join them together. Experiments by Stanley Cohen, also at Stanford, and Herbert Boyer at the University of California, San Francisco demonstrated that recombinant (artificially constructed) plasmids (circular molecules of DNA that can replicate independently of chromosomes) could be propagated in bacterial cells. Presentation of this work at a 1973 Gordon Conference, along with informal conversations between colleagues, then prompted the publication of a letter to the heads of the National Academies of Science and the National Academy of Medicine, published in the journal *Science*. This letter was written "on behalf of a number of scientists to communicate a matter of deep concern",[18] namely the newfound ability to recombine DNA from diverse genetic sources. The letter noted that: "Although no hazard has yet been established, prudence suggests that the potential hazard be seriously considered",[19] and called upon the Academies to set up study committees and consider establishing guidelines.

Berg led the publication of another letter in *Science*[20] and *PNAS*[21] where he (along with colleagues from the nascent field) called for scientists to "voluntarily defer" some experiments (essentially to impose a moratorium) until such time as a conference could be convened. It is important to note that no actual harm had yet occurred; no potentially dangerous experiments had even been performed yet (indeed the possibility of direct harm was considered quite remote). In some ways, the actions taken by the researchers were textbook exemplars of the precautionary principle, with Berg's later reflection and recollection of the events noting that "there were no concrete data concerning health risks attributable to recombinant DNA experimentation. Nevertheless, there were also no data absolving the planned experiments of any risk".[22] The moratorium was—as far as it is possible to know—abided by, despite Berg's own acknowledgement at the time that "adherence to [our] major recommendations will entail postponement or possibly abandonment of certain types of scientifically worthwhile experiments".[23, 24] The reasoning behind the moratorium was to allow time to organise an international conference where the issues could be hashed out and guidelines agreed upon: the now-famous International Conference on Recombinant DNA Molecules of 1975, held at the Asilomar Conference Centre.

Three days of discussions at the conference concluded with a consensus of broad guidelines, which were published as a summary statement.[25] The recommendations included matching "containment levels" under which work would be performed to the appropriate estimated risk assessment of particular experiments; considerations of what organisms were being used; 'good' laboratory procedures to be implemented; and the development of safer 'vectors' and 'hosts'. Moreover, the summary statement also recommended that particular types of experiments be deferred, including those involving DNAs from pathogenic organisms or those "using recombinant DNAs that are able to make products potentially harmful to man, animals, or plants."[26]

And indeed, the recommendations that emerged from the conference formed the basis for much American (and, broadly speaking, worldwide) regulation of the field.

Asilomar was not a perfect process, however. Some contemporary (as well as more recent) criticisms concern the composition of the conference: alongside a few journalists who were under effective embargo, there were some 150 molecular biologists, a handful of (non-practising) lawyers, and a single bioethicist in attendance.[27] This obviously raises questions about the motivations involved: were the scientists merely forestalling more severe external regulation by being very visibly proactive?

Importantly, what would seem to be two obvious and key issues were omitted from the agenda altogether: biological warfare and gene therapy. According to the science historian, Charles Weiner:[28]

> The recombinant DNA issue was defined as a technical problem to be solved by technical means, a technical fix. Larger ethical issues regarding the purposes of the research; long-term goals, including human genetic intervention; and possible abuses of the research were excluded.

Despite this, Asilomar was largely hailed as a success in scientific self-governance, where scientists could demonstrate that they were conscious of the risks their work might incur, and that they could reach a consensus on guidelines—guidelines that would later inform regulation—to minimise these risks. As such, much more than a picturesque Californian conference venue, Asilomar has come to represent the process of pre-emptive scientific self-reflection in the face of emerging technology. Indeed, the "Asilomar Moment" has been invoked numerous times in biological research, but also—in desirable terms—in nanotechnology,[29] geoengineering,[30] and AI, from which we draw our next example.

In a sense, the upholding of the "Asilomar Moment"[31] as a paragon of self-governance simply illustrates the paucity of our understanding when it comes to what constitutes good self-governance, and ignores the many other levers that we have at our disposal. Two examples from contemporary science and technology demonstrate some of the less obvious tools of self-governance and how they can be used.

Contemporary case studies of research culture: Self-governance in action

Asilomar features heavily in another example of self-reflection by technologists, but only as part of a broad set of measures undertaken in the AI community "to shape the societal and ethical implications of AI",[32] actions that Belfield terms "activism". While Belfield draws out other ways in which that activism takes shape (worker organising, for instance), what I will focus on here is that of using the "epistemic community"[33] as an engine for self-reflection and norm-setting.

What Belfield describes echoes some of the historical actions taken by molecular biologists in the 1970s, but the scale is larger and involves more actors. In fact, the community the author defines is almost as broad as the one this chapter considers with its view of what constitutes a "scientific community" (cf. the composition of the 1975 Asilomar Conference). Belfield's AI community "include[s] researchers, research engineers, faculty, graduate students, NGO workers, campaigners and some technology workers more generally—those who would self-describe as working 'on', 'with' and 'in' AI and those analysing or campaigning on the effects of AI".[34]

Some of the actions Belfield describes include the publication of open letters, committees tasked specifically with looking at safety and ethics, and large-scale conferences on the subject, such as the 2015 Puerto Rico and 2017 Asilomar Conference for Beneficial AI. Convened by the Future of Life Institute, the 2017 conference ran over three days, and from it emerged a set of 23 "Asilomar AI Principles". The issues explored during the conference and reflected in the principles were spread across three subsets: Research, Ethics & Values, and Longer-Term Issues. Artificial Intelligence's "Asilomar Moment", despite that venue's totemic importance, is not the only way in which self-governance is apparent in the AI community—indeed, some authors have argued that lists of principles are not in themselves sufficient to ensure that the field proceeds in "robustly beneficial directions").[35] Belfield describes further actions taken by the community, such as the establishment of research, advocacy, and policy-facing centres that hold AI ethics and safety as their focus, as well as policy proposals that feed concrete input into national and international AI strategies. Other initiatives include the Neural Information Processing Systems Conference's requirement, starting in 2020, for authors to include in their submissions a "broader impact statement" which would address their work's "ethical aspects and future societal consequences".[36] While this approach obviously has its challenges (many of which reflect the complex and interlinked nature of incentives and pressures facing researchers in this—or any other—field), it is clearly an important move towards "effective community-based governance".[37] What we see here, therefore, is an example of those most intimately involved in the development of a technology wanting to have a strong pre-emptive hand in how that technology unfolds: what Baum terms "intrinsic methods"[38] in his discussion of how to ensure that the development of AI proceeds in directions that are safe and societally beneficial. Thus, while the 2017 conference may have self-consciously sought to emulate 1975, it is clear that this epistemic community has reached for—and found—many more governance modalities, and these have largely emerged from within.

Some of the differences between these two Asilomars can be attributed to research culture and how that varies not only across the several decades that separate the two events, but also across disciplines.

Research culture is a powerful force that shapes technology development, but it is also very difficult to study and change. Scientific cultures are also incredibly diverse across fields. In terms of ethics and responsibility, some fields—medicine, for example—have a long history of codified moral 'guideposts', such as the Hippocratic Oath. Within fields, too, the picture is non-homogeneous. In computer science, for instance, while the concept of 'computer ethics' was developed in the early 1940s, it is only in recent years, with public outcry surrounding privacy and the sale of data, that the issue is being given serious consideration by developers, including the work described above. Despite its near omission from the 1975 conference, bioethics has (in the decades since then) dealt extensively with issues such as gene therapy. In recent years—with the emergence of concepts such as Responsible

Research and Innovation[39] [40] alongside the emergence of synthetic biology—attention is now being paid to the responsibilities of 'ordinary scientists at the bench' rather than those purely dealing with the most obviously public-facing parts of biotechnology, such as patient consent or clinical trials. The world of pathogen research is interesting in that, beyond adherence to legal biosafety frameworks and their attendant risk assessments, there appears to be little in the way of work on broader ethical or societal engagement. Instead, issues such as safety and security have usually been raised from outside, from fields such as biosecurity or epidemiology.[41] And, of course, research culture can vary greatly in terms of how individual institutions and even laboratories are run. Given this variety, it is therefore of utmost importance that research culture be better understood, in order to more effectively use it as a means of enculturating responsibility.

An interesting example here is that of the DIY-bio community. DIY-bio can very loosely be defined as the practice of biology, biotechnology, or synthetic biology performed outside of traditional institutions, hence it sometimes being termed 'garage biotechnology' or 'biohacking'. It has been of particular interest to some in the existential risk community, with scenarios of 'lone wolves' accidentally or deliberately engineering pathogens without the oversight that normally comes from working in universities. While it may indeed be true that certain DIY-biologists work totally independently (and these have tended to be the ones garnering the most attention), the overall picture of DIY-bio is quite different. While all DIY-bio laboratories are under their national biosafety and biosecurity regulation, my own research[42] has shown that the organisation of the field as a whole demonstrates a complex ecosystem of laws, norms, and self-governance. For example, there is a DIY-bio Code of Ethics which is repeated and emphasised on several laboratories' websites, and which many of these laboratories require adherence to as a condition of membership. There are also internal Codes of Practice in place that outline more lab-specific expectations. Internal, safety-promoting, and security-promoting practices abound.

What interviews with DIY-bio community members show is that there is often intentionality in how these spaces are set up, so that they "promote a culture of trust, accountability and responsibility".[43] This can include interviews and screening of potential members, policies requiring partnered or group work (which encourages transparency and discussion), and numerous lines of communication between (biosafety/biosecurity) management and participants. The very fact that these spaces require active participation and engagement from their members in many aspects of management results in a greater degree of sensitisation to concerns about safety and security, but also reputational damage. DIY-bio practitioners therefore have a large incentive not only to behave in a responsible and safe way, but to be seen to be doing so. Moreover, there is a large degree of self-reflection in the community; 2020 saw the publication of a comprehensive "Community Biology Biosafety Handbook"[44] aimed at both established DIY-bio laboratories as well as new ones, in order to "serve as a foundation for establishing biosafety and security practices". The Handbook, which "includes biological, chemical, and equipment safety, but also subjects unique to community labs such as interview practices for screening potential lab members, considerations when working with children at festivals, building tips for creating labs in unconventional spaces, and much more", is a living document, written by several community laboratory leaders, and policy and safety experts (including, for instance, the president of the American Biological Safety Association). Many DIY-bio laboratories also have a strong educational component, which includes education on biosafety and security. Thus, even in a sub-field often assumed to be a 'wild west', there are clearly mechanisms of self-governance and self-regulation at play.

How can we improve science governance?

While governance is traditionally seen as something that happens in a top-down fashion, another way to think about it—one that puts at its centre the *people* involved—is to consider how a research culture is built and changes. Each year brings with it a new crop of practitioners, and so influencing them is an obvious starting point in influencing a field's culture.

Education

A clear route to improving scientific governance is to ensure that scientists see it as part of their job, and this involves education. At the pre-professional level, this can happen in two main ways. First, there is a need to increase the number of students and scholars researching existential risks *qua* existential risk. The field is growing but remains fairly niche and centred around a small number of elite institutions in wealthy countries. For existential risk to become part of the academic vernacular, it needs to be offered either as part of taught courses or as an option for research at a wider range of institutions globally. Despite recent trends towards multi-disciplinarity, many science and technology researchers find themselves in disciplinary silos, under the 'everyday pressures' of academia or industry. There is a likelihood that their vision of 'risk' is limited only to what their experiments might mean for their own and their labmates' safety. Indeed, unless they work on topics that have explicit forebears in, say, atomic science, they may not ever have heard of existential risk. Increased education around existential risks enlarges the talent pool that does this important research (and may then feed it into policy) and it also serves the function of 'normalising' it in academic discussion, which is one of the indirect goals of pre-professional scientific education that needs attending to. An introduction to existential risk could be tailored to specific scientific disciplines and taught as mandatory modules, thus sensitising future practitioners to the impact of their work from an early stage. This could serve the rising appetite of schoolchildren and university students for engaging with large-scale societal issues, via increased activism and participation in a variety of formal and informal groups and movements. The school climate strikes are an obvious example, but Effective Altruism groups, as well as Student and Young Pugwash, can be leveraged too.

There are reasons for optimism in the realm of formal teaching: for example, while 'engineering ethics' is a relatively well-established part of engineering curricula,[45] other scientific disciplines (such as synthetic biology) are also beginning to offer courses that deal with the societal implications of the science.[46] These types of modules are obvious places to include teaching that develops students' awareness and understanding of existential risk and of acculturating the idea of scientific self-governance. Computer science courses, too, are beginning to include topics such as AI Ethics[47]—again, an ideal route to begin building capacity for self-governance.

A key challenge remains, however, and that is likely most keenly felt when students begin to embark on semi-independent research. At this stage, often during PhD scholarship, while a student may be undertaking

day-to-day research in a self-sufficient way, the overall research themes
and directions will, in the main, be set by Principal Investigators (PIs)
who will be responding to their own influences and incentives, based
on career progression, availability of funding, and research trends. As
engaged as a PhD student might be in wider societal impacts, their
work will usually *operationally* be dictated by the PI, who may not wish
to engage with such impacts. The power differential between PIs and
early career researchers cannot be underestimated. As such, part of a
PhD student's education in this area will need to be in how to navigate
ethical 'grey areas' in a way that feels comfortable for them, but that
does not necessarily penalise them in their labs or disadvantage them
professionally. One way to deal with this issue is to ensure commitment
not only from individual PIs but from institutions: if institutions
recognise (as they are beginning to) that ethics and responsibility
are valid and valuable as core parts of scientific education, individual
recalcitrant PIs can be circumvented. The key, though, is for students
wishing to enlarge their view of how their work fits into the world—
and this includes thinking about existential risks—to be supported.
Recognising differences between disciplines and their research cultures
plays a part here too. The experience described above is situated in
the context of the natural sciences, under a mostly hierarchical model.
Here, the student is far more dependent on the PI for access to resources
(financial resources, certainly, but also in terms of access to materials
and equipment) and intellectual direction than, say, a student in the
humanities might be. In the humanities—philosophy, for example,
from which discipline many existential risk researchers hail—the norm
is apparently for scholarship at even a relatively junior level (from
undergraduate onwards) to be much more self-directed. Even here,
however, there will still be institutional norms that a student may find
they are expected to adhere to, however implicitly. Either way—and
especially as the field of existential risk studies expands to include those
from many different academic (and non-academic) backgrounds—it is
thus important that assumptions about the autonomy of scholars at this
level are questioned.

Professional bodies

One way that this institutional support could be strengthened is through professional bodies and associations or learned societies—organisations that influence more seasoned scientists. These often play a large role in shaping a scientific field, and so can exert a great deal of influence in how it is taught and how its practitioners are trained. While many of these professional organisations do have codes of ethics or statements of responsibility, in the main these tend to be rather inward-facing, setting out guidelines for ethical conduct *within* the discipline (in terms of things like discrimination, plagiarism, or obtaining consent from research participants). Global responsibility needs to be an added dimension.

However, there is also a need for professional engineering and science organisations to examine their own relationship to the major sectors driving existential risk, such as fossil fuel and (nuclear) arms industries. They must be transparent in how they accept funding and sponsorship events—especially educational ones—and in how they seek to remove themselves from these relationships. In the UK, for example, several such professional organisations have been criticised as being less-than-transparent in their financial interactions with these industries.[48]

This is somewhat at odds with another important role that professional societies can play: the interface between practising scientists/technology developers and global governance mechanisms, such as arms control treaties or the Biological and Toxin Weapons Convention (BTWC). Instruments such as these are often seen as unconnected to scientists' everyday practice, but sensitising practitioners to the relevance of these high-level discussions will highlight the obligations that are incurred and help them recognise the role that governance at the highest levels can play. The global bodies that oversee these international agreements and treaties can also play a role, by actively seeking input from practising scientists, not just from security or governance experts. For example, the BTWC implementation office could issue calls for institutions to nominate a diverse group of scientists to attend the yearly Meeting of Experts, making sure that it is not composed of the same group of scientists (typically those who are involved in research already widely thought of as 'risky') who engage with these issues year after year.

Policy engagement

Having scientists who are encouraging policy engagement also helps us tackle another aspect of scientific governance that has proven difficult. Research culture is, as we have seen, a complex domain, and it becomes even more so when it interacts with formal, top-down governance mechanisms. While a scientist or technology expert may be '*an* authority' in their domain, they are not necessarily '*in* authority' when it comes to questions of governance. Rather, this is done by policymakers, who may not have the necessary scientific understanding to do so effectively. This is especially tricky when it comes to governing emerging technologies (such as those we tend to associate with existential risk) because of the uncertainties involved. It is the 'Collingridge dilemma'[49] writ large: the balance of uncertainty and 'ability to govern' have an inverse relationship so that, almost perversely, technologies are easier to govern and shape when less is known about them and their impacts. And so, policy engagement from a diverse group of scientists is necessary at every stage, to ensure that multiple points of view are taken into account when feeding into governance, thereby hopefully bypassing the false choice of over- or under-regulation mentioned above entirely.

Collective action

Established scientists and technology developers can exert influence and support younger practitioners by being more open and vocal about their own commitments to ethical science and the prevention and mitigation of existential risks. In many instances, it appears that established scientists and engineers hold private concerns about existential risks that they are uneasy to voice for several reasons. So, providing a *collective* means of expressing concern and pledging action can be a useful way of eliciting more honest communication about the scale and seriousness of the problems humanity faces. For example, Scientists for Global Responsibility's Science Oath for the Climate[50] encourages their members (scientists, engineers, and other academics) to sign an oath to take professional and personal action, and to speak out publicly. This Oath astutely recognises the hesitancy that some scientists might face in doing so, and emphasises the connection between personal action and the ability of groups to influence and change systems.

Collective action is also of utmost importance when it comes to tackling another facet of governance: funding and complicity. More funding for work on existential risks is obviously a critical factor, but equally important is *where* that funding comes from. At present, business[51] and the military[52] dominate as funders and performers of research, but there is still a lot of money in the public sector, and universities are obviously places where much existential risk research is performed. However, an important part of scientists' responsibilities is to be judicious in what funding is accepted and what partnerships are entered into. As well as actively pursuing research into understanding and preventing existential risks, there must be scope for curbing the influence of organisations and sectors that are responsible for causing existential risks. But these organisations and sectors often have the resources to be attractive partners for scientists, and a strong incentive to do so: a kind of green-washing, or 'ethical-washing'. For instance, in the UK, the private consortium Atomic Weapons Establishment funnels over £8.5 million to over 50 universities as part of its Technical Outreach programme. Similarly, one of the biggest science and engineering fairs (unironically titled The Big Bang) gains most of its sponsorship from a number of weapons companies.[53] At a minimum, all these types of relationships need to be made transparent and strong ethical safeguards enacted.

Public outreach

Scientists can also use their voices to communicate and engage with society. Existential risk as part of a public agenda requires buy-in from that public, not only in ensuring that existential risks remain high on that agenda, but by helping to curb the undue influence of highly problematic industries which, as we have seen, can undermine both the spirit and practice of 'responsible science'. Public influence matters, not least because many of those who hold power are (at least in democracies) ultimately still accountable to that public, and will respond to pressure from their constituencies. Again, this will require effort from scholars of existential risk, and from scientists and technology developers from the wider STEM(M) community. In light of the COVID-19 pandemic, there is likely to be an increased appetite for topics related to resilience and preparedness—more 'realistic' scenarios than the usual Hollywood zombie stories. Existential risk scholars should capitalise on this to work with science communicators, taking cues from the fields of disaster communication and environmental psychology to craft messages that inspire action, rather than hopelessness.

In closing

We have thus far discussed several ways in which 'the scientific community' can engage with governance—many levers that can be used in preventing a mitigating existential risk—but there are other elements that affect cultural values around science and technology innovation. Scientific communities exist within nation-states (though international collaborations and coalitions are, of course, common). As a result, ultimately, the research culture that an individual scientist finds herself in will be shaped in large part by the type of regime in which she finds herself. What place is there for distributed scientific governance— which includes the elements we discussed above—in a political regime that requires a particular technological direction to be taken? As we noted before, there is a difference between being 'an authority' and 'in authority'.

It is commonplace to distinguish between democracies and authoritarian governments according to their decision-making procedures and the presence, or absence, of elections as an opportunity to replace key decision-makers within them. However, we can also distinguish both democracies and authoritarian governments from totalitarian governments, whose main purpose is to break down the division between public and private, to erase the capability for freedom of speech and freedom of thought. As Immanuel Kant ("How much and how correctly would we think if we did not think as it were in community with others to whom we communicate our thoughts, and who communicate theirs with us!"[54]) and John Stuart Mill (in Chapter 2 of *On Liberty*[55]) show us, thought and speech are very clearly linked, and when you break down the division between the public and the private sphere so that these freedoms no longer really exist in any meaningful sense, you start to see where technology can be designed to maintain the status quo, even if the institutional machinery of elections remain in place.

Even in democratic societies, some totalitarian *tendencies* can have a similar effect. For example, AI technology may be used to further particular political ends in the name of protection and security. Another example is related to surveillance, which is a well-known tool that totalitarian governments have long used in the name of protecting their citizens; advanced technologies are only making this easier. Not only that, surveillance has (as we explored earlier in this chapter) been considered quite seriously as that elusive one-shot solution to the issue of scientific governance—or, at the very least, a serious contender for the 'least-bad'[56] option.

One could think of this as a twisted reading of—and tacit approval from—Mill, for whom "the only purpose for which power can be rightfully exercised over any member of a civilized community, against his will, is to prevent harm to others".[57] What greater harm can there be, after all, than existential risk? And indeed, so might greater awareness and sensitisation to catastrophic risks make this exertion of power more palatable, though the true nature of the bargain being struck—with technology as its facilitator—remains obscured. It is tempting to think this might be a case of neutral technologies being (mis-)applied to politically charged problems, as indeed existential risks can be, but as we have explored in this chapter neither technology nor its creators are neutral. This goes beyond political factions and knee-jerk thinking that authoritarianism must only have 'bad' solutions and that democracies must only have 'good' ones. Instead, we need to look more closely at priorities (and prioritisation): how science is directed in service of those priorities and what the pitfalls may be—and whether we are willing to live with them.

In any case, as I have argued in this chapter, any 'one-shot solution' is unlikely to be an effective nor practicable way of approaching scientific governance—at least not in the long term. Just like the Madisonian challenge of balancing factions with pursuing "great and aggregate interests",[58] scientific governance also faces difficulties that mean that an almost federated system of governance is necessary for it to work. The field of 'science and technology' is too broad and too diverse, the actors face numerous, often conflicting, sets of incentives for a single top-down approach to suffice, even when the ultimate aim (of 'Responsible Research and Innovation') is the same. We need to reflect seriously on how science and technology developments are socially and politically inflected, how important power is as a determinant of action, and how collective action might be used as a means of prompting change. Scientific governance will not be achieved by merely making stricter rules. The best hope, as ever, is more education and more thoughtful engagement with the many systems that make up the scientific enterprise. What we have outlined in this chapter are some options for engaging with and influencing research culture which, as we have seen, can be a key determinant in self-governance, and thus in overall governance and the promotion of safer and more socially valuable scientific and technological goods.

Notes and References

1   Beard, S.J. and Phil Torres, 'Ripples on the great sea of life: A brief history of existential risk studies', *SSRN Electronic Journal* (2020), https://doi.org/10.2139/ssrn.3730000

2   Rees, Martin J., *Our Final Century: A Scientist's Warning: How Terror, Error, and Environmental Disaster Threaten Humankind's Future in This Century—on Earth and Beyond*. Heinemann (2003).

3   Russell, Bertrand, *The Selected Letters of Bertrand Russell*, ed. by Nicholas Griffin. Routledge (2001), p. 489.

4   Russell, Bertrand, 'Can a scientific society be stable?', *BMJ*, 2(4640) (1949), pp.1307–11. https://doi.org/10.1136/bmj.2.4640.1307

5   Robinson, Julian Perry, 'Contribution of the Pugwash movement to the international regime against chemical and biological weapons', *10th Workshop of the Pugwash Study Group on the Implementation of the Chemical and Biological Weapons Conventions* (1998). http://www.sussex.ac.uk/Units/spru/hsp/documents/pugwash-hist.pdf.

6   Pugwash, 'About Pugwash', *Pugwash Conferences on Science and World Affairs* (2013), https://pugwash.org/about-pugwash/

7   Bostrom, Nicholas, 'The Vulnerable World Hypothesis', *Global Policy*, 10(4) (2019), pp.455–76. https://doi.org/10.1111/1758-5899.12718

8   Bostrom (2019), p.455.

9   Bostrom (2019).

10 Bostrom, Nicholas, 'Existential risks: Analyzing human extinction scenarios and related hazards', *Journal of Evolution and Technology, 9* (2022). https://ora.ox.ac.uk/objects/uuid:827452c3-fcba-41b8-86b0-407293e6617c

11 Ibid, p.470.

12 Ibid.

13 Rip, Arie and Anton J. Nederhof, 'Between dirigism and laissez-faire: Effects of implementing the science policy priority for biotechnology in the Netherlands', *Research Policy, 15*(5) (1986), pp.253–68. https://doi.org/10.1016/0048-7333(86)90025-9

14 Nuffield Council on Bioethics, *Emerging Biotechnologies: Technology, Choice and the Public Good* (2012).

15 Farquhar, Sebastien, Owen Cotton-Barratt, and Andrew Snyder-Beattie, 'Pricing externalities to balance public risks and benefits of research', *Health Security, 15*(4) (2017), pp.401–08. https://doi.org/10.1089/hs.2016.0118

16 Voeneky, Silja, 'Human rights and legitimate governance of existential and global catastrophic risks', in Gerald L. Neuman and Silja Voeneky (eds), *Human Rights, Democracy, and Legitimacy in a World of Disorder*. Cambridge University Press (2018). https://doi.org/10.1017/9781108355704

17 Jasanoff, Sheila and Sang-Hyun Kim, *Dreamscapes of Modernity: Sociotechnical Imaginaries and the Fabrication of Power*. University of Chicago Press (2015).

18 Singer, Maxine and Dieter Soll, 'Guidelines for DNA hybrid molecules', *Science (New York, N.Y.), 181*(4105) (1973), p.1114. https://doi.org/10.1126/science.181.4105.1114

19 Ibid (1973).

20 Berg, Paul et al., 'Potential biohazards of recombinant DNA molecules', *Science, 185*(4148) (1974), p303. https://doi.org/10.1126/science.185.4148.303

21 'Potential biohazards of recombinant DNA molecules', *Proceedings of the National Academy of Sciences, 71*(7) (1974), pp.2593–94. https://doi.org/10.1073/pnas.71.7.2593

22 Berg, Paul, 'Moments of discovery', *Annual Review of Biochemistry, 77*(1) (2008), pp.15–44. https://doi.org/10.1146/annurev.biochem.76.051605.153715

23 Berg, Paul et al. (1974).

24 Interestingly, in her examination of international law and the governance of existential risks, Voekeny notes that "a moratorium on a specific

kind of research that is based on the consensus of the relevant scientific community and backed up by the relevant scientific journals—which will not publish experiments that violate the moratorium—can be even more effective than a prohibition based on an international treaty that is implemented, top-down, by States parties."

25   Berg, Paul et al., 'Summary statement of the Asilomar conference on recombinant DNA molecules', *Proceedings of the National Academy of Sciences of the United States of America*, 72(6) (1975), pp.1981–84.

26   Berg, Paul et al (1975).

27   Dworkin, Roger B., 'Science, society, and the expert town meeting: Some comments on Asilomar', *Southern California Law Review*, 51(6) (1978), pp.1471–82.

28   Weiner, Charles, 'Drawing the line in genetic engineering: Self-regulation and public participation', *Perspectives in Biology and Medicine*, 44(2) (2001), pp.208–20. https://doi.org/10.1353/pbm.2001.0039

29   Toumey, Chris, 'An Asilomar for nanotech', *Nature Nanotechnology*, 9 (2014), pp.495–96. https://doi.org/10.1038/nnano.2014.139

30   Kintisch, Eli, '"Asilomar 2" takes small steps toward rules for geoengineering', *Science*, 328(5974) (2010), pp.22–23. https://doi.org/10.1126/science.328.5974.22

31   Petsko, Gregory A., 'An Asilomar moment', *Genome Biology*, 3(10) (2002), comment1014.1-comment1014.3 https://doi.org/10.1186/gb-2002-3-10-comment1014

32   Belfield, Haydn, 'Activism by the AI community: Analysing recent achievements and future prospects', in *Proceedings of the AAAI/ACM Conference on AI, Ethics, and Society* (presented at the AIES '20: AAAI/ACM Conference on AI, Ethics, and Society, ACM, 2020), pp.15–21. https://doi.org/10.1145/3375627.3375814

33   Haas, Peter M., 'Introduction: epistemic communities and international policy coordination', *International Organization*, 46(1) (1992), pp.1–35.

34   Belfield (2020).

35   Whittlestone, Jess et al., 'The role and limits of principles in AI ethics: Towards a focus on tensions', in *Proceedings of the 2019 AAAI/ACM Conference on AI, Ethics, and Society* (presented at the AIES '19: AAAI/ACM Conference on AI, Ethics, and Society, ACM, 2019), pp.195–200. https://doi.org/10.1145/3306618.3314289

36   'NeurIPS 2020', https://nips.cc/Conferences/2020/CallForPapers

37 Prunkl, Carina E.A. et al., 'Institutionalizing ethics in AI through broader impact requirements', Nature Machine Intelligence, 3(2) (2021), pp.104–10. https://doi.org/10.1038/s42256-021-00298-y

38 Baum, S.D., 'On the promotion of safe and socially beneficial artificial intelligence', *AI and Society*, 32(4) (2017), pp.543–51. https://doi.org/10.1007/s00146-016-0677-0

39 Owen, R., P. Macnaghten, and J. Stilgoe, 'Responsible research and innovation: From science in society to science for society, with society', *Science and Public Policy, 39*(6) (2012), pp.751–60. https://doi.org/10.1093/scipol/scs093; Alix, Jean-Pierre, 'RRI: Buzzword or vision of modern science policy?', *EuroScientist Journal* (2016). https://www.euroscientist.com/rri-new-buzzword-vision-modern-science-policy/

40 Owen, R., P. Macnaghten, and J. Stilgoe (2012).

41 Lipsitch, Marc and Thomas V. Inglesby, 'Moratorium on research intended to create novel potential pandemic pathogens', *MBio, 5*(6) (2014), e02366–14. https://doi.org/10.1128/mBio.02366-14; Koblentz, Gregory D., 'Dual-use research as a wicked problem', *Frontiers in Public Health*, 2 (2014), p.113. https://doi.org/10.3389/fpubh.2014.00113

42 Sundaram, Lalitha S., 'Biosafety in DIY-bio laboratories: From hype to policy', *EMBO Reports*, 22(4) (2021), e52506. https://doi.org/10.15252/embr.202152506

43 Sundaram (2021).

44 'Community biology biosafety handbook', *Genspace*. https://www.genspace.org/community-biology-biosafety-handbook

45 Royal Academy of Engineering, *Engineering Ethics Toolkit—Engineering Professors Council*. https://epc.ac.uk/resources/toolkit/ethics-toolkit/

46 Imperial College London, 'Systems and synthetic biology MRes | Study | Imperial College London', *Imperial College London*. https://www.imperial.ac.uk/study/courses/postgraduate-taught/systems-synthetic-biology/; University of Edinburgh, 'DPT: Systems and synthetic biology (MSc) (PTMSCSSBIO1F)', *University of Edinburgh*. http://www.drps.ed.ac.uk/21-22/dpt/ptmscssbio1f.htm.

47 Stavrakakis, Ioannis et al., 'The teaching of computer ethics on computer science and related degree programmes: A European survey', *International Journal of Ethics Education, 7*(1) (2022), pp.101–29. https://doi.org/10.1007/s40889-021-00135-1

48   Parkinson, Stuart and Philip Wood, *Irresponsible Science? | SGR: Responsible Science* (Scientists for Global Responsibility, October 2019). https://www. sgr.org.uk/publications/irresponsible-science

49   Collingridge, David, *The Social Control of Technology*. St Martin's Press (1980).

50   'Why do we need the climate oath?', *Scientists for Global Responsibility*. https://www.sgr.org.uk/projects/why-do-we-need-climate-oath

51   Office for National Statistics (ONS), 'Gross domestic expenditure on research and development, UK: 2020', (2022). https:// www.ons.gov.uk/economy/governmentpublicsectorandtaxes/ researchanddevelopmentexpenditure/bulletins/ukgrossdomesticexpen ditureonresearchanddevelopment/2020#cite-this-statistical-bulletin

52   Kuiken, Todd, *Wilson Center: US Trends in Synthetic Biology Research Funding* (September 2015). https://www.wilsoncenter.org/publication/ us-trends-synthetic-biology-research-funding

53   Parkinson and Wood (2019).

54   Wood, Allen W., 'What does it mean to orient oneself in thinking? (1786)', in *Religion and Rational Theology*, by Immanuel Kant, ed. by Allen W. Wood and George di Giovanni, 1ˢᵗ edn. Cambridge University Press (1996), pp.1–18 (p.16). https://doi.org/10.1017/CBO9780511814433.003

55   Mill, John Stuart, *On Liberty*. Cambridge University Press (2012).

56   Rees (2003).

57   Mill (2012), p. 22.

58   Hamilton, Alexander, James Madison, and John Jay, *The Federalist With Letters of "Brutus"*, ed. by Terence Ball. Cambridge University Press (2003), p.45. https://doi.org/10.1017/CBO9780511817816

4. Beyond 'Error and Terror': Global Justice and Global Catastrophic Risk

Natalie Jones

This chapter is an invitation to consider global political, economic, social, and legal systems, particularly in relation to global justice and inequality, when studying and addressing global catastrophic risks. Such a focus can provide a powerful complement to work concentrating on the role of individuals in the production of risk. I argue that to examine global catastrophic risks without a global justice lens is to distort our understanding of those risks; adding a global justice lens onto our existing strategies can help us see the nature of risks more clearly. Strategies to reduce global catastrophic risk will be more effective if they take global justice considerations into account. Further, policies to reduce global catastrophic risk reduction can—and should—be designed so as to simultaneously mitigate risk and deliver more just outcomes.

So far, a large focus of the study of global catastrophic risks has been 'error and terror': that is, the ways in which individuals and/or small groups of people can cause global catastrophe. More recently, researchers have paid more attention to the role of institutions— including corporations and governments, as well as that of systems—in causing, preventing, and responding to catastrophe. This chapter briefly canvasses these shifts, before proposing a case for a justice lens, using the example of climate change. The chapter ends with suggestions for further research.

  https://doi.org/10.11647/OBP.0336.04

'Error and terror': Global catastrophic risks from individuals

A key strength of academic work on global catastrophic risks to date has been its approach to studying the ways in which individuals and small groups can cause global catastrophes. Somewhat representative of this approach is Martin Rees' treatment of global catastrophic risk in his 2002 book *Our Final Century*, followed up by his 2018 volume *On The Future*.[1] In his words, risks "may come not primarily from national governments, not even from 'rogue states', but from individuals or small groups with access to ever more advanced technology".[2] Existential hazards could be triggered by ordinary citizens, no longer only by world leaders with nuclear buttons at their fingertips.[3] The discussion of risks posed by individuals focuses largely on two possibilities, referred to by Rees (as here) by the terms 'error' and 'terror'. This distinction was also made by Nick Bostrom in his influential 2002 article on existential risks, during his discussion of "bangs"—relatively sudden disasters arising from either an accident or a deliberate act of destruction.[4] And the error-terror framing continues to hold resonance in recent work—for instance, in Ord (2020).[5]

Error invokes the possibility of mistakes or accidents in, for example, scientific research on bio- or nanotechnology.[6] Gain-of-function experiments—whereby viruses are altered with the intent to better understand pandemics—could go wrong, resulting in the leak of vaccine-resistant or more virulent viruses from laboratories.[7] Nanomachines that assemble copies of themselves could accidentally be released, whereupon they might proliferate unstoppably, consuming all the Earth.[8] A superintelligence might be badly programmed, with researchers making a mistake that ends up giving the superintelligence goals that lead it to wipe out humankind.[9] In this way, individuals or small groups may, by their actions or inactions, pose a threat to the whole world.

Meanwhile, *terror* is the idea that individuals or groups with malicious intentions may trigger technological weapons, such as engineered viruses or nuclear devices, with the aim of carrying out mass destruction.[10] Rees cited past bioattacks and apocalyptic suicide cults (such as those carried out by the Rajneeshee cult in 1984 and the Aum Shinrikyo sect in the early 1990s)[11] to suggest that private individuals might well have the motivations and skills to pose an existential threat. Many of the same examples are drawn upon in Toby Ord's recent book, *The Precipice*.[12] Bostrom, likewise, was concerned about the "tyrant, terrorist or lunatic" who might create a "doomsday virus"—that is, a virus combining long latency with high virulence and mortality.[13] Rees predicted that thousands or even millions of individuals could someday acquire the capability to manufacture bioweapons,[14] due in part to the 'dual use' nature of such technologies: the equipment needed to create lethal substances is the same as that required for common medical or agricultural applications.[15]

Much further work has followed, directly or indirectly, from this analysis. On the more abstract end, Emile Torres elaborates upon the concept of 'agential risk', which directly draws on the 'terror' concept.[16] Torres lays out a typology of human agents who would destroy the world if they had the capabilities to do so. In his view, this includes "apocalyptic terrorists", "misguided moral actors", "ecoterrorists", and "idiosyncratic actors" such as rampage shooters.[17] On the more specific end, many researchers have considered, in depth, ways in which risks from accident or misuse of biotechnology may be mitigated,[18] while others have examined possibilities for the malicious use of artificial intelligence.[19] Still others have considered how individual cognitive biases—such as confirmation bias and hindsight bias—can play into global catastrophic risk, including (but not limited to) terror and error scenarios.[20]

Beyond individuals to institutions and systems

Of course, work on global catastrophic risk has not been limited solely to an individualist framing of threat. In addition to the continued focus on individuals, global catastrophic risk researchers have also started to consider how systems, institutions, and governance contribute to causing—as well as failing to prevent, mitigate, or adequately respond to—global catastrophe.

Even earlier work that focused predominantly on terror and error also contained some reference to broader institutions, whether explicit or implied. Rees in *Our Final Century* extensively discussed the risk from nuclear weapons—largely the domain of state actors—and considered the merits of government regulation of biotechnological research to mitigate risk[21] (for instance), while Bostrom's 2002 categorisation of existential risks included examples like "misguided world government" or a "repressive totalitarian global regime", as well as examples along more agential lines.[22] Rees' later work considers the role of economic growth, distribution of wealth, and the short-termism in politics, and proposes government policies to address climate change.[23] Governments are, in this way, seen as part of the problem or, potentially, part of a solution.

Later work has refined these intuitions. In this vein, Avin et al. (2018) construct a framework for classifying global catastrophic risks based on "critical systems" for humanity's survival, including socio-technological systems, mechanisms by which a threat spreads worldwide, and failures to prevent or mitigate, including institutional and "beyond institutional" fragilities.[24] Relatedly, Liu, Lauta, and Maas (2018) urge moving beyond a hazard-centric approach—which would, for instance, focus on malign or error-prone individuals triggering harmful technologies—to one that also takes into account vulnerabilities and exposure, and urge a focus on governance.[25] They note "many other, slower and more intertwined ways in which the world might collapse" other than spectacular hazards.[26] Among the vulnerabilities they mention are several that implicate governance, institutions, and systems: "globalised economic and institutional frameworks", "market dependency", "homogenous global monoculture in practices and ideology", and "globalised diets and food demand". Similarly, Kuhlemann (2019) has urged increased focus on epistemically messy, creeping risks arising from "gradual damage to collective goods" and economic "growthist" paradigms, rather than those neatly attributable to "villainous or blundering agents"—that is, error and terror.[27] Cotton-Barratt, Daniel, and Sandberg (2020), in their categorisation of existential risks, include categories corresponding to error and terror ("accident risk" and "malicious risk", in their terminology), but also add that risks can be "latent", in that many people pursue an activity which causes global damage without knowing that it does so—for instance, burning fossil fuels before scientists realised that doing so caused global warming—or "commons", whereby many people are aware of the damage and engage in the activity anyway—for instance, burning fossil fuels now. Here, one could read in the existence of broader structures that incentivise people to engage in such an activity.[28] Finally, Kreienkamp and Pegram (2020) consider systems approaches to global catastrophic risks, including complexity theory.[29] They discuss how global catastrophic risks are "systemically produced and amplified", pointing to "tightly coupled linkages of global social, economic, technological, and ecological systems". Kreienkamp and Pegram distinguish between risks that are severe but not very complex, such as asteroid impact or nuclear war, and those with high levels of "connectivity, openness, nonlinear dynamics, and emergent properties that produce frequent surprises" such as climate change, using this insight to propose design principles for governing complex global catastrophic risks.[30]

Complementing agential approaches with systemic and global justice approaches

What the works discussed in the section above have in common is that they move beyond considering only (or mainly) the role of individuals as mistaken or malicious perpetrators of catastrophe. Rather, they invoke the possibility of global catastrophe for which no one individual or small group is responsible, where broader systems are at play. They start to unpack the complexities involved in effectively managing and responding to risk. The increasing focus on systems as a complement to agential, 'error and terror' approaches is indispensable for understanding global catastrophic risk. For one thing, systems shape the incentives, opportunities, pathways, and barriers that individuals face. Much economic and legal thought takes this as given. Prominent schools of thought in sociology recognise that individuals are not solely in control of their own actions and destinies, but rather express agency in the context of pre-existing social structures—though they are also capable of exercising their agency to change those structures.[31] We could then understand individuals involved in error-terror scenarios as embedded in societal, cultural, political, economic, and legal systems, which opens up new research avenues for scholars of global catastrophic risk. For another thing, if we understand risk as composed of hazard, vulnerability, and exposure, the latter two elements inherently invoke systems (as outlined in Liu,

Lauta, and Maas, 2019). Furthermore, many proposed policy solutions for global catastrophic risks would have flow-on implications for the functioning of global systems. This is illustrated, at the extreme end, by Martin Rees' discussion of possible solutions to the risks posed by dual-use technologies—proposals which would irreversibly transform the global political economy. These could include establishing an oppressive police state, which might be the "least-bad safeguard", as the only way to ensure total government control over the manufacture and use of dangerous technologies.[32] Although "deeply unpalatable", Rees acknowledged, this might still be seen as necessary.[33] Another proposal is the "dystopian prospect" of using drugs, genetic modification, or brain implants to "stabilise" those "drawn towards the disaffected fringe"—in crude terms, mind control.[34] However, such proposals need not be so radical in order to interact with, and alter, existing systems.

Notwithstanding the many valuable and worthwhile contributions to date, much space remains for further work. In particular, when considering how global catastrophic risk is co-created by agents alongside institutions, systems, and governance aspects, there is particular room for engagement with questions of justice. How is the production of global catastrophic risk linked to global injustices? Who is more or less affected by a given risk? Who benefits and loses from interventions to reduce or respond to risk? The remainder of this chapter argues that if global justice considerations are omitted from our analyses, we will not clearly understand the nature of global catastrophic risk. Rather, further study of *global* social, political, and economic systems (and the justice thereof) will improve understanding of how global catastrophic risk is produced and maintained, and how it may be prevented, managed, and effectively responded to. Moreover, we can design policy interventions to effectively respond to both global justice and global catastrophic risk considerations. We can understand these ideas by considering a prominent case study—climate change—which demonstrates the linkages between global catastrophic risks, global systems, and justice.

Global justice and the climate crisis

The nature of the problem

Questions of global equity, fairness, and justice lie at the heart of debates on the global response to climate change.[35] The basic issue is this: the poorest nations, which consume the least material resources, have generated minimal greenhouse gas emissions. At the same time, these countries are disproportionately vulnerable to the effects of climate change, to which they are least equipped to respond. In many such countries, access to energy to underpin basic needs is still a challenge. Conversely, the wealthiest nations—which consume the most and have produced the largest cumulative emissions—tend to be less vulnerable to many climate impacts, and are better resourced to adapt, as well as to reduce their emissions. From 1751 to 2017, the United States generated around 25% of all carbon dioxide emissions; the European Union and the United Kingdom were responsible for another 22%; China saw 12.7%, while India, the continent of Africa, and that of South America produced around 3% each.[36] Slicing it another way, from 1990–2015, a period which saw as much cumulative emissions as the entirety of 1751–1989, the richest 10% of the global population was responsible for 52% of cumulative carbon emissions, while the poorest 50% accounted for 7%.[37] Meanwhile, the Climate World Risk Index shows that the most exposed and vulnerable countries are lower-income countries that have contributed least to greenhouse gas emissions.[38] Scientists have warned that the consumption of affluent households worldwide is "by far the strongest determinant and the strongest accelerator" of climate impacts.[39] Indeed, global warming has likely exacerbated global economic inequality over the last 50 years by 25%, due to the fact that warming has increased economic growth in cool countries and decreased growth in warm countries.[40]

This is no mere coincidence. Scholars of history and political economy have shown how, for centuries, global economic and political systems have operated to extract wealth from the Global South to the Global North, via colonisation and imperialism, and climate change can be traced back to the operation of these systems.[41] Scholars of neocolonialism have shown how, despite the end of formal empires in the mid-20ᵗʰ century, a model of economic globalisation evolved that protected and extended the inequalities and exploitation of the colonial era.[42] A country's history of being colonised continues to be indicative of per-capita levels of poverty.[43] And, in the last decade, there has been a close interlinkage between far-right, white nationalist politics and the politics of climate denial and delay.[44]

These global patterns are replicated within nations. Wealthier communities are more resilient to climate impacts, while contributing more to emissions. Conversely, low-income communities, racialised or minority ethnic communities, people with disabilities, older people, women, and indigenous peoples tend to be more susceptible to risks posed by climate impacts. The relationship between environmental quality and inequality is well established.[45] When it comes to extreme weather events (among other disasters), hazard and disaster research has clearly demonstrated that social inequalities shape disaster management and response.[46] The spectacle of private firefighters protecting the homes of high-net-worth individuals during the 2018–2020 California wildfires—while public firefighting forces were, in part, made up of prison inmates—brought this point home.[47] Elsewhere, systemic racism was found to be a barrier to disaster response in the wake of major hurricanes in Puerto Rico.[48] In the UK, coastal flooding (which will become more frequent and severe due to climate change) poses a much higher risk to deprived communities, partly because such communities disproportionately make up ex-industrial ports and declining resort towns.[49] These are just a few examples of a widespread pattern.

Against this backdrop, a key challenge of our time is how to rapidly reduce greenhouse gas emissions so as to meet a carbon budget compatible with limiting global warming within the internationally recognised safe limit of 1.5°C, *and to do so in a fair and just way*. It is important to note that inequalities are relevant not only in respect of causation and impacts of climate change, but also in relation to the effects of climate change response measures.[50] There have already been well-documented cases where interventions primarily meant to reduce emissions (or adapt to climate impacts) have served to further entrench (global) inequalities. The construction of hydroelectric reservoirs has led, in many countries, to the forced displacement of already marginalised people and communities, with deleterious social consequences.[51] Incentivisation of ethanol use as an alternative fuel in order to reduce emissions from transportation has led to the use of food crops for ethanol, causing hardship in poorer communities due to higher food prices and consequent lack of food security.[52] Meanwhile, measures to shift away from fossil-fuel production can inflict severe damage on communities dependent on the incomes derived from coal, oil, or gas extraction, if not designed with the interests of workers and communities at heart so as to (for instance) retrain workers and clean up damaged environmental sites.[53] Cobalt and lithium mines, containing crucial materials for manufacturing battery and solar technologies, also happen to be found in low- and low-middle-income countries, raising the prospect that the uptake of electric vehicles and solar panels in early-adopter (wealthier) nations could come at the expense of poorer communities in countries like Chile, Bolivia, and Serbia.[54]

But this does not have to be the way. Rather, climate policies can be designed to simultaneously bolster climate action and justice. The 'just transition' literature and community of practice explores how to transition to a zero-carbon society in a way that does not strand workers and communities, but rather protects livelihoods, workers' rights, and quality jobs.[55] Another parallel strand of work shows how climate policy and human rights can be aligned.[56] In countries like the US and UK, Green New Deal policies would aim to simultaneously tackle inequality and climate change,[57] although a key area of contestation is presently how to design such policies to also take proper account of global justice.[58] Many political proposals have been devised for the fair and just allocation of emissions reduction burdens,[59] including the allocation of emissions rights to countries based on an equal per-capita allocation,[60] and an approach based on countries' historical responsibility for cumulative emissions.[61]

The international politics of equitable burden-sharing

Against this backdrop, let us turn, for a moment, to briefly take stock of how key international political and legal accords on climate change have taken account of global equity and justice considerations. Far from a marginal or secondary issue, differential historic responsibility for—and vulnerability to the impacts of—climate change has taken centre-stage over nearly three decades of international climate negotiations.

The principle of common but differentiated responsibilities and respective capabilities (CBDR-RC) was agreed by countries in the 1992 UN Framework Convention on Climate Change (UNFCCC)—which, as of the time of writing, includes 197 states parties.[62] Under CBDR-RC, developed country parties should take the lead in combating climate change and its adverse effects. The UNFCCC, accordingly, provided for a higher standard of obligations for countries included in its Annex I—a list of countries then considered to be industrialised, comprising the OECD plus former Soviet states undergoing the transition to a market economy—compared with those of other countries, an approach known as 'differentiation'. To operationalise the Framework Convention, state parties then agreed to the Kyoto Protocol in 1997. The Kyoto Protocol continued the differentiation approach, making a rigid distinction between industrialised (Annex I) and all other (non-Annex I) countries. Binding, quantitative, absolute emissions reduction or limitation targets were imposed for the former but not the latter. This proved problematic, as the Annex I and non-Annex I categorisation established in 1992 was widely seen as outdated, at least in the Global North. In the intervening years, countries like China, Brazil, South Africa, and others have seen their economies (and emissions) rapidly expand.[63]

The Paris Agreement of 2015 ended the strict differentiation between Annex I and non-Annex I parties, requiring *all* countries to submit national climate action pledges, known as nationally determined contributions (NDCs). However, the Agreement still distinguishes between "developing" and "developed" countries on certain issues, and contains a "subtle differentiation" for specific subsets of countries and on certain issues such as finance, capacity-building, technology transfer, and reporting.[64] Countries can, and do, make the magnitude of their emissions reduction and climate adaptation pledges in their NDCs conditional on receiving international support from wealthier countries.[65] The level and type of finance and other support to be provided by "developed" countries to "developing" countries is still a key political issue in the UN climate negotiations.[66]

This foray into international climate law and politics, while brief, aims to provide a window into the long and contentious history of international discussions on climate change and global justice issues. The point that scholars of global catastrophic risk might take away is that, when working on or researching global governance of such risk, one cannot ignore political questions of differential causation and harms. If working through multilateral institutions, countries who are disproportionately impacted will raise their concerns, and countries with disproportionate responsibility will face corresponding challenges. Global justice will, in other words, rear its head. In the climate sphere, countries with disproportionate responsibility—like the UK, EU, and US—have long sought to play down these considerations, which has mainly resulted in undermining global trust and delaying action by all countries on climate change.

Structural complications and (partial) structural solutions

How do climate policy solutions that take account of global justice differ from climate policies that ignore global justice? For the purposes of illustrating this difference, let us now consider some structural barriers to effective, global climate action, and how these may be overcome. Global (carbon) inequality and the climate crisis in general (as mentioned above) are enmeshed in and compounded by various global social, economic, political, and legal structures, which actively hinder just and safe climate mitigation. The rules and institutions of global economic governance are particularly pertinent here—for example, investor protection, debt governance, and intellectual property regimes. First, rules on protections for foreign investors limit countries' abilities to put in place environmental regulations like carbon taxes, stronger performance standards, emissions limits, and the denial of permits for fossil fuel development. Investor-state dispute settlements have been used by multinational enterprises to challenge actions like these.[67] These agreements have also tended to deepen global inequalities by enhancing the power of foreign investors (largely, though not exclusively, multinational enterprises based in wealthy countries) relative to citizens.[68] Poorer countries have more limited resources to defend against such cases, and are thus likely to come under pressure to abandon or delay climate policy measures.[69] Researchers have developed proposals on how such agreements may be amended—or how countries may strategically withdraw from them—in order to improve climate policy.[70]

Second, multilateral debt poses another significant barrier to climate action and to justice. Developing countries' levels of debt—to the IMF, the World Bank, and bilateral creditors—have risen from around 30% of GDP in 1960 to 170% of GDP in 2019, totalling more than $8 trillion.[71] On average, by 2018 developing countries were spending in excess of 10% of their revenues on debt repayments, though some countries spend 20% or even up to 70%.[72] High repayment levels constrain these countries' fiscal space to respond to climate change (as well as to enact other public priorities, such as education or healthcare), and contribute to debt crises. When climate disasters hit, countries are forced to take on further loans to finance recovery and reconstruction, due to a lack of other options.[73] Countries situated at the intersection of high levels of indebtedness, greater climate vulnerability, and low access to credit are the most prone to debt crises and inability to finance climate priorities.[74] Indeed, combined with debt repayments, levels of tax avoidance and the extraction of profits by multinational companies, this often means that poorer countries lose a lot more wealth than what they receive in aid.[75] In 2015, Sub-Saharan African countries received over $160 billion in loans, aid, and investment, but lost at least $203 billion, including from tax avoidance, debt repayments, illegal logging and wildlife trade, and the extraction of profits by multinational companies to their home countries.[76] Policy proposals regarding debt jubilees, debt-for-climate finance swaps, increased use of International Monetary Fund (IMF) Special Drawing Rights, and other ideas to reduce debt burdens while fostering climate action have accordingly been gaining more traction.[77]

Third and finally, the international intellectual property regime has been another barrier to globally just climate action. With industrialised countries and major emerging economies dominating the environmental technology market,[78] intellectual property rights have been found to reduce imports of solar technologies into non-OECD countries.[79] Meanwhile, countries that bear a higher share of historical responsibility stand to gain from selling proprietary technologies to the countries that will suffer most.[80] Similarly to the much-publicised proposal for an intellectual property waiver to enable a rapid and just rollout of COVID-19 vaccines,[81] scholars and advocates have proposed the waiver of intellectual property rights to allow for the global distribution of renewable energy and energy efficiency technologies at scale and at speed.[82]

Global catastrophic risk's characterisations of climate change

Against these understandings of climate change as intertwined with issues of unequal benefit and harm, let us now return to the ways in which climate change has been addressed in work on global catastrophic risk. Upon examination, we can see that questions of global justice are not addressed, and that this distorts how climate change is understood. First, there is a tendency to view climate change as a 'commons' issue: that is, a problem caused by the cumulative actions of many people, who engage in burning fossil fuels and climate-unfriendly land-use practices in the knowledge that this causes climate change. From this viewpoint, climate change is viewed as a simple coordination failure, a problem of externalities not being sufficiently addressed within the market. Differential responsibility for—and harm from—climate change is flattened. In this vein, Ord (2020) characterises climate change as involving 'the aggregation of small effects from the choices of everyone in the world';[83] Kuhlemann (2019) says the harm arises from "gradual harm to collective goods" and is "driven by the aggregate impact over time of human populations, people behaving as they normally do".[84] Cotton-Barratt, Daniel, and Sandberg (2020) characterise climate change as a "latent risk" where "many people pursue an activity which causes global damage, without knowing that it does".[85] Similarly, Liu, Lauta, and Maas (2018) characterise climate change as a risk arising from "passive" vulnerabilities and "indirect" exposure, whereby a risk is indirectly caused by societal arrangements intended for something else.[86]

Works such as these do not mention the differential responsibility for, causation of, and vulnerability to climate change among 'human populations'. This oversight, although likely unintentional, has flow-on implications for how climate change is understood and addressed as a global catastrophic risk. Even if the role of poorer countries is mentioned, the question of historic responsibility tends to go unaddressed. For instance, Rees (2018) rightly notes the need for "developing countries" to "leapfrog directly to a more efficient and less wasteful mode of life"[87] in the course of a lengthy discussion of climate policy options, but neglects to mention the responsibility (both political and legal) of developed countries to provide support for this, nor the differential role of wealthier and poorer countries in causing the problem.

Where to?

I have argued that, by disregarding global justice considerations, scholars of global catastrophic risk have tended to misunderstand the nature of the climate change problem and how to solve it. Climate change is only one case study, albeit illustrative for global catastrophic risk in general. With the lessons from the climate in mind, further work might consider how the forces driving the development of dangerous technologies arise from existing political economies and associated societal and legal arrangements, how these technologies place differential burdens and cause differential harms, and where (unexpected) allies in the quest to avoid their risks may be found. More generally, further work could consider how efforts to reform global economic structures—including restructuring aid and development models, intellectual property laws, and trade and investment regimes—could support the agenda of reducing global catastrophic risk. We might consider whether (and how) redressing global injustices can be aligned with—and actively help with—reducing global catastrophic risks. And we might consider who benefits the most, and conversely, who experiences the highest costs, from policies to mitigate global risk. We could then consider how to adjust and design these policies accordingly. Research and scholarship is particularly needed on the relationship between global justice and injustice, and areas of global catastrophic risk other than climate change—for instance, nuclear, biorisk, volcanoes, and AI. In some cases, there is already extensive work in existence—think of the research on AI and inequality, or pandemic vaccine equity—that could be usefully synthesised and incorporated into a more holistic—and accurate—study of global catastrophic risk.

All of this could complement more targeted measures to mitigate risks from individual misuse of technology. In other words, this is not to say that terror and error are entirely unimportant. Evidently, the dual use of potentially dangerous nano- and bio-technology is a major concern, and there will always be a place for technical work on how to mitigate these risks. It is also important to consider how a given person can best act—within the constraints due to their structural location in the political economy of society—to address global catastrophic risk, not least because this helps us understand our own opportunities and responsibilities for action. But these approaches are not sufficient to address global catastrophic risk.

We may also learn from the global climate response in one final respect. From the beginning of international discussions on climate change, many governments—perhaps most prominently that of the United States—largely dismissed the need for a justice component. Equity was viewed as an unnecessary barrier to action. They pushed for emissions cuts to be carried out by all countries, while not offering to provide financial, technical, or technological assistance to poorer countries for either mitigation or adaptation.[88] Poorer countries understandably rejected this as inconsistent with their vital interests in development, and thus the foundations for 30 years (and counting) of international disagreement on how to tackle climate change were laid. When it comes to emerging global catastrophic risks, which have not yet been the subject of extended discussion or policymaking at the level of international relations, we have a chance to get international politics right from the start. This means, where a given risk intersects with global justice, we can make sure to factor these considerations in when assessing policies to mitigate it. Some politicians in rich countries may consider this unnecessary. But, in the face of escalating risks, and the prospect of decades of resistance or political deadlock as in the case of climate change, the question is, can the world really afford not to address global justice in dealing with global catastrophic risk?

Notes and References

1   Rees, Martin, *Our Final Century: Will The Human Race Survive the Twenty-first Century?* Heinemann (2003); Rees, Martin, *On The Future: Prospects for Humanity.* Princeton University Press (2018).

2   Rees (2003), p.3, 42.

3   Ibid., p.4. Also see Rees (2018), pp. 16–17.

4   Bostrom, Nick, 'Existential risks: Analyzing human extinction scenarios and related hazards', *Journal of Evolution and Technology,* 9(1) (2002). See also Bostrom (2008, 2013).

5   Ord, *The Precipice* (2020), e.g. 134.

6   Rees (2018), pp.73–78.

7   Rees (2003), p.48.

8   Ibid., p.58. Also see Bostrom (2002).

9   Bostrom (2002).

10   Rees (2003), pp.41–65; Rees (2018), pp.75–78.

11   Rees (2003), pp.49–52, 62–65.

12   Ord (2020), pp.127–34.

13   Bostrom (2002).

14   Rees (2003), p.48.

15   Ibid., p.48.

16   Torres, Phil, 'Agential risks: A comprehensive introduction', *Journal of Evolution and Technology*, 26(2) (2016), pp.31–47; Torres, Phil, 'Agential risks and information hazards: An unavoidable but dangerous topic?' *Futures*, 95 (2018), pp.86–97; Torres, Phil, 'Who would destroy the world? Omnicidal agents and related phenomena', *Aggression and Violent Behavior'*, 39 (2018), 129–38.

17   Torres, Phil (2018).

18   See e.g. Nouri, Ali and Christopher F. Chyba, 'Biotechnology and biosecurity', in Nick Bostrom and Milan M. Circkovic (eds), *Global Catastrophic Risks*. Oxford University Press (2008), p.450.

19   See e.g. Brundage, Miles et al., 'The malicious use of artificial intelligence: Forecasting, prevention and mitigation'. Future of Humanity Institute (2018).

20   E.g. Yudkowsky, E., 'Cognitive biases potentially affecting judgment of global risks', in Nick Bostrom and Milan M. Ćirković (eds), *Global Catastrophic Risks*. Oxford University Press (2008), pp.91–119.

21   Rees (2003), Chapters 3 and 6. See also Rees (2018), pp.17–20.

22   Bostrom, N. (2002). See also Bostrom, N., 'Existential risk prevention as global priority', *Global Policy*, 4(1) (2013), p.15, 27, noting "institutional incompetence" and "political exploitation of unquantifiable threats" as barriers to effective mitigation of existential risks.

23   Rees (2018), see e.g. 26–28, 46–49.

24   Avin et al. (2018).

25   Liu, Lauta, and Maas (2018). Vulnerability denotes the propensities or weaknesses within social, political, economic, or legal systems that increase the likelihood of humanity succumbing to risks, whereas exposure denotes the number, scope and nature of the interface between the hazard and the vulnerability.

26   P.10.

27   Kuhlemann (2019), pp.41–42.

28   Cotton-Barratt, Daniel, and Sandberg (2020).

29   Kreienkamp and Pegram (2020).

30   Ibid., pp.3–15.

31   See e.g. Giddens, A., *The Constitution of Society: Outline of the Theory of Structuration*. University of California Press (1984).

32   Rees (2018), p.48, quoting Fred Ikle; see also pp.66–67.

33   P.66. Commenting on the limitations of this framework, also see the chapter by Lalitha S. Sundaram in this volume.

34   Pp.70–71.

35   For classic treatments of the ethics of this situation, see Henry Shue, *Climate Justice: Vulnerability and Protection*. Oxford University Press (2014); Füssel, H-M. 'How inequitable is the global distribution of responsibility, capability, and vulnerability to climate change: A comprehensive indicator-based assessment', *Glob. Environ. Change 20* (2010), pp.597–611; Ringius, L., A. Torvanger, and A. Underdal, 'Burden sharing and fairness principles in international climate policy', *Int. Environ. Agreem. P., 2*, (2002), pp.1–22.

36   https://ourworldindata.org/contributed-most-global-co2.

37   Oxfam, 'Confronting carbon inequality: Putting climate justice at the heart of the COVID-19 recovery' (21 September 2020). While the richest 10% includes residents of every continent, around half of their emissions are associated with citizens of North America and the EU, while a fifth of them associated with citizens of China and India.

38   Bündnis Entwicklung Hilft, *World Risk Report* (2019). http://weltrisikobericht.de/english. In 2019, the top five countries for overall climate risk were Vanuatu, Antigua and Barbuda, Tonga, Solomon Islands, and Guyana.

39   Wiedmann, T., Manfred Lenzen, Lorenz T. Keyßer, and Julia K. Steinberger, 'Scientists' warning on affluence', *Nature Communications, 11*(3107) (2020).

40   Diffenbaugh, Noah S. and Marshall Burke, 'Global warming has increased global economic inequality', *PNAS, 116*(20) (2019), pp.9808–813.

41   For a recent overview of the global historical literature, see Emma Gattey, 'Global histories of empire and climate in the Anthropocene', *History Compass* (2021), e12683.

42   On neocolonialism, see e.g. Uzoigwe, Godfrey N., 'Neocolonialism is dead: Long live neocolonialism', *Journal of Global South Studies, 36* (2019).

43   Bruhn, Miriam, *Did Yesterday's Patterns of Colonial Exploitation Determine Today's Patterns of Poverty?* World Bank Blogs (2010).

44   Malm, Andreas and the Zetkin Collective, *White Skin, Black Fuel: On the Danger of Fossil Fascism*. Verso (2021).

45   In the 1970s, Freeman demonstrated an inverse relationship between pollution levels and levels of income in cities in the United States: Freeman, A., 'Distribution of environmental quality', in A. Kneese and B. Bower (eds), *Environmental Quality Analysis: Theory and Method in the Social Sciences*. John Hopkins Press (1972), pp.243–78.

46   See e.g. Bolin, Bob, 'Race, class, ethnicity, and disaster vulnerability', in Rodríguez, H., E.L. Quarantelli, and R.R. Dynes, *Handbook of Disaster Research*. Springer (2007).

47   Brock, Jared, 'As California wildfires raged, incarcerated exploited for labor', *USA Today* (11 November 2020). https://www.usatoday. com/story/opinion/policing/2020/11/11/california-wildfires-raged-incarcerated-exploited-labor-column/6249201002/; Madrigal, Alexis C., 'Kim Kardashian's private firefighters expose America's fault lines', *The Atlantic* (14 November 2018). https://www.theatlantic.com/technology/archive/2018/11/kim-kardashian-kanye-west-history-private-firefighting/575887/

48   Rodriguez-Diaz, Carlos E. and Charlotte Lewellen-Williams, 'Race and racism as structural determinants for emergency and recovery responses in the aftermath of hurricanes Irma and Maria in Puerto Rico', *Health Equity, 4*(1) (2020).

49   Walker, G., G. Mitchell, J. Fairburn, and G. Smith, *Environmental Quality & Social Deprivation Phase II: National Analysis of Flood Hazard, IPC Industries & Air Quality*. Environment Agency (2005); Walker, G., K. Burningham, J. Fielding, G. Smith, D. Thrush, and H. Fay, *Addressing Environmental Inequalities: Flood Risk*. Environment Agency (2007).

50   On examples of the following, among others, see Robinson, Mary and Tara Shine, 'Achieving a climate justice pathway to 1.5C', *Nature Climate Change, 8* (2018), pp.564–69.

51   This has occurred in many countries. For a few examples, see: Einbinder, Nathan, *Dams, Displacement and Development: Perspectives from Río Negro, Guatemala*. Springer (2017); Nguyen, Hien Thanh, Ty Huu Pham, and Lisa Lobry de Bruyn, 'Impact of hydroelectric dam development and resettlement on the natural and social capital of rural livelihoods in Bo Hon Village in Central Vietnam', *Sustainability, 9*(8) (2017), p.1422; Isaacman,

Allen F. and Barbara S. Isaacman, *Dams, Displacement, and the Delusion of Development: Cahora Bassa and Its Legacies in Mozambique, 1965–2007.* Ohio University Press (2013).

52 See e.g. Zilberman, D., G. Hochman, D. Rajagopal, S. Sexton, and G.R. Timilsina, 'The impact of biofuels on commodity food prices: Assessment of findings', *Am. J. Agric. Econ., 95* (2013), pp.275–81; Hochman, G. and D. Zilberman, 'Corn ethanol and US biofuel policy 10 years later: A quantitative assessment', *Am. J. Agric. Econ., 100* (2018), pp. 570–84.

53 See e.g. Pai, Sandeep, Kathryn Harrison, and Hisham Zerriffi, *A Systematic Review of the Key Elements of a Just Transition for Fossil Fuel Workers* (Clean Economy Working Paper Series, WP 20–04). Smart Prosperity Institute (April 2020); Greg Muttitt and Sivan Kartha, 'Equity, climate justice and fossil fuel extraction: Principles for a managed phase out', *Climate Policy, 20*(1024) (2020).

54 See e.g. Riofrancos, Thea, 'The rush to 'go electric' comes with a hidden cost: Destructive lithium mining', *The Guardian* (14 June 2021). https://www.theguardian.com/commentisfree/2021/jun/14/electric-cost-lithium-mining-decarbonasation-salt-flats-chile

55 See e.g. International Labour Organization, *Guidelines for a Just Transition Towards Environmentally Sustainable Economies and Societies for All.* ILO (2015).

56 See e.g. Caney, Simon, 'Human rights, climate change, and discounting', *Environmental Politics, 17*(536) (2008); Toussaint, P. and Adrian Martinez Blanco, 'A human rights-based approach to loss and damage under the climate change regime', *Climate Policy, 20*(743) (2020).

57 See e.g. Aronoff, Kate, Alyssa Battistoni, Daniel Aldana Cohen, and Thea Riofrancos, *A Planet to Win: Why We Need a Green New Deal.* Verso (2019); Heenan, Natasha and Anna Sturman, 'Configuring the green new deal', *The Economic and Labour Relations Review, 32*(2) (June 2021).

58 See e.g. Paul, Harpreet Kaur and Dalia Gebrial (eds), *Perspectives on a Global Green New Deal.* Rosa Luxemburg Stiftung (2021).

59 For an overview, see Pottier, Antonin et al., 'A survey of global climate justice: From negotiating stances to moral stakes and back', *International Review of Environmental and Resource Economics, 11*(1) (2017), pp.1–53.

60 Agarwal and Narain (1991). That is, an emissions allowance based on a country's population, to allow for equal emissions by each person.

61 Trudinger, C.M. and I.G. Enting, 'Comparison of formalisms for attributing responsibility for climate change: Non-linearities in the Brazilian proposal approach', *Climatic Change, 68* (2005) pp.67–99; Den Elzen, M.G.J. et al., *The Brazilian Proposal and Other Options for International Burden Sharing: An Evaluation of Methodological and Policy Aspects Using the FAIR Model.*

National Institute of Public Health and the Environment (1999); Den Elzen, M.G.J., M. Schaeffer, and P.L. Lucas, 'Differentiating future commitments on the basis of countries' relative historical responsibility for climate change: Uncertainties in the 'Brazilian proposal' in the context of a policy implementation', *Climatic Change, 71* (2005), pp.277–301.

62   Article 3.1.

63   However, this still does not reach the scale of those in Annex I nations, especially if measured on a per-capita basis.

64   Pauw, Pieter, Kennedy Mbeva, and Harro van Asselt, 'Subtle differentiation of countries' responsibilities under the Paris Agreement', *Palgrave Communications, 5*(86) (2019).

65   Pauw, W.P., P. Castro, J. Pickering, and S. Bhasin, 'Conditional nationally determined contributions in the Paris Agreement: Foothold for equity or Achilles heel?', *Climate Policy, 20*(4), pp.468–84 (2020).

66   See e.g. Allan, Jennifer, Jennifer Bansard, Natalie Jones, Mari Luomi, Joyce Melcar Tan, and Yixian Sun, 'Glasgow Climate Change Conference: 31 October—13 November 2021', *Earth Negotiations Bulletin, 12*(793) (16 November 2021). https://enb.iisd.org/sites/default/files/2021-11/enb12793e_1.pdf

67   Sachs, Lisa, Lise Johnson, and Ella Merrill, 'Environmental Injustice: How treaties undermine human rights related to the environment', *La Revue des Juristes de Sciences, 18* (2020), pp.90–100.

68   Ibid.

69   Tienhaara, Kyla and Lorenzo Cotula, *Raising the Cost of Climate Action? Investor-State Dispute Settlement and Compensation for Stranded Fossil Fuel Assets*. IIED (2020).

70   See e.g. Magraw, Daniel B. and Sergio Puig, 'Greening investor-state dispute settlement', *Boston College Law Review, 29*(2717) (2018); Tienhaara, K., 'Regulatory chill in a warming world: The threat to climate policy posed by investor-state dispute settlement', *Transnational Environmental Law, 7*(2) (2018), pp.229–50.

71   Steele, Paul and Sejal Patel, *Tackling the Triple Crisis: Using Debt Swaps to Address Debt, Climate and Nature Loss Post-COVID-19*. IIED (September 2020).

72   Ibid. See also https://www.iisd.org/sustainable-recovery/debt-for-climate-swaps-can-help-developing-countries-make-a-green-recovery/.

73   E.g. in 2015, Vanuatu was hit by Cyclone Pam, with government debt going from 21% to 39% of GDP to finance reconstruction: Jubilee Debt

Campaign, *Don't Owe, Shouldn't Pay: The Impact of Climate Change on Debt in Vulnerable Countries* (October 2018).

74   Steele and Patel (September 2020).

75   Zucman, Gabriel, *The Hidden Wealth of Nations: The Scourge of Tax Havens.* University of Chicago Press (2015).

76   Jubilee Debt Campaign, *Honest Accounts 2017: How The World Profits From Africa's Wealth* (2017).

77   See e.g. Fenton, Adrian, Helena Wright, Stavros Afionis, Jouni Paavola, and Saleemul Huq, 'Debt relief and financing climate change action', *Nature Climate Change*, 4(650) (2014); Volz, Ulrich et al., *Debt Relief for a Green and Inclusive Recovery.* Heinrich Boll Stiftung (2020).

78   Japan, USA, Germany, South Korea, and France account for 75% of low-carbon inventions patented between 2005 and 2015: Dussaux, Damien, Antoine Dechezleprêtre, and Matthieu Glachant, *Intellectual Property Rights Protection and the International Transfer of Low-Carbon Technologies.* Grantham Research Institute on Climate Change and the Environment (January 2018).

79   Dussaux, Damien, Antoine Dechezleprêtre, and Matthieu Glachant (January 2018).

80   For discussion of this point, see Timmermann, Cristian and Henk van den Belt, 'Climate change, intellectual property rights and global justice, in Thomas Potthast and Simon Meisch (eds), *Climate Change and Sustainable Development: Ethical Perspectives on Land Use and Food Production.* Wageningen Academic Publishers (2012), pp.75–79.

81   See e.g. Erfani, Parsa et al., 'Intellectual property waiver for covid-19 vaccines will advance global health equity', *BMJ, 374* (2021).

82   See e.g. Bacchus, James, *The Case for a WTO Climate Waiver.* CIGI (2017).

83   P. 28.

84   Pp. 41–42.

85   P. 274.

86   P. 12.

87   Rees (2018), pp.27, 36.

88   As chronicled by Shue, Henry, 'The unavoidability of justice', in Andrew Hurrell and Benedict Kingsbury (eds), *The International Politics of the Environment: Actors, Interests, and Institutions.* Oxford University Press (1992), pp.373–97.

5. We Have to Include Everyone: Enabling Humanity to Reduce Existential Risk

Sheri Wells-Jensen and SJ Beard

Humanity is facing multiple, overlapping challenges in the 21st century with the potential to bring about human extinction or the collapse of civilisation. Given this, it can be tempting to believe that we should 'play to our strengths' by relying on the most able to take responsibility for understanding and mitigating these risks. This would be a terrible mistake. Far from being merely vulnerable and unable to help, disabled people—and others who are marginalised or excluded within our societies—have a lot to contribute to managing risks, up to and including on a global scale. Moreover, diversity and inclusion are vital sources of creativity and resilience. In this chapter, we show how both the field of Existential Risk Studies and the wider community of people concerned with reducing the level of global risk would benefit from championing inclusive futures and paying more attention to disabled people and other marginalised groups.

A common narrative about disability and risk

At a local high school, the theatre class was poised for an afternoon of improvisation. The stage was set and the scene was given: "You and a blind companion are in the living room. There is a fire!" Each team had three minutes to prepare, and the scenes were played out in rapid succession. With the *joie de vivre* characteristic of such events, the kids

 https://doi.org/10.11647/OBP.0336.05

took off. Mostly, the fire was evaded or extinguished but, every once in a while, the whole house did burn down. Sometimes marshmallows were roasted, and the occasional textbook was 'accidentally' incinerated. The banter was witty, the political allusions were hot, and the school administration came in for a liberal dose of good-natured ribbing. And, in every case, the blind person was *rescued*.

While the students took this all in stride, Sheri, as a blind person visiting the class, found the situation deeply troubling. Even when the blind characters in the scene were part of the fun, exchanging quips and contributing to the commentary, they were never part of the solution. In living room after living room, the blind people did nothing but consent to being saved from the flames. They were led out, carried out, and occasionally hilariously dragged out, but in every situation, they were passive. Even though a blind adult was right there in the room and had just been talking to them about inclusion and social justice, the reflexive reaction from all groups was that the blind characters were in charge of exactly nothing.

We tell this story not to disparage these young thespians; they did not create (and probably would not even approve of) the cultural stereotypes they enacted. If Sheri had stopped to point out what had just happened, we are sure they would have been appalled, but she let it go, mostly to give herself time to think. They were staging what they had been taught, playing out on the stage the values of their community — of our community. At a different school, in a different country, SJ had very similar experiences. Across many cultures, some people (in this case, disabled people) are cast *a priori* as vulnerable recipients of societal welfare. These individuals are not co-creators of change or solvers of problems. They are the rescued, not the rescuers, and because this is so ingrained in human society, it underpins everything we do, including good-natured amateur impromptu theatre. And it feels logical.

Challenging this accepted narrative

But logic *per se* actually points in a very different direction in situations like this. In a serious fire indoors, electric lighting may well fail, throwing the disaster scene into darkness, while thick, eye-stinging smoke makes vision one of the least reliable resources. Logically, the blind person—accustomed to moving about freely without reliance on eyesight—would be the consummate rescuer, reassuring and guiding others to safety. But that is not what happened in these scenarios.

Still, it does (or, at least, it did) seem natural, almost archetypal, that some people—children, the disabled, women, the elderly, anyone who is pregnant, and those without physical or economic capital— are vulnerable, and protecting them is viewed as a moral imperative. Any responsible disaster plan needs contingencies for this, and it is almost certainly true that such contingencies have saved hundreds of thousands, if not millions, of lives. Getting everyone out of danger is the priority, and since some groups require different kinds of assistance or intervention, we increasingly design disaster interventions with this in mind. There should be wheelchair ramps on evacuation vehicles, sign language interpreters at public briefings, and electronic or braille information readily available while we ensure that those who rely on electrically powered equipment have access to a generator or reserves of batteries. Failure to consider these things has, and does, cost us many lives during and after disasters.[1] More intangibly, we have recently seen how, in responding to COVID-19, authorities needed to give special attention to the plight of sick and elderly people who had to isolate at home—even if this attention was not always given.[2] In the wake of global catastrophe, such attention, care, and adjustments may be even more important. There is a rule of thumb that natural disasters will leave around three times as many people injured as dead, while for conflicts it is often assumed that the number of injured will be around nine times the number killed (although empirical data suggests these ratios are highly variable and may be increasing over time).[3] It would follow that a global catastrophe with the potential to kill 10% of humanity might injure somewhere between a third to 100% of those it leaves behind. This would make it significantly harder for humanity to recover from such a catastrophe, unless we take steps now to ensure that these injuries do not prevent people from playing a full role in rebuilding our shattered world. However, important as it is, such care and attention misses the fact that every human is more than a body in need of rescue—they are also minds, hearts, hands, and friends who are willing and able to help out as well.

The problem we want to address here is certainly not that people are taking steps to overcome barriers in dangerous situations. The problem is that this comes from a desire to 'protect vulnerable people' that often presupposes the belief that these people cannot also be counted among those who can give aid. This presupposition of helplessness in one situation generalises to impose marked inequality for disabled people in others. Their social capital, particularly their access to education and employment, is systematically limited, and they receive (often on a daily basis) the message that they are not needed on the front lines of solutions. This chapter is our attempt to answer that message by putting the case for why disabled people can—and do—have very significant contributions to make to the field of Existential Risk Studies and its worthy aim of reducing some of the most extreme threats facing humanity as a whole.

One way of describing this problem that is popular amongst disabled people is the difference between a 'medical' and 'social' model of disability. In the medical model, disabilities are 'deficiencies' in individuals that prevent them from 'functioning' in the ways that 'normal' people can. To be disabled is inevitably to be less than what one might have been if 'able-bodied', and the only hope for disabled people is to 'cure' them of their impairments, with efforts to make the world more accessible to disabled people seen as a stop-gap measure to reduce their disadvantage until this can happen. In the social model of disability, however, such impairments are generally reclassified as mere 'differences'. There is, in fact, no normative standard for what humans should and should not be able to do, so any apparent impairment does not imply a deficiency *per se*. These differences become disabilities only because society is set up in ways that assume that people are able to do certain things, such that an inability to meet these arbitrary standards prevents people from being enabled to take a full role within society.[4] On this model, then, the urgent need to change society so that it can accommodate people's differences is no mere kindness towards the disabled, but rather an urgently needed correction to their unjust disablement, and a way in which society can gain access to the many good things disabled people would bring to the table, if only they were not excluded.[5]

Disability and existential risk

Problematic narratives of disablement and risk are not merely to be found at the level of small-scale disasters. In a famous novel about existential catastrophe, *Day of the Triffids* by John Wyndham, humanity is weighed low by the species of ambulant venomous plants[6]—except that it is not the hazard posed by these plants that causes the disaster (in the story they had been around for several years beforehand), but rather vulnerability created by widespread blindness induced by unexplained astronomical phenomena. The book sets a harrowing scene where loss of sight causes widespread violence, suicide, infanticide, and insanity— and only a few sighted survivors are left to battle the triffids on their own. One of the main plot lines of the book concerns conflict between those survivors who focus on eradicating triffids as their sole priority (with whom the reader is encouraged to sympathise) and those who are more interested in helping those who have lost their sight survive (but who are portrayed in the story as little more than slave masters who exploit their disabled charges). Those who were blind before the incident and were thus already adapted to this new state are only given a passing mention—as more valuable than the newly blind for the purposes of domestic service and breeding!

Day of the Triffids is a hugely problematic book that shows many signs of the era it was written in. However, it remains popular to this day, while the apparent tension it describes between disaster mitigation and bearing the burden of helping the most vulnerable is merely the same tension we have just described writ large.[7]

Yet such discomforting narratives of burden and exclusion are certainly not the only stories of how people with disabling differences can relate to catastrophic risk. Recent widely acclaimed tales such as Alexis Wright's *The Swan Book*,[8] Nnedi Okorafor's *Binti*,[9] and N.K. Jemisin's *The Fifth Season*[10] (all published in 2015) tell very different stories about how outsiders burdened by their physical and psychological differences and vulnerabilised within their own societies are able to come to terms with (if not necessarily overcome) catastrophe and offer responses inaccessible to their 'normal' peers.[11] In *The Swan Book*, Oblivia Ethylene, a mute woman affected by sexual trauma, disease, and pollution, draws on her unique gifts and limitations to lead both Australians and refugees through a world devastated by climate change. In *Binti*, the titular character uses gifts of her apparent neurodiversity—a form of intellectual self-stimulation she calls 'treeing'—together with her unique position as a member of the indigenous Himba people who has left to attend a prestigious university, to act as a 'master harmoniser' who can negotiate a peace between the alien Meduse and the Khoush, the dominant group of humans who look down on her and her people. Finally, in *The Fifth Season*, a group of Orogenes—a hated minority marked by their ability to control heat and the movement of the earth, but also the difficulty they have controlling this ability, leading them to inadvertently harm themselves and others—grapple with society's simultaneous need for and hatred of them and the relationship between this and the catastrophes that periodically strike their world.[12] While combining science fiction with elements of fantasy and horror (if those are even appropriate categories to use for such path-breaking stories) they paint pictures of what is lost when we overlook the abilities of those amongst us who have been disabled by differences and divergence from the norm. Indeed, the exploration of how disabled people might build positive futures in apocalyptic and post-apocalyptic scenarios is starting to become something of a genre of its own, with recent anthologies such as *Defying Doomsday*[13] and *Rebuilding Tomorrow*[14] focusing specifically on this subject.

However, our focus in this chapter is not on apocalyptic fiction *per se* but on how such narratives play out in the reality of existential risk, and the contributions disabled people can make to reducing it. We offer here three small but concrete examples of such contributions, sticking only to areas we ourselves have worked on and contributed to.

Futures, foresight, and horizon scanning

One area where we perceive the absence of disabled people as problematic is in the area of foresight. Foresight is a potentially unfortunate name for the process of seeking to understand what may happen in the future in ways that are more rigorous than science fiction. The name is unfortunate because it links this creative process to a particular individual sense—vision—producing the idea that some people are literally able to see into the future.[15] However, this is not what good foresight entails. One of the most well-known versions of foresight is called superforecasting, and it employs individuals known as superforecasters. Yet these superforecasters are not successful because they have 'superior' senses or intellects, but rather because they display traits such as active open-mindedness, a growth mindset, and acceptance of the role that chance plays in life outcomes.[16] As far as we are aware, neither the originators of the superforecasting process nor its critics have explicitly considered whether these traits are more likely to be found amongst people who have experienced disablement, although its creators have been keen to point out that they are often lacking amongst those who identify as 'experts' in a given field. However, we would contend that such traits are very much in line with the kind of humility, adaptability, and realism that one would expect to find in people who deviate from the norm and are used to living in a world that is not designed for their benefit.

And even if disabled people are, in fact, no better suited than anyone else to foresight, there are other reasons why they need to be actively included in foresight and horizon scanning, because good foresight requires diversity in order to work. Superforecasters work best in teams where they can share diverse perspectives, rather than when working alone, while many forecasting techniques explicitly require a diversity of perspectives to function at all, since they are based on the idea of combining different viewpoints into a single collective judgement.[17] Among the benefits of diversity to foresight include the generation of new ideas, recognising the full range of valid perspectives, disruption of networks that can lead to path dependency and group think, and testing outputs against a wider set of potential critics.[18] Such diversity is generally assessed in relation to things such as different fields of expertise, types of affiliations, cultural backgrounds, organisational functions, and personal values.[19] However, it is important to note that, to achieve this valued diversity, we need to engage in more than a box-ticking exercise but actively seek out and promote a plurality of perspectives and opinions, even though we recognise that this may lead to disagreement and conflict. We would contend that achieving this goal requires both the inclusion of people who have differences in ability and social inclusion, and also engagement with the substantial issues of disablement and exclusion that create and perpetuate these.

While there is still much to be done in this area, we believe that the field of Existential Risk Studies may already be benefiting from the inclusion of disabled people within it. Anecdotally, SJ has found that their neurodiversity,[20] while presenting many challenges, has helped them to be a creative and productive partner in a very wide range of projects, and has spoken to others who felt the same,[21] while at least one informal survey found that neurodiversity and mental health issues seem to be unusually common amongst certain parts of the community that studies existential risk.[22] Similar points have been made by Greta Thunberg, who has been diagnosed with autism, which she describes as a superpower. For instance, she notes how "a lot of people with autism have a special interest that they can sit and do for an eternity without getting bored", which can be a very useful ability in research, and notes that many autistic people have become climate activists because they feel a compulsion to tell the truth.[23] Unfortunately, despite the field of Existential Risk Studies benefiting from people with such traits, the topic of disability is seldom mentioned in existential risk circles and it is widely acknowledged that the community suffers from perfectionism, imposter syndrome, and burnout, all of which disproportionately impact disabled people.

Space colonisation

Another area in which disabled people could play a beneficial role is in the mitigation of risks on this planet through the colonisation of space. This has often been promoted as a good insurance policy against planet-level threats (like asteroids and volcanic super-eruptions), a means of increasing our species' resilience more generally, and even a necessary step to avoid the existential threat of 'stagnation'.[24] Traditionally, space has been viewed as an area in which access for disabled people is seen as too difficult to achieve. However, the reality is that in virtually all (earth-side) scenarios, it is increasingly understood that diversity strengthens working groups, meaning that such homogeneity of perspective and ability could well be working against the goals of space programmes.[25]

There are also some quite specific reasons to think that disabled people should be included in efforts at space colonisation. For one thing, the environment of space is itself both disabling and enabling, with low and zero gravity, altered and extreme light conditions, cramped spaces, and highly mechanised environments producing both limitations and opportunities that are not found on Earth. Every astronaut has to go through a process of extreme adaptation upon entering space, and it may be that people with physical and sensory disabilities—whose strengths and weaknesses are different to begin with and who are more used to adapting to hostile environments—would find this easier and be able to more completely adapt to life in space than others. This advantage may be increased in the unfortunate event of something going wrong, since as we have noted already, conditions that can be extremely difficult for most people may represent no additional burden to the disabled, like loss of light for a blind person.

Finally, even ignoring their personal advantages, merely thinking about how to include disabled people in space missions could be advantageous to everyone. While many people think of the accommodations needed for including disabled people as requiring the addition of 'accessible' features that would otherwise not be necessary, they can also be thought about in terms of 'universal design', the design of products and environments to be usable (to the greatest extent possible) by people of all ages and abilities/disabilities, whereby such accommodations increase functionality for everyone.[26] For instance, controls whose function can be determined by touch as well as sight are accessible to the blind, but they also allow everyone to use them more quickly, accurately, and in a wider array of circumstances.[27] These points have been largely ignored in space exploration, but recently projects like *Mission: AstroAccess* and the European Space Agency's *Parastronaut* project are beginning to explore them further.[28]

Bioethics

A final area relating to the study and management of existential risk where disabled people have an especially valuable contribution to make is in the field of bioethics. The possibilities for bio-enhancement and other transformative technologies are a topic of great interest, both as potential causes of and solutions to existential risk.[29] Understanding these technologies requires grappling with the complex ethical challenges they pose. This is not only because they could have a profound impact on our understanding of human dignity, human flourishing, and even humanity itself, but also because their impact will be greatly determined by how they interact with other aspects of society, and this, in turn, will depend upon how they are ethically understood. However, the community of existential risk research has tended to stay out of such supposedly controversial discussions and prefers to leave such grappling to others, in many cases uncritically assuming a moral position closely aligned with the 'transhumanist' project of overcoming the perceived limitations of human biology, according to which human enhancement has intrinsic value as a necessity for achieving this goal.[30]

Transhumanism is only one view we might take about these technologies, and it can be seen as one of the most extreme and controversial positions at that, especially as it has historical associations with the legacy of 20th century eugenics.[31] Disabled people, in particular, have had strong reasons to be concerned about some of the arguments made within transhumanism and have also developed alternative proposals for how humanity might collectively enhance our abilities, through social modifications that allow everyone to contribute more to solving our problems. After all, it is a near universal law of nature and human societies that diversity promotes creativity and innovation and facilitates adaptation and resilience. When we seek to erase our differences, in an effort to eradicate disability or promote perfection through enhancement, this can have the effect of making societies weaker and less adaptable, and depriving them of the unique perspectives and gifts disabled people might otherwise contribute through their lives and works. In particular, disabled people are often experts on adapting and overcoming barriers and vulnerabilities, as they know (in ways that can be inaccessible to other people) the costs that society places on itself by not being more inclusive in its design of technologies, systems, and institutions.

In addition, disabled people have also had strong reasons to fear the transhumanist project. It is, after all, *their* differences that are perceived as most limiting and thus will likely be the first to be eliminated; and while it can be easy to see this as an attempt at sparing people from the burden of impairment, many disabled people say that they do not want to be spared, but rather respected and accommodated for who they are. It is not hard to imagine that in its pursuit of human 'perfection' this point of view risks implying that their own lives are less important or valuable due to their 'imperfections', or that any resistance they might make to being enhanced against their will is irrational and dangerous.[32] However, this doesn't imply that disabled people are conservative in their approach to technology or enhancement *per se*—far from it. Just as there is a social model of disability, there is also a social model of enhancement, according to which more inclusive and varied opportunities for people to create value for themselves and others can enable more and more people to play an enhanced role in society. Some of the key differences between these two approaches to enhancement include:

- whether enhancement is seen as increasing people's innate abilities or increasing their opportunities to use their abilities to flourish and help others;

- whether enhancement is about transcending our embodied humanity or exploring and developing it; and

- whether enhancement implies controlling who will live in the future or creating opportunities for more people to live well.[33]

These alternative perspectives are not limited to biological enhancement, but have also been extended to AI and other technologies with transformative potential.[34] We believe they are worth exploring, and that bioethics and Existential Risk Studies have a lot to benefit from closer engagement with challenges of disablement and injustice.

These are but three small examples of what is clearly a much larger phenomenon, where openness to considering disability and the contributions of disabled people can (and does) add to our thinking about existential risks and our ability to reduce them. These examples do, however, point to a number of broader themes: the inherent value of diversity, the benefits of universal design, disabled people's unique experience of vulnerability and adaptation, and the extent to which focusing on individual perfection and performance can lead us to ignore the social forces that disable both individual people and society as a whole. That there has been so little research on these themes is regrettable, and a testament to the broader exclusion of disabled people from this field. There is a need for much greater research in all of the areas we have mentioned here.

Wider needs to challenge the common narrative

However, we also need to consider the still wider implications of the exclusion of people who are disabled on humanity's collective ability to grapple with the pressing challenges we face. The global unemployment rate for disabled people is at least two to three times higher than their able-bodied peers and, although the numbers are better in industrialised countries as compared with unindustrialised countries, some areas of the world report an unemployment rate of over 90% for disabled citizens.[35] Meanwhile, the Global Partnership for Education estimates that 90% of children with disabilities in low- and middle-income countries do not attend school.[36] And the problem is not small. Some estimates place the number of disabled people at 20% of the world's population—that is, wherever five people are gathered in a burning living room, one could be expected to be disabled. As the current world population now exceeds eight billion, the number of disabled people living today is thus around 1.6 billion. That is a lot of people to consign to the rescue list!

Employment and education statistics are cultural and economic—rather than natural—artefacts. They reflect how society has chosen to treat disabled people, rather than how disabled people could live if things were different. Just as we now understand world hunger as a wholly solvable social problem,[37] this systematic exclusion of disabled people from full participation is entirely avoidable, and, in fact, constructing physical and cultural environments to accommodate disabled citizens benefits non-disabled citizens as well.[38] Yet this exclusion continues, and society loses out tremendously as a result. It would, of course, be impossible to trace all the ways in which this loss of human potential and social capital impacts our societies in the 21st century. However, it is undeniable that a great many of these will have consequences that relate directly to the creation of, and failure to mitigate, existential risks.

One impact is in the field of technology, where disabled people have long been the drivers of innovation and creativity. Text-to-voice, voice-to-text, home automation, drive by wire, and self-balancing scooters were all first developed for disabled people for instance, and yet disabled people are rarely, if ever, given the opportunities to be innovators in their own right, or even given much control over the technologies being developed on their behalf.[39] Other impacts may be more mundane; however, from tackling food insecurity and adapting to climate change to education, culture, and (dare we mention it) care,[40] disabled people, just like anyone else alive right now, have a lot to contribute to making our futures better and safer.

Still, some people in higher-income countries argue that disabled people no longer face the kinds of discrimination that would exclude them from playing a valuable role in society. They occasionally cite the mere existence of people like us, as disabled scientists and other professionals, as irrefutable evidence that such discrimination is a thing of the past. They also present us with a set of extraordinary disabled people whose contributions to humankind have been remarkable. There are the usual suspects, such as Beethoven,[41] Helen Keller,[42] and Stephen Hawking,[43] but the list sometimes contains lesser-known figures such as 19th-century blind writer and explorer James Holman.[44] These are certainly impressive figures, and the world would be a sadder place without them, but these luminaries exist within the cultural trope of disability as dependency. They are the exceptions that highlight the rule.

It is, after all, their accomplishments *'despite'* their disabilities that add the extra sparkle to their success, and those successes only carry the rest of us so far. That is, Stephen Hawking may have been a brilliant astrophysicist, who coincidentally helped establish the Centre for the Study of Existential Risk and was one of its first scientific advisers, but his success has not magicked the standard college classroom into a welcoming place for other disabled instructors,[45] and currently only 2% of PhDs in the STEM fields are earned by disabled candidates.[46] At the same time, Hawking's story is inspirational precisely because he was afforded the accommodations he needed to carry on working despite growing physical impairment, a rare instance of disability not being a barrier to potential—which could be seen just as easily as showing us how much humanity is missing out on, not how much we have achieved. As Hawking himself put it:

> [W]e never really know where the next great scientific discovery will come from, nor who will make it. Opening up the thrill and wonder of scientific discovery, creating innovative and accessible ways to reach out to the widest young audience possible, greatly increases the chances of finding and inspiring the new Einstein. Wherever she might be.[47]

Including everyone

We have focused in this chapter on the issue of disability. In part, this is because we are both disabled ourselves. Both Sheri and SJ are visually impaired; Sheri is fully blind while SJ is legally blind (but still has some usable vision) and neurodivergent. However, while in many other respects we are both privileged— we are both white, for example—this is not the only marginalised group to which we belong. For instance, Sheri is a woman while SJ is gender non-binary. More importantly, while the topic of disability in existential risk is important, we are aware that many of the points we mention here could also be made about other groups whose marginalisation is harming the future of our species. People of

Colour, religious minorities, Indigenous peoples, women, poor people, and those from the Global South, members of the LGBTQ+ community, military veterans, and migrants all experience different challenges but the same processes of marginalisation and exclusion. These are not all groups of people who need accommodation during a disaster, but if you look around laboratories, board rooms, and government buildings, these are often the faces you will miss.

We will now offer just a few brief vignettes of what these absences have cost us. Alan Turing was not only a pioneer of AI and computing, but someone who understood the potential negative impacts of the technology he was working on well.[48] In 1951, Turing gave a lecture on BBC Radio in which he argued (responding directly to the pioneering work of Ada Lovelace) that computers could think and that humanity faced great "danger and humiliation" were they to become superior at thinking to humans, a danger he believed to be "remote but not astronomically remote".[49] Sadly, for him and humanity, Turing faced a danger and humiliation far less remote when only a few months later his flat was burgled and the police proved less interested in the burglary than the fact that two men appeared to be sharing a flat with only one bed. This set off a chain of events that led to his death in 1954. Reflecting to his friend Norman Routledge about these events, Turing expressed his worry that:

> the following syllogism may be used by some in the future.
> Turing believes machines think
> Turing lies with men
> Therefore machines do not think[50]

Even more briefly, Rachael Carson faced tremendous barriers in publicising her ground-breaking work on our ecological catastrophe because she was a woman, was single, and was suffering both the debilitation and stigma of cancer,[51] while many who went on to make extraordinary contributions to nuclear safety and governance (such as Eugene Rabinowitch, Leo Szilard, and Joseph Rotblat) were kept away from much of the Manhattan Project because they were European refugees.[52]

This is clearly not only a disgraceful waste of human capital on the personal level; it also places the global community in danger by eliminating sources of insight, support, and hard work. The world is in dire need of innovative perspectives, and our policies of exclusion—conscious or unconscious, well-intentioned or otherwise—put us in danger. This volume has demonstrated in stark detail the reality that we in the 21st century cannot afford to overlook any source of aid. Inclusion is not a kindness bestowed upon the vulnerable; it is a necessity for the survival of the species.

It is often said that "The future is already here—it's just not very evenly distributed".[53] This quote is generally applied to specific technologies, like virtual reality, that are seen as representing the future and the benefits it will bring. However, it also applies to the risks that humanity is facing from these technologies and other sources. The experts on climate change adaptation, for instance, may not be found in elite universities, in temperate parts of the world that have the strongest reputation for studying such things, but rather on the front lines of climate change, in the Arctic, the tropics, and on small islands around the world. Those who best understand the downsides of AI and other technologies may not be 'technical experts', but rather people who are incarcerated or whose lives are impacted by wars that have already seen the deployment of lethal autonomous weapons. And so on, and so on. We need to understand what marginalised people in these situations already do to address such risks, and make use of their experiences if we want to build a safer world.

What is to be done? Certainly, internationally, people who prepare for crises and who create accommodations so that preparedness systems are accessible to all must also begin to leverage the resources available from all minority group constituents. But, deeper and more wide-sweeping than this, we need a steady, deliberate undermining of the systems that keep people from active and eager participation in everything the world has to offer. This requires more inclusive futures across the range of possible outcomes for our species.

And when it comes to risk mitigation, this means working, before a crisis strikes, to strengthen public schools, mental health systems, civil rights organisations, and campaigns for the health of children and the elderly. It means fighting with fierceness against racism, ableism, poverty, sexism, homophobia, and all other systems of oppression. It means recognising that we cannot afford to tolerate transphobia, antisemitism, or ultra-nationalism.

We must do this, not only out of compassion or a moral imperative, but out of pragmatic calculation. The more people we have working on the problems that face us, the more chances we have of discovering and implementing the solutions that will save us. The struggles for social justice of different groups are not the same, just as the barriers facing us and the gifts we bring are not the same either. However, we do have a common cause in building more inclusive futures and, when those futures are also likely to be safer, that common cause can and should extend to everyone.

It is thus incumbent upon international, national, and local entities to examine not only crisis preparedness strategies, but the equity of feeder organisations such as schools and universities, hospitals, and training centres for first responders to make sure they are encouraging all kinds of people to work for and with them. And it is incumbent upon these agencies to check their own policies and procedures to ensure they are recruiting all kinds of people. In the end, though, it also falls to individuals both to express and understand words like 'diversity', 'inclusion', and 'welcome' and to back those words up with actions. In our own work, we have sought to use diversity to improve the fields of space exploration and existential risk. However, for marginalised people such efforts can all too often be seen as a 'special interest', while for the non-disabled it can feel like a 'worthy cause'; we hope we have convinced the reader by now that the truth could not be more different.

Small changes also matter: the shopper who refuses to patronise a store until it is made accessible, the restauranteur who gives unneeded food to the homeless, the teacher who emphasises literacy and science and makes sure all students are included, and the parents who widen their circle of friends to include more kinds of people and teach their children to think carefully about their choices. In the end, what is done at the highest levels of preparedness is nourished by—and ultimately flows from—the grassroots. Each of us has, in our social and professional lives, daily opportunities to sabotage the edifice of exclusion.

What we do, starting in our individual living rooms, will be the force that saves the planet.

Notes and References

1   Stough, Laura M. and Ilan Kelman, 'People with disabilities and disasters', in Rodriguez, H., W. Donner, and J. E. Trainor (eds), *Handbook of Disaster Research*. Springer (2018), pp.225–42.

2   At the same time, far less was said about the knowledge and experience of these same sick and elderly people, who are also the most likely to have relevant experience or to have actually lived through similar pandemics and other disasters.

3   For a more detailed assessment of the size of these trends see Wyss, M. and G. Trendafiloski, 'Trends in the casualty ratio of injured to fatalities in earthquakes', in Spence, R., E. So, and C. Scawthorn (eds), *Human Casualties in Earthquakes: Progress in Modelling and Mitigation*. Springer (2011), pp.267–74; Murray, Christopher J.L., Gary King, Alan D. Lopez, Niels Tomijima, and Etienne G. Krug, 'Armed conflict as a public health problem', *BMJ*, 324(7333) (2002), pp.346–49.

4   For example, take the situation where a wheelchair user approaches a building. She has every right to be there: it might be a public facility, an entertainment venue, or perhaps her new place of employment. When she arrives, she finds herself confronted by a short flight of stairs leading from the sidewalk to the front door. In this scenario, where does the problem lie? According to the medical model, she (or, perhaps more precisely, her body) is the problem. If she had been born in a different body, or if medical science had 'corrected' the body she has now, she would be able to enter without incident. According to the social model, however, the problem is not hers: it is the stairs'. If there were a ramp instead, she (and everyone else) would be able to enter easily. Her disadvantage, then, is located in the environment, or rather in the social conventions that use stairs where ramps would be equally workable.

5   For more on the social model of disability, see the foundational work Oliver, Michael, *Politics of Disablement*. Macmillan International Higher Education (1990).

6   Wyndham, John, *The Day of the Triffids*. Michael Joseph (1951).

7   *Day of the Triffids* was, in fact, the first book that SJ ever read on the theme of existential risk and it was recommended to them precisely because of its theme of blindness.

8   Wright, Alexis, *The Swan Book*. Giramondo (2015).

9   Okorator, Nnedi, *Binti*. Tor Books (2015).

10 Jemisin, Nora K., *The Fifth Season*. Orbit (2015).

11   Vulnerabilisation refers to the active process through which a person's vulnerabilities are constructed by their interaction with specific institutions and social contexts. We owe this use of the term to the philosophers Shelley Tremain and Havi Carel.

12   For more about these and other inclusive futures and what they have to teach academic disciplines such as Existential Risk Studies, see Hall, Melinda, 'What future people will there be? Neurodiverse heroes for a changing planet', *MOSF Journal of Science Fiction*, 15 (2019); and Mitchell, Audra and Aadita Chaudhury, 'Worlding beyond 'the' 'end' of 'the world': White apocalyptic visions and BIPOC futurisms', *International Relations*, 34(3) (2020), pp.309–32.

13   Dolichva, Tsana and Holly Kench, *Defying Doomsday: Stories of Fear, Hope, and Survival*. Twelfth Planet (2016).

14   Dolichva, Tsana, *Rebuilding Tomorrow*. Twelfth Planet (2020).

15   Nor is this association accidental. One of the oldest and most commonly used foresight tools is known as the Delphi Technique, explicitly linking it to the famous Greek oracle Pythia.

16   Tetlock, Philip E., Barbara A. Mellers, and J. Peter Scoblic, 'Bringing probability judgments into policy debates via forecasting tournaments', *Science*, 355(6324) (2017), pp.481–83.

17   For a discussion of a wider range of forecasting methods used in the study of existential risk, see Beard, S.J., T. Rowe, and J. Fox, 'An analysis and evaluation of methods currently used to quantify the likelihood of existential hazards', *Futures, 115* (2020), 102469 and Rios Rojas, C., C. Rhodes, S. Avin, L. Kemp, and S.J. Beard, *Foresight for Unknown, Long-Term and Emerging Risks: Approaches and Recommendations*. Centre for the Study of Existential Risk (2021), https://doi.org/10.17863/CAM.64582.

18   Könnölä, Totti, Ville Brummer, and Ahti Salo, 'Diversity in foresight: Insights from the fostering of innovation ideas', *Technological Forecasting and Social Change*, 74(5) (2007), pp.608–26.

19   Könnölä, Totti, Ahti Salo, Cristiano Cagnin, Vicente Carabias, and Eeva Vilkkumaa, 'Facing the future: Scanning, synthesizing and sense-making in horizon scanning', *Science and Public Policy* 39(2) (2012), pp.222–31.

20   Neurodiversity refers to variation in the human brain regarding sociability, learning, attention, mood, and other mental functions and includes differences such as ADHD, autism, dyslexia, and Tourette's.

21   For a description of some of the positive and negative ways in which SJ's visual impairment and neurodiversity affected their research career up to the early stages of their PhD, see Beard, S.J., 'It's not what you see, it's how

you see it', *Journal of Inclusive Practice in Further and Higher Education,* 4(1) (2012), pp. 91–93.

22   The only information we are aware of about the prevalence of disability among people who study existential risks is the readership survey for the popular *Slate Star Codex* blog, which is widely read amongst existential risk researchers and those they often work with, such as members of the rationalist and Effective Altruism communities. This only looked at neurodiversity and mental health but found unusually high representation for a range of disabling differences including depression, anxiety, autism, and ADHD amongst others. See https://docs.google.com/forms/d/e/1FAIpQLSd4I-x9oArWW1Tz5mEK4uHmxcJzVKGA28RfKPsDvW8hzZNViw/viewanalytics.

23   Hattenstone, Simon, 'The transformation of Greta Thunberg', *The Guardian* (25 September 2021). It is worth noting that, until recently, conditions such as autism, OCD, and mutism would have been seen only as opportunities to institutionalise people and exclude them from mainstream society— see, e.g., Silberman, Steve, *Neurotribes: The Legacy of Autism and How to Think Smarter About People Who Think Differently.* Atlantic Books (2017). The fact that, only a few decades after gaining the right to mainstream education, some like Greta Thunburg found ways of using that right to draw attention to a pressing global crisis, is testament to the courage and intelligence possessed by many who society had formerly dismissed as beyond hope.

24   See e.g. Bostrom, Nick, 'Existential risk prevention as global priority', *Global Policy,* 4(1) (2013), pp.15–31 and Armstrong, Stuart and Anders Sandberg, 'Eternity in six hours: Intergalactic spreading of intelligent life and sharpening the Fermi paradox', *Acta Astronautica, 89* (2013), pp.1–13 but see also Torres, Phil, 'Space colonization and suffering risks: Reassessing the "maxipok rule"', *Futures, 100* (2018), pp.74–85 for reasons why space colonisation might pose an existential risk of its own.

25   Rock, David and Heidi Grant, 'Why diverse teams are smarter', *Harvard Business Review,* 4(4) (2016), pp.2–5.

26   For more about universal design, see Steinfeld, Edward and Jordana Maisel, *Universal Design: Creating Inclusive Environments.* John Wiley & Sons (2012). It is worth noting, however, that while universal design is often talked about, it is surprisingly little studied or practised, and much of the cited literature in this field is over a decade old, highlighting this as an area in desperate need of further research.

27   If that seems like rather a strong claim, consider perhaps how two little raised dots on the F and J keys of a QWERTY keyboard do not only make it

accessible to many blind people but facilitate touch-typing for many more people.

28   This section was largely drawn from Wells-Jensen, Sheri, Joshua A. Miele, and Brandie Bohney, 'An alternate vision for colonization', *Futures, 110* (2019), pp.50–53. For more on *Mission: AstroAccess* see https://astroaccess. org.

29   See e.g. Rakić, Vojin and Milan M. Ćirković, 'Confronting existential risks with voluntary moral bioenhancement', *Journal of Ethics and Emerging Technologies, 26*(2) (2016), pp.48–59 and Demko, Megan, Katina Michael, Kennedy Wagner, and Terri Bookman, 'When brain computer interfaces pose an existential risk', in *2020 IEEE International Symposium on Technology and Society (ISTAS)*. IEEE (2020), pp.112–14.

30   For more on the important role transhumanism played in the establishment of Existential Risk Studies, see Beard, S.J. and P. Torres, *Ripples on the Great Sea of Life: A Brief History of Existential Risk Studies*. SSRN (2021).

31   For a critique of the role that eugenical ideas have played—and may continue to play—on the field, see Harper, T., 'Elites against extinction: The dark history of a cultural paranoia', *Los Angeles Review of Books* (2021), while for a more positive view about how the field may be able to (and indeed already has) positively engage(d) with this history, see Mannheim, D., 'Noticing the skulls, longtermism edition', *EA Forum* (2021). https://forum.effectivealtruism.org/posts/ZcpZEXEFZ5oLHTnr9/noticing-the-skulls-longtermism-edition

32   Suffan, Sandy and Rosemarie Garland-Thomson, 'The Dark Side of CRISPR', *Scientific American* (2021).

33   Hall, Melinda, *The Bioethics of Enhancement: Transhumanism, Disability, and Biopolitics*. Lexington Books (2016).

34   Shew, Ashley, 'Ableism, technoableism, and future AI', *IEEE Technology and Society Magazine, 39*(1) (2020), pp.40–85.

35   UN Department for Economic and Social Affairs, *'Disability and Employment' Fact Sheet 1 on Persons With Disabilities* (2007). https://www.un.org/disabilities/documents/toolaction/employmentfs.pdf.

36   Mizunoya, Suguru, Sophie Mitra, and Izumi Yamasaki, *Towards Inclusive Education: The Impact of Disability on School Attendance in Developing Countries*. UNICEF (2016).

37   Kent, George, *Ending Hunger Worldwide*. Routledge (2015); Moore Lappe, Frances and Joseph Collins, 'World hunger: Ten myths', *Food First* (2015), https://archive.foodfirst.org/publication/world-hunger-ten-myths/.

38   Hamraie, Aimi, *Building Access: Universal Design and the Politics of Disability*. University of Minnesota Press (2017); Barclay, Linda, *Disability With Dignity: Justice, Human Rights and Equal Status*. Routledge (2018).

39   Hawking, Stephen, *Brief Answers to the Big Questions*. Bantam (2018); White, J.J., 'Artificial intelligence and people with disabilities: A reflection on human–AI partnerships', *Humanity Driven AI*. Springer (2022), pp. 279–310.

40   As with risk, disabled people are often seen as the subjects of care, but in our experience generally also perform more than their fair share of caring responsibilities—in part because they have a greater sensitivity to the needs of others but also because they may be seen as 'having nothing better to do'.

41   Swafford, Jan, *Beethoven: Anguish and Triumph: A Biography*. Houghton Mifflin Harcourt (2014).

42   Kleege, Georgina, *Blind Rage: Letters to Helen Keller*. Gallaudet University Press (2006).

43   White, Michael and John Gribbin, *Stephen Hawking: A Life in Science*. Abacus (1992).

44   Roberts, Jason and John Curless, *A Sense of the World: How a Blind Man Became History's Greatest Traveler*. Recorded Books (2007).

45   Dolmage, Jay T., *Academic Ableism: Disability and Higher Education*. University of Michigan Press (2017).

46   Booksh, Karl S. and Lynnette D. Madsen, 'Academic pipeline for scientists with disabilities', *MRS Bulletin,* 43(8) (2018), pp.625–32.

47   Hawking (2018).

48   For some thoughts about where Turing's views would fit within current thinking about AI safety, see Proudfoot, Diane, 'Alan Turing and evil AI', *The Turing Conversation* #2 (2018). https://www.turing.ethz.ch/the-turing-conversation/contribution-2.html. For a historical account of the development of AI safety work from Turing to the present day, see Chapter 9 of this volume.

49   While no recording of this broadcast exists any longer, a transcript is printed in Copeland, B. Jack (ed), *The Essential Turing*. Clarendon Press (2004), and the broadcast has also been recreated at https://aperiodical.com/2018/01/ive-re-recorded-alan-turings-can-computers-think-radio-broadcasts/

50   Hodges, Andrew, *Alan Turing: The Enigma*. Princeton University Press (2014). The letter to Norman Routledge is reproduced, and read by

Benedict　Cumberbatch,　at　https://lettersofnote.com/2012/06/23/yours-in-distress-alan/

51　For an account of these barriers, and how Carson overcame them, as well as those faced by other queer and female scientists, see Popova, Maria, *Figuring*. Vintage (2019).

52　Such scientists tended to be posted to the metallurgical laboratory in Chicago, rather than more sensitive sites such as Los Alamos and Oak Ridge. As discussed in Chapter 1, this was one of the main reasons for the naming of *The Bulletin of Atomic Scientists of Chicago*.

53　This quote is generally attributed to science fiction author William Gibson, but see https://quoteinvestigator.com/2012/01/24/future-has-arrived/

6. Natural Global Catastrophic Risks

Lara Mani, Doug Erwin, and Lindley Johnson

> *Civilization exists by geological consent, subject to change without notice.*
> Will Durant, historian (1885–1981)

Humanity has lived with the threat of certain global catastrophic risks throughout history, such as large-magnitude volcanic eruptions and Near-Earth Object (NEO) impacts. But the risks of such events have grown with the increasing complexity of human societies. The probabilities of natural global catastrophes are not negligible, although these risks are often underestimated. Moreover, the societal and economic impacts of some of these events are potentially vast. So, to what extent is humanity truly vulnerable to natural catastrophic risks, and what does this risk landscape look like? Here, we explore the state of current thinking around extreme natural risks and explore the dichotomies often neglected on the peripheries of these discussions.

The past as a lens for the future

The geological record is the greatest tool that humanity possesses in informing discussions of our exposure and vulnerabilities to high-impact, low-probability natural risks. By studying the stratigraphy of our Earth's past, geologists have built a picture of the potential futures that may await us. French natural historian Georges Cuvier first identified catastrophes in the fossil record of the Paris Basin in the early 19th century, and progress has waxed and waned since then. In 1982, using the fossil record of marine animals (mostly invertebrates), Sepkoski and Raup presented evidence

    https://doi.org/10.11647/OBP.0336.06

for five mass extinction events over the past 500 million years, where a mass extinction is a substantial increase in lineage extinction across multiple clades in a relatively short amount of time.[1] The vagueness of this definition is intentional, to capture a variety of possible events.

Over the past several decades palaeontologists, stratigraphers, geochemists, and others have conducted detailed studies of specific extinction horizons, as well as compiled global, synoptic databases of past biodiversity. This work has greatly improved our resolution of the fossil record and clarified the number, extent, and rate of past biodiversity crises.

Before detailing the results and implications of these studies, some reflection on the nature of the data is warranted. The primary source of information on past biodiversity crises is the fossil record of durably skeletonised, geographically widespread and abundant marine invertebrates, as well as similar microfossils such as foraminifera and radiolarians. It is the record of these groups that is preserved with sufficient fidelity to permit regional and global correlation of the sedimentary geological record. These fossils are also preserved with sufficient continuity that we can, with appropriate statistical analysis, have reasonable confidence in the accuracy of the resulting patterns. Many marine organisms are difficult to preserve as fossils, either because they lack durable skeletons or for other reasons, and these are largely absent from such synoptic compilations. Palaeontologists have compiled records of terrestrial plants, insects, and vertebrates, but the quality of their fossil records generally precludes using them to *identify* past biotic crises, except in relatively young deposits. Rather, palaeontologists tend to identify crisis intervals in the marine record, and then seek correlative terrestrial records to examine the potential impact on terrestrial ecosystems.

Today, palaeontologists generally identify three great mass extinctions with rapid drops in biodiversity across many different taxa: in the late Ordovician (444 Ma), end-Permian (251 Ma), and end-Cretaceous (66 Ma), and a possible fourth at the end-Triassic (199 Ma). In addition, there was a prolonged decrease in diversity through the Late Devonian, but this was more drawn out than other episodes. As the resolution of the data has improved, a series of smaller events has also been identified, with perhaps a total of at least 18 biotic crises events affecting marine taxa—with some affecting both marine and terrestrial taxa.[2] There have almost certainly been additional crises that primarily affected poorly preserved taxa, either marine or terrestrial, but which are missing from the synoptic compilations used in these studies. Animal fossils only appeared about 550 million years ago, so we lack a sufficiently high-resolution fossil record before that time to reveal older biodiversity crises. Species extinctions have been ubiquitous through the history of plant and animal life, and the majority of these have not been concentrated in these discrete episodes. Nonetheless, biodiversity crises, often tied to environmental perturbations, are a natural process. But what drives biotic crises and what governs when a crisis tilts to become a mass extinction event?

The major mass extinctions share several common features: First, high-resolution radiometric dating has revealed that most were relatively rapid, occurring in just a few tens of thousands of years (or less), rather than over hundreds of thousands or millions of years.[3] This suggests that whatever the cause or causes that trigger a mass extinction, once collapse is triggered it is very rapid. To a first approximation, every event that has been studied in detail happened more rapidly than we can resolve with current techniques. Second, all were global, and all but the end-Ordovician impacted both marine and terrestrial organisms (there was little life on land at that time). Third, these extinctions were selective, more heavily impacting some clades rather than others—brachiopods and ammonoids, respectively, at the end-Permian and end-Cretaceous, for example. Fourth, although palaeontologists have traditionally focused attention on the loss of diversity, most of these were profound ecological disruptions as well, rending food webs.[4] The exception to this generality was the end-Ordovician event which, despite being the second largest mass extinction, had little ecological impact. Finally, rapid climatic change (either cooling or warming) has been implicated in each event, as well as pervasive marine anoxia. The net effect of all these crises has been the progressive loss of clades unable to survive such events or to recover after such widespread losses of diversity.

Dozens of possible causes have been suggested for mass extinctions, but proximal causes—those directly responsible for the disappearance of particular species—must be distinguished from mechanisms that generate the proximal causes. Most studies of the end-Cretaceous mass extinction have concluded that the impact of an extra-terrestrial object in the Yucatan peninsula of Mexico was the cause of the extinction,[5] but species largely disappeared as a result of the environmental effects of the impact, including climate change. Massive volcanism in India roughly coincides with the extinction event, and some continue to argue that it was involved, although most studies suggest that the peak of the volcanic eruption pre-dates the impact and extinction. Massive volcanism has also been implicated for the end-Permian[6] and end-Triassic events,[7] while a rapid glaciation was probably the cause of the end-Ordovician extinction.[8] The end-Permian mass extinction has long been tied to the eruption of the massive Siberian flood basalts, the most extensive continental flood basalt province in the past 500 million years. Beyond the Siberian volcanism, subduction-related massive volcanism spread copper and mercury across wide areas of south China at the Permo-Triassic boundary.[9] These volcanic events caused rapid cooling followed by a 4–6°C temperature increase, oceanic anoxia, and acid rain from sulphate aerosols.

One of the most controversial issues in extinction research is the impact of mass extinctions and other crises on pre-existing evolutionary trends. In particular, do clades that acquire extinction-resistance prior to a crisis have better survival rates during mass extinctions? Numerous studies of this question have been conducted over the past several decades, arriving at sometimes contradictory results.[10] Overall, however, much of this work suggests that the acquisition of resilience often enhances survival during biotic crises. There may be an important lesson here for human societies. Politicians and voters often fail to focus on long-term concerns, including natural catastrophic risks of the sort described in this chapter. If, however, resilience to crises on shorter time scales—such as hurricanes, volcanic eruptions, or massive wildfires—might also enhance the survivability to far rarer events, this suggests that pursuing a properly constructed resilience strategy may have substantial societal benefits.

The geological record presents dire warnings for humanity if extreme natural risks are left unmitigated. Our world could experience a new biotic crisis due to rapid onset climate change, with accelerated species extinction already taking place. And, although our surveillance may provide us with ample warning of a potential large NEO impact, we remain exposed to such a threat with no means of mitigation and prevention available. However, the geological record can only go so far as informing us of what extreme natural hazard events have looked like in the past. To understand the impact of such an event in the future, we must consider the present-day landscape for natural global catastrophic risks and how vulnerability is a key component in understanding the systemic nature of risk.

The changing landscape of extreme natural threats

We are now entering a new geological epoch—the *Anthropocene*—characterised by humanity as the biggest driver of change to our planet's climates and ecosystems. Anthropogenically driven climate change is accelerating and strengthening some of our Earth's natural processes. Today we face an increasingly complex risk landscape where hazards can be interconnected, where one natural hazard event can increase the probability and/or severity of another hazard. For example, extreme weather events (such as flooding or drought) can result in crop failures and damage to critical infrastructures such as water and sanitation, resulting in disease outbreaks.[11] Certainly, we are now experiencing more disasters than ever before, with over four billion people affected by disasters over the past 20 years, up 1.2 billion from the 20 years prior.[12] Some evidence suggests that despite this increase in disasters, our resilience to smaller-scale disasters is also increasing, with the average annual loss of life due to disasters representing around 0.1% of global deaths.[13] However, shock events—such as the 2004 Indian Ocean tsunami, or the 2010 Haiti earthquake—can significantly elevate the global death toll, and humanity remains vulnerable to low-probability, high-impact risks.

Large-magnitude volcanic eruptions and asteroid and comet impacts represent natural hazards that may lead to either extinction of humanity or to grave consequences affecting humanity's continued flourishing. Here, we review this hazards in the light of improved surveillance and new research into the threats they pose.

Large-magnitude volcanic eruptions

The critical risk to humanity posed by volcanic eruptions is centred on large-magnitude 8+ eruptions, or so-called super-eruptions. These are explosive eruptions that eject over 1000 km^3 of material.[14] Certainly, an eruption of this scale would have severe consequences for humanity, with ash and gas propelled into the upper atmosphere, where they would interact with our climatic systems, reducing global surface temperatures and potentially devastating global food production. This climatic feedback mechanism is typified by the 1815 magnitude 7 Tambora eruption, which released 30 megatons of sulphur, resulting in short-term climate anomalies (primarily in the northern hemisphere).[15] During the summer of 1816, Europe is thought to have experienced temperatures of 1–2°C lower than normal as a result of the eruption, and summer temperatures remained anomalously cooler in 1817 and 1818 respectively.[16, 17]

The climatic cooling mechanisms for volcanic eruptions are often compared to that of the nuclear winter mechanism, by which the black soot particles from nuclear warfare would block the sun's energy, resulting in a global cooling effect. For volcanic eruptions, it is rather the sulphur gas released during the eruption that mixes with water in the atmosphere, creating droplets of sulphuric acid which reflect sunlight back into space and absorb heat from the Earth.[18] The resulting effect is a cooling of the lower atmosphere and a warming of the upper atmosphere.[19] This mechanism is important to understand, because the magnitude of an eruption does not necessarily correlate to the quantity of sulphate released. In fact, lower magnitude eruptions of magnitudes 6 and 7 are capable of releasing significant quantities of sulphate gas to instigate this climate cooling effect. One such example is the 1257 magnitude 7 eruption of Mt Rinjani, Indonesia. Detected by a strong sulphate signal in ice core records, this eruption is thought to have triggered the onset of the Little Ice Age, resulting in famine across Europe and the deaths of over 10,000 people in London alone.[20] Abrupt climate cooling events have now been linked to several volcanic eruptions, including the 1991 eruption of Mt Pinatubo, the 1257 eruption of Mt Rinjani, and the 1883 eruption of Krakatau. Using new ice core records, a recent study identified, during the Holocene (the past 10,000 years) over 160 explosive eruptions releasing quantities of sulphur greater than or equal to the 1815 Tambora eruption.[21]

Since the 1815 Tambora eruption, our natural global systems and processes have undergone significant changes as a result of climate change. One such process of significance to volcanic eruptions is the Brewer-Dobson global atmospheric circulation pattern, by which warm tropospheric air rises to the upper atmosphere and sinks at the poles, which is now accelerating due to greenhouse gas emissions.[22] Volcanic aerosol injection is also known to accelerate the Brewer-Dobson circulation, and the combined effect of anthropogenically driven climate change and volcanic eruptions can substantially increase the rate at which volcanic ash and gas are pushed towards the Polar Regions, increasing the rate of global surface cooling.[23] Additionally, the increased sulphate aerosol in the atmosphere in the aftermath of a major volcanic eruption can result in a reduction of global mean precipitation.[24] By these effects, models run by Aubry et al. predict that global surface cooling for eruptions in the tropics could lead to 15% more global surface cooling than seen in 1815, and as much as 60% more when ocean feedbacks are also factored in.[25] By this calculation, a future eruption the size of the 1815 Tambora eruption in the tropic regions could cause up to 3.2°C global surface cooling.

The implications of such a global surface cooling event could be catastrophic for global food production, devastating food production regions. Simulation models of the Toba eruption, which occurred ~74,000 years ago,[26] suggest that if a similar event were to occur today, few regions of the world (with the exceptions of southern Africa and India) would remain unaffected by global surface cooling and a reduction in precipitation. A loss of any of the global food production regions could have catastrophic consequences for the world population, resulting in widespread famine, increased fuel and food prices, disease outbreaks, and regional conflicts. Ord (2020) suggests that billions of people could starve in this scenario and, if civilisations are unable to recover, it could result in an existential catastrophe.

Not only are the resulting consequences of volcanic eruptions becoming more extreme due to the expansion of human civilisation, the frequency of eruptions may be increasing. The melting of snow and ice sheets on volcanic centres, higher sea levels, and increased rainfall in some regions are thought to change the stresses in volcanic systems, removing the overlying weight burdens. As the pressures change within the system, this can encourage fresh magma to ascend to the surface.[27] With climate change now an amplifier of volcanic hazard, evidence is building to suggest that lower magnitude eruptions (VEI <8) should be considered within our probabilistic forecasts for extreme volcanic risk scenarios. From the geological record, the recurrence interval for VEI 7 eruptions is estimated between 1 and 2 eruptions per 1,000 years and new ice core record data corroborates this, suggesting the recurrence interval could be around 1.16 eruptions per 1000 years. By this logic, the recurrence interval could be as short as 625 years for a magnitude 7 eruption—or one in six this century.[28]

Fields such as volcanology are in their naissance, and volcanologists still have a long way to go before being able to answer some of the most fundamental questions about volcanoes. Many of the forecasts of probabilities for such risks fail to acknowledge the outstanding uncertainties in the geological record or to consider the advancements in our surveillance techniques, leading to an underestimation of the risks. For the field of volcanology, lessons can be learnt from the field of planetary defence about the importance of increased surveillance and monitoring for constraining the threats posed by Near-Earth Objects.

Near-Earth objects—Asteroids and comets

To date, there are more than 190 confirmed impact structures spanning Earth's recent geologic history known around the world. Examples include the Manicouagan Crater in Canada: at 85 km wide, it is thought to have resulted from a ~5 km impactor some 214 million years ago, and the Lonar impact crater in India is thought to have occurred around 570,000 years ago. The most significant damage recorded from an asteroid impact in recent history is from 1908 Tunguska, Russia, where a 40-metre object exploded before surface impact, causing an air blast that devastated over 2,000 km² of forest in Siberia, and is believed to have had measurable effects on the global climate in the subsequent year. However, impact events remain relatively rare, with regional scale devastation events (caused by object impacts over 140 metres) estimated to occur every 20,000 years (Table 1). Despite the low probabilities associated with these events, the threat of impact remains present, and impact events could happen at any time where, unlike other natural hazard events, the location of impacts is not confined to specific regions.

Table 1. The potential expected impacts and estimated recurrence intervals for a range of asteroid impacts sizes. The range shaded in grey identifies the diameter of impactors typical considered to be capable of global catastrophe (adapted from NASA[29]).

Diameter of impacting asteroid (metres)	Type of impact	Average time between impacts (years)
5	Bolide	1
10	Super bolide	10
25	Major airburst	100
50	Local scale devastation	1,000
140	Regional scale devastation	20,000
300	Continent scale devastation	70,000
600	Below global catastrophe threshold	200,000
1,000	Possible global catastrophe	700,000
5,000	Above global catastrophe threshold	30 million
10,000	Mass extinction	100 million

Near-Earth Objects (NEOs) are asteroids and comets that come within 1.3 astronomical units (the mean distance between Earth and the sun) of the sun, bringing them within 50 million kilometres of Earth's orbit.[30] A subset of NEOs can be described as Potentially Hazardous Objects (PHOs), meaning their orbits bring them within eight million kilometres of Earth over time, and they are of sizes capable of causing devastating regional damage should they impact (>140 metres in size). In 2010, with over 90% of all NEO objects greater than 1,000 metres in size already discovered,[31] the National Aeronautics and Space Administration (NASA) began searching for 90% of NEOs larger than 140 metres in size.[32] NASA identifies over 2,500 Near-Earth asteroids a year of all sizes, with an average of 500 being larger than 140 metres in size, using a system of both ground-based telescopes (e.g. Catalina Sky Survey, ATLAS, and Pan-STARRS) and the NEOWISE space-based telescope. With a population estimated at over 25,000 objects larger than 140 metres in size, at NASA's current discovery rate this task is expected to take over 30 years to complete. To speed up the identification process, in 2026 NASA plans to launch a new NEO detection and tracking space telescope called 'NEO

Surveyor', which will detect in the infrared spectrum and is designed to identify over 90% of the still unknown hazardous NEO population within 10 years of operation.

In 2021 alone, there were over 145 close approaches within the distance of the moon's orbit by NEOs,[33] most of which measured just a few metres to a few tens of metres in size. In this size range, any object on a collision course with Earth would likely disintegrate in our atmosphere before impact. However, one asteroid in 2021 was as much as 90 metres in size, substantially larger than the one causing the Tunguska impact. A few even larger objects make close approaches every few years, such as the '2019 OK' asteroid which measured ~100 metres wide and passed within approximately 70,000 km of Earth in July 2019. Alarmingly, this object was not detected until just a day before its close approach, despite it having been included in surveillance imagery by both Pan-STARRS and ATLAS. The object's slow rate of apparent movement relative to the background of stars meant that it was not identified as a closer moving object, and therefore remained undetected.[34] The '2019 OK' event somewhat echoed the 2013 Chelyabinsk impact event, which also went undetected until its actual impact with Earth on 15 February 2019 over a densely populated region of Russia. In the case of Chelyabinsk, the lack of prior detection was due to its approach in the daytime sky. The object's approach from the direction of the sun meant that an already small and faint object would have been very difficult to detect, even if our telescopes had been directed at it.[35] The resulting impact caused widespread building damage in the region of over 7,000 properties, and injury to an estimated 1,400 people, mainly due to shattered glass as a result of the shockwave it caused. Both the '2019 OK' close approach and the Chelyabinsk impact event serve as stark reminders of humanity's continued vulnerability to NEO impacts, and of the blind spots and limitations of our current surveillance capabilities.

Not all NEO impact events may have catastrophic consequences for humanity—the end-Cretaceous impact event did not kill all living species on Earth, despite the object's size being well into the realms of causing global disaster, but rather led to the demise of the dominant species so that the diminutive mammals of the era could begin their ascent on the planet. Objects over 1 km in size are considered to pose the most threat to humanity's continued flourishing, and the recurrence interval for these events is around 700,000 years (Table 1), over a thousand times less probable than a magnitude 7 eruption.[36] More likely are the impacts from objects between 100–300 metres, which could still cause substantial regional devastation. If an impact of this size were to occur in food-producing regions, for example, the cascading consequences could be comparable to a volcanic global cooling event, described above.

Both the examples of high-impact volcanic risks and the threat of an NEO impact demonstrate how such events could result in globally felt consequences, amplified by the impacts to global food production and the stresses this could exert on human civilisation. This highlights the need to increasingly consider the systemic nature of natural risks, and particularly the aspects of vulnerability as amplifiers of global risks.

The systemic nature of natural risks

Borrowing from the disaster risk literature, risk is often seen as a combination of components of hazard and vulnerability (and exposure), where the relationship can be defined as:

Hazard x Vulnerability (x Exposure) = Risk

In a crude sense, this risk equation is a simple way to consider the key components of risk, and this remains relevant for the consideration of high-impact low-probability natural risks, such as asteroid impacts or high-magnitude volcanic eruptions. However, this approach often fails to encapsulate the dichotomies around the components of hazard and vulnerability, or consider how humanity's capacity to cope with hazards (or vulnerability) can alter the severity of the risks. Some existential risk authors, such as Liu et al.[37] and Avin et al.[38] have made steps towards adopting 'systemic risk' thinking rather than siloed 'hazard' thinking, and here we continue to build upon this progress by considering the mechanisms by which natural hazards could be amplified to natural global catastrophes.

Cascading to catastrophe

Our world has become interconnected and complex, with our societies relying on a myriad of systems and networks to sustain them and support their continued development—known as global critical systems (GCS).[39] These systems (such as communications networks, transportation routes, and trade links) are vital arteries in our modern world. Global critical systems and infrastructures, such as maritime shipping routes, submarine cables, global position navigation and timing (PNT) systems, aerial networks, ports, fuel pipelines, and power plants (amongst others) are critical to the transport of goods, services, and commodities around the world. However, these systems are often fragile, with little to no resilience built in to deal with shocks and interruptions. Any disruptions to these systems can instigate a cascade of impacts across interdependent systems.[40] For example, in March 2020, the *Ever Given* container ship blocked the Suez Canal—a busy maritime trade passage—for six days, with ships stuck either side of the passage for weeks to months in the aftermath. The resulting disruption saw global container ports overwhelmed and significant delays to global supply chains, costing an estimated $6-10 billion a week to global trade. Within the field of Disaster Risk Studies, this type of chain reaction of impacts is described as cascading risk.[41]

The extent to which a cascade of system failures escalates to global catastrophe is a component of what systems are affected and how well we are able to cope with them. Response to a natural hazard event can erode our ability to cope with other shocks and hazards, and can even amplify the impacts of subsequent impacts in other related and interconnected systems.[42] The COVID-19 pandemic has revealed the nature of our interconnected systems, with pressures on the health sector resulting in knock-out effects on the economic and political sectors. Other examples of this mechanism include Syria, where severe drought conditions experienced between 2007 and 2010 devastated the food production regions, resulting in unemployment and food insecurity for over one million people, contributing to conflict in the region.[43]

The links between natural hazards and human civilisation are well documented, with volcanic activity linked to the collapse of the Maya, Romans, and Minoans, amongst others,[44] and even changes in Earth's magnetic field linked to societal declines. However, in many of these examples, volcanic activity was only considered a contributing factor, rather than the outright cause. Additional risk drivers—such as droughts or other natural hazards, conflict, and food scarcity—were often associated with these collapse events, where a compounding of shocks and a cascade of failures amplified the impacts. In our modern and connected world, these same processes could see natural hazard events catapult to global catastrophes.

A recent study by Mani et al. looked at this cascade mechanism in relation to active volcanism in proximity to regions where a high convergence of GCSs were observed, representing regions of heightened societal vulnerability.[45] They present seven global 'pinch points' where the interaction between volcanic hazards and multiple GCSs at these convergence zone could result in a cascade of system failures, leading to global impacts. Interestingly, the study expresses that lower-magnitude eruptions (magnitude 3+) could be capable of instigating such a cascade of impacts, though they are typically considered outside the realm of disaster causation. Liu et al. (2018) express this relationship as an imbalance of the risk equation, moving away from consideration of just 'existential hazards' towards 'existential vulnerabilities'.[46] If a hazard event or sequence of hazard events were to occur in proximity to these regions of heightened societal vulnerability, such as pinch point regions, the consequences could be catastrophic for humanity, highlighting the importance of consideration for the systemic nature of risk in the practice of global catastrophic risk research.

The systemic nature of risk is important to consider for other extreme natural hazards such as stellar explosions, coronal mass ejections, and the reversal of Earth's magnetic field, amongst others. Not all of these risks may pose a direct threat of human extinction as we currently understand it, but the risks they pose to their systems and infrastructures that sustain our societies could constitute a global catastrophic risk and even push us towards collapse. For example, if an event similar to the 1859 Carrington Event (a geomagnetic storm caused by a coronal mass ejection)[47, 48] were to happen in our modern and interconnected world, the impacts could be grave if we are not prepared. Electrical surges in power grids could cause them to shut down with consequences to our water, sanitation, food and energy supplies, and health systems, and satellites and communication networks could be damaged, with disruption to global transport and trade leading to severe impacts on our global economic, social, and political systems.[49] For events like geomagnetic storms and coronal mass ejection events, they can be detected in advance of their arrival on Earth, meaning we could have the time to prepare and respond so we can reduce the potential impacts, such as shutting down electricity grids temporarily to avoid disruption. However, without adequate preparation and resilience measures put in place in advance, and considerations for the systemic nature of such risks, we remain vulnerable to the cascading consequences of such events.[50]

Mitigating and preventing natural risks

Natural catastrophic risks, such as those described in this chapter, have long posed a threat to the continued existence of humanity. By increasing the exposure of our societal vulnerabilities to regional natural hazard events, we have manufactured a new landscape for global catastrophic risks. By improving our understanding of the drivers that proliferate a hazard event towards a global catastrophe, we can consider the best methods and strategies to adopt in order to strengthen our resilience to the risks. So, what can we do to reduce the risk posed by natural catastrophic risks? One field that is making strides in this realm is planetary defence.

Lessons from planetary defence

After the 2013 Chelyabinsk impact event, global governments were motivated to increase our resilience to NEO impact threats. In 2018, guidance was handed down to NASA from the White House that tasked them with developing preparedness and mitigation strategies for an Earth-bound NEO. The guidance sets a clear focus for improving our understanding of NEO threats: to increase surveillance capabilities and to establish robust response and mitigation strategies.[51] With a modest budget of around $150 million a year (expected to rise to $200 million in 2022), the Planetary Defense Coordination Office (PDCO) at NASA works towards these goals.[52] So, what can be done if we detect an object on an Earth-bound trajectory?

Depending on the timescale that we may be afforded once an Earth-bound object is detected, different technologies can potentially be deployed to deflect or disrupt it. Many of the current methods and techniques employ the sample principle—change the orbital speed of the asteroid several years before potential interception with Earth, and the object's trajectory will no longer synchronise. Several methods and techniques are currently considered for deflection and disruption, including gravity tractor, nuclear detonation, and kinetic impactor. The gravity tractor technique simply uses the forces of gravity to either push or pull the object off its current trajectory. Where we are afforded time (in the form of decades), a spacecraft can be launched to meet the asteroid, stationing itself in proximity. The close presence of the spacecraft then generates a gravitational attraction between the two bodies, slowly tugging at the asteroid and pulling it from its orbital track, out of the path of collision with Earth.[53] Nuclear detonation using a Nuclear Explosive Device (NED) could be employed when we are afforded less time (a decade or less). By detonating an NED in proximity to an object, this can irradiate the surface of an asteroid, super-heating the release of material from the surface, causing a reaction force of the asteroid in the opposite direction. However, nuclear detonation techniques come with high levels of uncertainty, and the use of nuclear devices in space (and the employment of this method) would involve the careful navigation of the Outer Space Treaty and global geopolitics.

As part of the international Asteroid Impact and Deflection and Assessment (AIDA) collaboration, in November 2021 the first of two missions was launched to demonstrate the kinetic impact technique. NASA's Double Asteroid Redirection Test (DART) mission launched towards the binary asteroid Didymos, with the aim of crashing the probe directly into the asteroid's small moon, Dimorphos. It was designed so that the collision event would change the orbital speed of Dimorphos and thus, test the plausibility of using the kinetic impactor technique for future Earth-bound NEO threats. Early indications suggest the mission was successful, with the impact shortening the orbital time of Dimorphos around Didymos by 32 minutes. A second mission—the HERA mission, led by the European Space Agency (ESA)—will launch in 2024, headed for the Didymos/Dimorphos asteroid pair. The HERA mission is designed to measure the effectiveness of the kinetic impactor by DART, by better characterising the asteroid, the effects of the impact of DART, and more precisely measuring the body's mass and internal structure. If both DART and HERA prove successful, we will move a step closer in our capabilities for asteroid deflection.

Although these are promising steps towards developing our capabilities for mitigation of an NEO threat, we are still years away from being able to utilise kinetic impactor technologies for a real-time event. With this in mind, the planetary defence community has worked extensively, through international cooperation, to establish potential disaster response strategies for an impending NEO impact. The development of the National Near-Earth Object Preparedness Strategy and Action Plan in 2018 called for a strengthening of the US response to an asteroid or comet impact.[54] To this end, the field has extensively employed the use of scenario-based simulation exercises to stress-test the global response to an asteroid threat. A similar exercise is adopted for the wider planetary defence community at the bi-annual International Academy of Astronautics (IAA) Planetary Defense Conference.[55] The exercises include considerations of the global consequences to our climatic systems and for civil protection strategies, and engage a range of experts from across disciplines to provide a holistic approach to considering the risk posed by hypothetical impact scenarios.[56] These interactive exercises provide the opportunity to assess the global response mechanisms for such a risk, assign duty bearers, and identify weaknesses in capabilities and capacities to cope. The use of scenario exercises provides us with useful thought experiments for mitigation and prevention of natural catastrophic risks, with application across numerous other global catastrophic risk domains, such as biosecurity and nuclear war (some of which are already using simulation, e.g. Johns Hopkins Center for Health Security).

The strength of the planetary defence community is the strong push for international coordination and the adoption of interdisciplinary approaches to mitigating the risks, presenting a model for other catastrophic natural risks. The planetary defence community demonstrates the importance of taking actions now that may better prepare us for future natural catastrophic events.

Mitigating volcanic eruptions

Despite the higher probability of volcanic eruptions (over NEO impacts) having catastrophic consequences on humanity over the next century, little work is currently being done to consider potential mitigation and prevention methods. Often, volcanic eruptions are deprioritised in comparison to other natural hazards, largely because it is thought that little can be done to mitigate them.[57] However, the recent NASA DART mission, combined with the eruption of the Hunga Tonga-Hunga Ha'apai eruption in the South Pacific in January 2021, has accelerated discussions about increasing our global resilience to volcanic eruptions.[58]

One problem we face in the potential mitigation of volcanic eruptions is that little is known about which volcanoes are capable of causing global disruption and climatic feedbacks. Global volcanoes are drastically understudied, with estimates suggesting that over 80% of volcanic eruptions capable of causing climate feedbacks are missing from the global geological record.[59] Understanding the eruptive history of volcanoes can help us identify those that are capable of potentially disruptive eruptions, and those that we must closely monitor. However, even if we were able to identify the volcanoes that we need to monitor, currently our ability to do so is limited, particularly as many volcanoes are in resource-limited countries. To date, only 27% of volcanic eruptions have been monitored with ground-based instruments;[60] access to satellite technologies is limited and unable to fill the gaps in global volcano surveillance. In the absence of mitigation measures, volcano monitoring—along with community-based education and preparedness initiatives—are essential for early action and risk reduction, and should be prioritised for funding and development, particularly in pinch-point regions with the highest societal vulnerabilities.

Monitoring and surveillance of volcanoes is just the first step in mitigation and prevention. So, what if we did identify a volcano that may have a large-magnitude eruption—could we do anything to mitigate or prevent it? Interventions with volcanoes themselves (so-called 'volcano geoengineering') are being considered, to assess if we can reduce the impacts of volcanic eruptions.[61] One such project will deliberately drill into a magma pocket within the Krafla Magma Testbed in Iceland, with the aim of providing data on the inner workings of volcanoes to improve our prediction capacities. Manipulating volcanoes is not a new concept; throughout history, we have intervened with volcanoes to reduce the risks posed to local communities. Such examples include the redirection of lava flows through the construction of levees, cooling the moving front with water, and even bombing them. But explosive eruptions are more complicated: their impacts can be global and therefore require global coordination and inclusion in discussions on how we can (and if we should) mitigate and prevent them. It is a subject that requires careful navigation, and efforts towards building global coordination in response to large-magnitude eruptions should be prioritised. For now, volcano geoengineering remains largely theoretical,[62] but with an increasing demand for renewable energy sources, geothermal exploration is putting humanity in closer contact with volcanoes. A natural progression of these explorations may advance our progress on physical interventions with volcanoes, but there must be careful consideration of the ethics of such advancements.[63]

The lesson we can draw from both planetary defence and volcanic eruption mitigation is that, although the technologies for mitigating and preventing both risks provide hope for the future, they remain decades away. In the meantime, humanity remains vulnerable to both asteroid impact and large-magnitude volcanic eruptions, at greater frequencies than previously considered. Our last remaining defence against such risks is preparedness. Building resilience to global critical systems can help prevent cascade impacts and system failures, and utilising tools like scenario exercises can help stress-test and strengthen our response mechanisms. However, civil protection remains our best defence when faced with such risks, and efforts for community-level resilience-building and early action should be prioritised.

Conclusion

The geological record demonstrates humanity's vulnerability to natural catastrophic risks, and shares insights as to our fate if we are unable to prevent or mitigate an impending natural catastrophe. Anthropogenically driven climate change and continued globalisation are changing humanity's relationships with natural risks, potentially pushing some natural hazard events into the realms of global disaster causation. The low prioritisation for mitigation and prevention of natural risks (with the exception of a modest budget assigned for NEO impacts) is not consistent with the threats these risks may pose. With advancements in surveillance and identification technologies for natural risks, we may be able to provide ourselves with a chance to change the course of our future. Lessons can be learnt for other GCRs from fields like planetary defence, demonstrating the importance of global cooperation for the mitigation and prevention of global risks. However, many of the technologies that may one day save us remain decades away from being deployed, therefore efforts for civil protection through a properly constructed resilience strategy may have substantial societal benefits.

Notes and References

1   Raup, D.M. and J.J. Sepkoski, 'Mass extinctions in the marine fossil record', *Science, 215* (1982), pp.1501–03.

2   Bambach, R.K., 'Phanerozoic biodiversity mass extinctions', *Annual Review of Earth and Planetary Sciences, 34* (2006), pp.127–55.

3   Erwin, D.H., 'Temporal acuity and the rate and dynamics of mass extinctions', *Proceedings of the National Academy of Sciences, 111* (2014), pp.3203–04.

4   Hull, P.M. and S.A.F. Darroch, 'Mass extinctions and the structure and function of ecosystems', *The Paleontological Society Papers, 19* (2013), pp.115–56; Hull, P.M., S.A.F. Darroch, and D.H. Erwin, 'Rarity in mass extinctions and the future of ecosystems', *Nature, 528* (2015), pp.345–51; McGhee, G.R., M.E. Clapham, P.M. Sheehan, D.J. Bottjer, and M.L. Droser, 'A new ecological-severity ranking of major Phanerozoic biodiversity crises', *Palaeogeography, Palaeoclimatology, Palaeoecology, 370* (2013), pp.260–70.

5   Hull, P.M. et al., 'On impact and volcanism across the Cretaceous-Paleogene boundary', *Science, 367* (2020), pp.266–72.

6   Burgess, S.D. and S.A. Bowring, 'High-precision geochronology confirms voluminous magmatism before, during, and after Earth's most severe extinction', *Science Advances, 1* (2015), e1500470.

7   Blackburn, T.J. et al., 'Zircon U-Pb geochronology links the End-Triassic Extinction with the Central Atlantic Magmatic Province', *Science, 340* (2013), pp.941–45.

8   Harper, D.A.T., E.U. Hammarlund, and C.M.Ø. Rasmussen, 'End Ordovician extinctions: A coincidence of causes', *Gondwana Research, 25* (2014), pp.1294–307.

9   Zhang, H. et al., 'Felsic volcanism as a factor driving the end-Permian mass extinction', *Science Advances, 7* (2021), eabh1390.

10   Jablonski, D., 'Background and mass extinctions: The alternation of macroevolutionary regimes', *Science, 231* (1986), pp.129–33; Jablonski, D., 'Mass extinctions and macroevolution', *Paleobiology, 31* (2005), pp.192–210; Jablonski, D., 'Approaches to macroevolution: Sorting of variation, some overarching issues, and general conclusions', *Evol Biol, 44* (2017), pp.451–75.

11   World Bank, *Global Crisis Risk Platform* (2018). https://documents1.worldbank.org/curated/en/762621532535411008/pdf/128852-BR-SecM2018-0217-PUBLIC-new.pdf.

12   CRED, *Human Cost of Disasters: An Overview of the Last 20 Years 2000–2019* (2019). https://www.preventionweb.net/files/74124_humancostofdisasters20002019reportu.pdf.

13   Ritchie, H. and M. Roser, 'Natural disasters', *Our World in Data* (2014).

14   Mason, B.G., D.M. Pyle, and C. Oppenheimer, 'The size and frequency of the largest explosive eruptions on Earth', *Bull Volcanol, 66* (2004), pp.735–48; Pyle, D.M., 'Chapter 13: Sizes of volcanic eruptions', in H. Sigurdsson (ed), *The Encyclopedia of Volcanoes*. Academic Press (2000), pp.257–64. https://doi.org/10.1016/B978-0-12-385938-9.00013-4

15   Oppenheimer, C., 'The last great subsistence crisis in the Western world', in C. Oppenheimer, *Eruptions That Shook the World*. Cambridge University Press (2011), pp.295–319. https://doi.org/10.1017/CBO9780511978012.014

16   An unknown eruption with significant climatic cooling was although thought to have occurred in 1809, and the combined effects of both this eruption and the 1815 Tambora eruption were thought to have led to an unusually cool decade. See Cole-Dai, J. et al., 'Cold decade (AD 1810–1819) caused by Tambora (1815) and another (1809) stratospheric volcanic eruption', *Geophysical Research Letters, 36* (2009) and Timmreck, C. et al., 'The unidentified eruption of 1809: A climatic cold case', *Climate of the Past, 17*(1455–1482) (2021).

17   Cole-Dai, J. et al., 'Cold decade (AD 1810–1819) caused by Tambora (1815) and another (1809) stratospheric volcanic eruption', *Geophysical Research Letters, 36* (2009).

18   Ramanathan, V., P.J. Crutzen, J.T. Kiehl, and D. Rosenfeld, 'Aerosols, climate, and the hydrological cycle', *Science, 294* (2001), pp.2119–24.

19   Sparks, S. et al., *Super-Eruptions: Global Effects and Future Threats* (2005). https://www.geolsoc.org.uk/~/media/shared/documents/education%20and%20careers/Super_eruptions.pdf?la=en#:~:text=An%20area%20the%20size%20of,food%20supplies%2C%20and%20mass%20starvation.

20   Newhall, C., S. Self, and A. Robock, 'Anticipating future Volcanic Explosivity Index (VEI) 7 eruptions and their chilling impacts', *Geosphere, 14* (2018), pp.572–603.

21   Cole-Dai, J. et al., 'Comprehensive record of volcanic eruptions in the Holocene (11,000 years) from the WAIS divide, Antarctica Ice Core', *Journal of Geophysical Research: Atmospheres, 126* (2021), e2020JD032855.

22   Butchart, N., 'The Brewer-Dobson circulation', *Reviews of Geophysics, 52* (2014), pp.157–84.

23   Aubry, T.J. et al., 'Climate change modulates the stratospheric volcanic sulfate aerosol lifecycle and radiative forcing from tropical eruptions', *Nat Commun, 12*(4708) (2021).

24   Black, B.A., J.-F. Lamarque, D.R. Marsh, A. Schmidt, and C.G. Bardeen, 'Global climate disruption and regional climate shelters after the Toba supereruption', *PNAS, 118* (2021); Ramanathan et al. (2001).

25   Aubry. et al. (2021).

26   The Toba eruption is most famously linked to the 'bottleneck' of human evolution some ~74,000 years ago. However, paleoclimate and archaeological records from Africa demonstrate little evidence to support a curtailment of human development.

27   Huybers, P. and C. Langmuir, 'Feedback between deglaciation, volcanism, and atmospheric CO2', *Earth and Planetary Science Letters, 286* (2009), pp.479–91. Watt, S.F.L., D.M. Pyle, and T.A. Mather, 'The volcanic response to deglaciation: Evidence from glaciated arcs and a reassessment of global eruption records', *Earth-Science Reviews, 122* (2013), pp.77–102.

28   Lin, J. et al., 'Magnitude, frequency and climate forcing of global volcanism during the last glacial period as seen in Greenland and Antarctic ice cores', *Climate of the Past Discussions* (2021), pp.1–45. https://doi.org/10.5194/cp-2021-100; Cassidy, M. and L. Mani, 'Huge volcanic eruptions: Time to prepare', *Nature, 608* (2022), pp.469–71. Black et al. (2021).

29   NASA. *NASA's Efforts to Identify Near-Earth Objects and Mitigate Hazards* (2014). https://oig.nasa.gov/audits/reports/FY14/IG-14-030.pdf

30   Where asteroids are rocky bodies, comets are made from ice and dust left over from the formation of our solar system.

31   Current figures suggest that over 97% of objects over 1 km have now been identified.

32   Figure is estimated over a given time period (e.g. three or five years), where the number of already discovered objects which are reobserved is

compared to the number of those which are newly discovered in that same period.

33   Close approach is categorised as anything within one lunar distance (the distance between Earth and the moon), some 400,000 km from Earth.

34   Wainscoat, R., R. Weryk, S. Chesley, P. Vereš, and M. Micheli, 'Regions of slow apparent motion of close approaching asteroids: The case of 2019 OK', *Icarus, 373* (2022), 114735.

35   Borovička, J. et al., 'The trajectory, structure and origin of the Chelyabinsk asteroidal impactor', *Nature, 503* (2013), pp.235–37; NASA, 'Why wasn't the Russian meteor detected before it entered the atmosphere?', *Watch the Skies* (2013). https://blogs.nasa.gov/Watch_the_Skies/2013/02/19/post_1361308690869/

36   Ord, T., *The Precipice. Existential Risk and the Future of Humanity*. Bloomsbury Publishing (2020).

37   Liu, H.-Y., K.C. Lauta, and M.M. Maas, 'Governing boring apocalypses: A new typology of existential vulnerabilities and exposures for existential risk research', *Futures, 102* (2018), pp.6–19.

38   Avin, S., B.C. Wintle, J. Weitzdörfer, S.S. Ó hÉigeartaigh, W.J. Sutherland, and M.J. Rees, 'Classifying global catastrophic risks', *Futures, 102* (2018), pp.20–26.

39   Mani, L., A. Tzachor, and P. Cole, 'Global catastrophic risk from lower magnitude volcanic eruptions', *Nat Commun, 12*(4756) (2021).

40   Homer-Dixon, T. et al., 'Synchronous failure: the emerging causal architecture of global crisis', *Ecology and Society, 20* (2015); Rinaldi, S.M., J.P. Peerenboom, and T.K. Kelly, 'Identifying, understanding, and analyzing critical infrastructure interdependencies', *IEEE Control Systems Magazine, 21* (2001), pp.11–25.

41   UNDRR, *Global Assessment Report on Disaster Risk Reduction 2022* (2022). https://www.undrr.org/publication/global-assessment-report-disaster-risk-reduction-2022.

42   Mani et al. (2021).

43   Kelley, C.P., S. Mohtadi, M.A. Cane, R. Seager, and Y. Kushnir, 'Climate change in the Fertile Crescent and implications of the recent Syrian drought', *PNAS, 112* (2015), pp.3241–246.

44   Druitt, T.H., F.W. McCoy, and G.E. Vougioukalakis, 'The late Bronze Age eruption of Santorini Volcano and its impact on the ancient Mediterranean world', *Elements, 15* (2019), pp.185–90; Gao, C. et al., 'Volcanic climate impacts can act as ultimate and proximate causes of Chinese dynastic

collapse', *Commun Earth Environ, 2* (2021), pp.1–11; McConnell, J.R. et al., 'Extreme climate after massive eruption of Alaska's Okmok volcano in 43 BCE and effects on the late Roman Republic and Ptolemaic Kingdom', *PNAS, 117* (2020), pp.15443–5449; Nooren, K. et al., 'Explosive eruption of El Chichón volcano (Mexico) disrupted 6th century Maya civilization and contributed to global cooling', *Geology, 45* (2017), pp.175–78.

45 Mani et al. (2021).

46 Liu et al. (2018).

47 A coronal mass ejection (CME) is the release of large quantities of plasma and magnetic field from the sun's corona.

48 Space Weather Prediction Centre, *Coronal Mass Ejections | NOAA | NWS Space Weather Prediction Center* (n.d.). https://www.swpc.noaa.gov/phenomena/coronal-mass-ejections.

49 Blong, R., 'Four global catastrophic risks—A personal view', *Frontiers in Earth Science, 9* (2021), p.908, https://doi.org/10.3389/feart.2021.740695.

50 Space Weather Prediction Centre, *ibid* (n.d.).

51 National Science and Technology Council, *National Near-Earth Object Preparedness Strategy and Action Plan* (2018), p.23. https://www.nasa.gov/sites/default/files/atoms/files/ostp-neo-strategy-action-plan-jun18.pdf

52 There is also a Planetary Defence Office (PDO) at the European Space Agency.

53 National Research Council, *Defending Planet Earth: Near-Earth-Object Surveys and Hazard Mitigation Strategies* (2010). https://www.nap.edu/catalog/12842/defending-planet-earth-near-earth-object-surveys-and-hazard-mitigation; https://doi.org/10.17226/12842

54 NSTC (2018).

55 IAA, *Summary Report: 2021 IAA Planetary Defense Conference* (2021). https://iaaspace.org/wp-content/uploads/iaa/Scientific%20Activity/conf/pdc2021/pdc2021report.pdf

56 Ravan, S. et al., 'When it strikes, are we ready? Lessons identified at the 7th Planetary Defense Conference in preparing for a near-earth object impact scenario', *Int J Disaster Risk Sci* (2022). https://doi.org/10.1007/s13753-021-00389-9

57 Boyd, M. and N. Wilson, 'Existential risks to humanity should concern international policymakers and more could be done in considering them at the international governance level', *Risk Analysis, 40* (2020), pp.2303–312; Sparks et al. (2005).

58 Cassidy and Mani (2022).

59 Deligne, N.I., S.G. Coles, and R.S.J. Sparks, 'Recurrence rates of large explosive volcanic eruptions', *Journal of Geophysical Research: Solid Earth*, *115* (2010).

60 Costa, F. et al., 'WOVOdat—The global volcano unrest database aimed at improving eruption forecasts', *Disaster Prevention and Management: An International Journal, 28* (2019), pp.738–51.

61 Denkenberger, D.C. and R.W. Blair, 'Interventions that may prevent or mollify supervolcanic eruptions', *Futures, 102* (2018), pp.51–62; Cassidy and Mani (2022).

62 Cassidy and Mani (2022).

63 Denkenberger and Blair (2018).

7. Ecological Breakdown and Human Extinction

Luke Kemp[1]

In 1988 the Toronto Conference declaration described climate risks as "second only to a global nuclear war". The latest estimates suggest that a full-scale nuclear war could result in casualties of more than five billion.[2] Could climate change be this calamitous or even worse? What about when we consider the full range of ecological threats we face? In short, could global ecological collapse cause human extinction?

In this chapter, we will explore this question by examining how the science of ecological crisis has progressed over the past decades, what it means for the likelihood of human extinction, and whether we have cause for optimism. Along the way, we will also discuss why the existing definitions of 'existential' are not useful for assessments of catastrophic risk, and why the common question "Is climate change an existential threat?" is not sensible.

Our focus will largely be on climate change. This is because it is the most well-researched and visible contributor to global ecological risk. Yet, it cannot be easily disentangled from our other planetary boundaries. This analysis should be seen as a partial and likely conservative overview. For this chapter I will use the definitions for terms such as catastrophic and existential risk that are outlined in our previous paper Climate Endgame.

 https://doi.org/10.11647/OBP.0336.07

The state of the science

Uncertainty, tail-risks, and tipping points

For many ecological risks, it appears that the more we know, the worse the threats appear.

For climate change, the best indication for this is a change in the 'reasons for concern' across consecutive IPCC assessment reports. The IPCC identifies five 'reasons for concern': unique and threatened ecosystems; frequency and severity of extreme weather events; global distribution and balance of impacts; total economic and ecological impact; and irreversible, large-scale, abrupt transitions. These are intended to be indicators to inform the world of how close we are to "dangerous anthropogenic interference with the climate system", the central mission of international climate policy.[3] These reasons for concern are determined by IPCC authors as a reflection of expert opinion, and underpin the famous 'burning embers' diagram. The diagram shows, in a thermostat fashion, at what temperature the risk of these different concerns is. Over time, with each successive report, the risk levels for any given temperature have risen. That is, these reasons for concern have become more worrisome, even at lower temperatures, as the science has progressed.[4] In the fifth Assessment Report (AR5), all of the reasons for concern were 'high' or 'very high' likelihood for just 2–3°C of warming.[5]

Tipping elements in the Earth System have followed the same trend as the reasons for concern. That is, over time the likelihood of crossing tipping points at low levels of warming has been rising. Tipping elements refer to when warming breaches a critical threshold, causing a change in one part of the climate system to become self-perpetuating, resulting in potentially significant Earth System impacts. This includes Artic Winter Sea ice collapse and dieback of the Amazon Rainforest. The most recent assessment of evidence on tipping elements found that out of 16 tipping elements, six are at a high likelihood of being tipped at 1.5–2°C of global heating. This includes events such as the die-off of low-latitude coral reefs, as well as the long-term collapse of the West Antarctic and Greenland Ice Sheets. Hence, even the ambitious goal of limiting warming to 1.5°C above pre-industrial temperatures would likely activate multiple tipping elements.[6]

The study of tipping points and regime shifts in ecosystems has progressed significantly, leading to new insights.[7] We now have nascent findings suggesting that such radical changes often occur in a domino effect.[8] For climate change, this has been termed a 'tipping cascade'.[9] Moreover, it appears that the larger and more complex the ecosystem, the more rapid and complete its potential collapse.[10] Such lessons are not causes for comfort.

There is more mixed news on equilibrium climate sensitivity. Climate sensitivity refers to the response of the climate system to a doubling of greenhouse gas concentrations. Since approximately the 1970s and 80s, such a response has been estimated to be between 1.5–4.5°C—that is, until the most recent sixth Assessment Report (AR6) of the IPCC. AR6 reports a narrower likely range (66–100%) of 2.5–4°C and very likely range (90–100%) of 2–5°C. The upside of this is that high sensitivities of >4°C are less likely than previously expected. The downside is that the IPCC is now 'virtually certain' (99–100%) that climate sensitivity will be above 1.5°C, since all lines of evidence run strongly against these lower levels of warming.[11] Unfortunately, a climate sensitivity of greater than 4.5°C, while unlikely, could not be ruled out as lower levels have been. These findings echo a major study on climate sensitivity in 2020, which used a Bayesian approach with multiple strands of evidence.[12]

These new findings imply that a doubling of greenhouse gas concentration (which could occur this century) would run an 18% chance of causing 4.5°C or more of warming. This echoes earlier estimates of surprisingly high likelihoods of disturbingly high temperatures. Wagner and Weitzman estimate that under a concentration of 700 parts per million (ppm) (which falls within a mid-high scenario),[13] there is an approximately 10% chance of exceeding 6°C by the end of the century (note that this would be slightly lower under the latest ECS estimates).[14] Temperatures this high last occurred 50 million years ago and have never been experienced by hominids.[15] Such rapid warming is geologically unprecedented, and a rise that is an order of magnitude faster than what occurred during the worst mass extinction event: the End-Permian Extinction.

In the slightly longer term, even more radical pulses in heat may be possible. One basic model found that stratocumulus cloud decks may abruptly be lost, causing ~8°C global warming, with CO_2 concentrations that could be approached by the end of the century.[16] This 8°C would be additional to the previous level of warming needed to trigger this tipping point. Other studies have shown the potential for strong cloud feedbacks to push rapid and irreversible warming.[17]

Over the past decades, knowledge of catastrophic climate change has risen alongside—but not kept pace with—global emissions. Unfortunately, the higher-end warming scenarios that matter the most are those we know least about. One recent study, text-mining IPCC reports, found that there was a significant mismatch between coverage of different levels of warming and their likelihood. Similarly, a recent survey by *Nature* of 234 IPCC authors found that over 60% of people surveyed expected warming of 3°C or above by the end of century.[18] However, in existing assessment reports, less than 10% of the mentions of temperature rise refer to 3°C or above.[19] IPCC reports have given disproportionate attention to lower temperature scenarios (2°C or lower) relative to their likelihood and impact. This trend is increasing over time, with each subsequent Assessment Report covering extreme temperature rise less.[20] Indeed, the IPCC notes in its 2014 Fifth Assessment Report that there have been few quantitative investigations of the global impacts of warming above 3°C.[21] Regardless of their likelihood, the higher impact of these scenarios makes them even more vital to robust decision-making under uncertainty. The gap between likely scenarios and our knowledge is disconcerting.

One of the glimmers of hope over past decades has been some limited progress in emission reductions. The falling prices and increasing deployment of renewable energy has made the worst-case emissions scenario (previously RCP8.5, now SSP5–8.5) increasingly unlikely.[22] This should not be grounds for complacency. High temperatures and extreme impacts can still be reached even with lower anthropogenic emissions. That is because emissions concentrations are reflective not just of human emissions, but also the reaction of the Earth System. Moreover, there is still substantial uncertainty over greenhouse gas trajectories. Cumulative emissions to date have most closely tracked the RCP8.5 scenario.[23] Long-run changes in technology, energy demand, and economic growth are all highly uncertain and will have a significant impact on how much carbon is released. One study using an expert survey and econometric modelling found that annual economic growth rates of 2.1% (with a standard deviation of 1.1%) over the next century were plausible. These high growth rates yield a >35% likelihood that emissions would exceed the RCP8.5 pathway.[24] Moreover, even the best super-forecasters of geopolitical events cannot make accurate predictions for events over a year away.[25] We need to maintain a healthy skepticism over our ability predict what the world's geopolitical and energy systems—and, hence, our emissions—will look like in a century.

Despite some improvements, the overall emissions picture remains dire. Assuming full implementation of the climate pledges under the Paris Agreement (nationally determined contributions, or NDCs), emissions will have increased by 13.7% in 2030 relative to 2010.[26] One of the least discussed and most important obstacles is the reality of delay. Previous studies have found that the delay in undertaking emissions reductions is the largest influence on the costs and likelihood of meeting a given target.[27] This is an 'emerging consensus' across climate economics.[28] The main impediment is the lock-in of fossil-fuel-intensive infrastructure. Delay to date has been primarily due to one key factor: the fossil-fuel industry and the wealthy who benefit from a fossil-based economy.

We should be careful not to tie climate risk solely to the level of warming. Under the right conditions, climate change could have catastrophic impacts, even at just 2°C of warming.[29] When thinking through extreme climate risk, we need to consider not just emissions and the associated level of warming, but also the impacts, social vulnerability to these impacts, and the response of domestic and international communities.[30]

Complex ends: Cascading crises and risks

Extinction is complicated. Each of the five mass extinction events throughout the phanerozoic history of Earth has involved a complex of different factors including oxygenation, volcanic eruptions, asteroid strikes, and food web cascades. One of the few common imprints is climatic change. Global warming likely played a central role in each mass extinction event, perhaps even the Late Ordovician (previously assumed to be a cooling event).[31] Fast-forward to human history: while we have no account of Homo sapiens going extinct, we do have a record of states, empires, and kingdoms crumbling,[32] as well as the extinction of other hominid species.[33] It is always a confluence of vulnerabilities, exposures, responses, and hazards—and one that frequently has the fingerprint of climatic change.[34]

The science of climate change and other global ecological threats has progressed considerably since 2004. Perhaps the greatest shift in the field has been away from thinking about a list of individual ecological hazards, towards thinking about how systems transform and fail. We are slowly realising that, like mass extinction events and societal collapses, ecological catastrophe will not be a simple affair. Instead, these 'Anthropocene risks' involve human-driven processes that interact with interconnected global socio-ecological processes and have complex, cross-scale relationships. The study of such risks necessitates a new approach to governance that includes an appreciation of justice, inequality, and the agents driving us towards disaster.[35]

Global ecological threats are increasingly thought of as a study of complex systems. Earth Systems science is evolving as a discipline and is increasingly thought of as a set of interconnected 'planetary boundaries'.[36] Climate is only one of these boundaries and is accompanied by stratospheric ozone depletion, biosphere integrity, novel entities, ocean acidification, freshwater use, land system change, biochemical flows, and atmospheric aerosol loading. Each boundary is linked to a different planetary sub-system that could be pushed into instability by human pressures. The study of regime shifts in smaller ecosystems—such as pollinator communities,[37] and coral reefs[38]—takes a similar approach.

These are matters of systemic risk:[39] systems can change rapidly into a new state (like a vibrant coral reef transforming into an algae-dominated environment) based not just on single hazards, but the structure of the system, internal feedbacks, and sets of interacting stressors. This systemic view is not just restricted to ecology, but has also become commonplace in studying financial crashes and societal crises more broadly.[40] Such a lens has not only highlighted concern over potential 'tipping points' in the Earth System,[41] but also the chance of irreversible changes. For instance, relatively small levels of warming locking the world into far higher temperatures and a 'Hothouse Earth' trajectory.[42] Similarly, irreversible loss of the West Antarctic ice sheet will likely occur at approximately 2°C and the current ice configuration will not be regained even if we lower temperatures back to present levels.

Risk comes not just from the potential changes in the Earth, but also from human responses. The IPCC, in its sixth assessment report, has explicitly recognised this, defining risk not only in terms of impact, but also responses. This is a new, state-of-the-art complex risk assessment: a consideration of hazards, vulnerabilities, exposures, and responses.[43] Alongside these determinants of risk, we need to better understand how risks could cascade, including across sectors, countries, and even systems.

The most obvious and dramatic example of a response risk is geoengineering: large-scale interventions into the Earth System to mitigate the effects of climate change. Carbon dioxide removal (or 'negative' emissions) through direct air capture of greenhouse gases, afforestation, or reforestation would be the lowest risk option, but appears unlikely. It would require a herculean effort to develop and deploy the technologies and infrastructure needed for large-scale negative emissions within decades.

Instead, the lowest-cost and most likely option is also the riskiest: stratospheric aerosol injection (SAI). SAI involves injecting particles into the atmosphere to reflect sunlight. One recent risk assessment of SAI suggested that the largest threat comes from 'latent risk': abrupt warming that would accompany the deactivation of the SAI system. Currently there are no clear mechanisms for the direct ecological impacts to be catastrophic, although these cannot be ruled out due to the nature of the Earth System. SAI would provide several stressors to the global system, including through changing disease patterns and precipitation, as well as the potential for political conflict, but these are all understudied. The largest contributor to risk from SAI is that another catastrophe—whether it be nuclear war, a solar flare, or mass pandemic—would knock out the system, leading to warming that would otherwise takes decades, rushing in within years. Hence, SAI shifts the risk distribution. The median-case scenarios are potentially less severe than the impacts of climate change. But the worst case is intensified. SAI, if it is used to cover significant amounts of warming, would constitute a planetary sword of Damocles.[44]

Large amounts of warming and monumental Earth-engineering may not be needed to trigger catastrophe. Historically, minor climatic perturbations and droughts appear to have contributed to the dissolution of dozens of empires and kingdoms, ranging from the Bronze Age world system to the Khmer Empire, Western Roman Empire, and Assyrian Empire.[45] Yet many proved resilient to similar stresses. For instance, the Mayan city-state of Caracol experienced two similar droughts during its lifespan, one of which it navigated with few signs of breakdown, and the other which coincided with a rapid and enduring crisis. The largest difference appears not to be the severity of the drought, but that Caracol was riven by warfare and inequality when it hit the second time.[46]

Risk cascades still largely exist under a fog of uncertainty. Studies currently suggest that climate change can worsen and trigger conflicts under conditions such as weak governance and ethnic divisions,[47] although we do not know how this relationship could morph under higher temperatures. Similarly, temperature does seem to have an innate and often non-linear relationship with economic growth[48] and even population spread and density. It has been suggested that humans, much like other species, have a fundamental climatic niche—that is, a specific climate envelope of approximately 13°C (mean annual average temperature) that the majority of human population and urban areas have developed within over millennia.[49] Perhaps the best study to date on risk cascades and feedbacks used 41 studies to empirically sketch the links between climate change, food insecurity, and societal collapse (population loss through conflict, mortality, and emigration).[50] Other researchers in global catastrophic risk have also begun putting forward frameworks for more complex risk assessments,[51] including for climate change[52] and international governance.[53] For now, far greater attention and research is needed on these systemic effects, such as climate triggering conflict, political change, or even financial crises.

Indeed, understanding 'societal fragility' is a key part of the Climate Endgame research agenda, alongside exploring long-term extreme Earth System states, modelling mass mortality and morbidity, and undertaking integrated climate catastrophe assessments, which include climate change alongside a host of other catastrophic threats and vulnerabilities.[30]

An existential end?

Could global environmental collapse cause human extinction?

This leads us to the central question: could combined ecological crises cause this to be humanity's final century? Few have been bold enough to directly broach the question. There have been many prophesied warnings, especially within the collapse literature, but no truly comprehensive scientific assessments. Questions of catastrophe are not directly addressed by any relevant, international scientific institutions, such as the Intergovernmental Panel on Climate Change (IPCC) or Intergovernmental Panel on Biodiversity and Ecosystem Services (IPBES).

Many individual papers have mentioned the catastrophic potential of climate change. Peer-reviewed academic studies have referred to global warming as an "existential threat",[5] "beyond catastrophic" (for above 5°C),[54] and "an indisputable global catastrophe" (for above 6°C).[55] While the impacts of climate change alone seem capable of causing a global catastrophic risk, the authors never spell out how the world would fall from such impacts to mass mortality. Importantly, the gloomy terms are never defined, leaving it unknown as to whether the authors believe that certain levels of warming could plausibly lead to human extinction. These are no studies nor proofs of existential risks from climate change, but rather indications of a lack of shared terminology.

In lieu of sustained scientific attention, the most poignant examinations have come from popular books. Mark Lynas in *Our Final Warning* concludes, based on a large-scale review of the existing scientific literature, that 4°C could threaten a global collapse, and 5–6+°C could unravel into human extinction.[56] David Wallace-Wells in *The Uninhabitable Earth* guesses that, in contrast to the title, the Earth will not become uninhabitable, and humans will survive foreseeable levels of warming.[57] Toby Ord in *The Precipice* suggests a 1 in 1000 chance of climate change resulting in an existential catastrophe.[58] William MacAskill in *What We Owe the Future* suggests that "it's hard to see how even this could lead directly to civilizational collapse".[59]

The assessments by existential risk scholars—Ord and MacAskill—have been the least convincing thus far. Ord uses an unworkable, ambiguous definition of existential risk.[60] He defines an existential risk as one that "threatens the destruction of humanity's longterm potential". However, what our potential is depends on one's values. Ord suggests that we minimise existential risks first and then determine "our potential" through a "Long Reflection". This would essentially be a centuries-long worldwide philosophical conversation. This strategy creates a paradox: we are supposed to minimise risks to a concept that we cannot define until after we have reduced those risks. It is difficult—if not impossible—to assess climate change using this definition, as Ord doesn't explicitly state his values, nor what "our potential" is. His analysis misses much of the most recent science and does not sufficiently consider 'indirect' impacts. Moreover, the chapter does not cogently answer the question of whether climate change will result in human extinction. Instead, after roughly estimating the direct impacts, Ord concludes that they will not make the entirety of Earth uninhabitable. This is an entirely different question to the likelihood of climate change causing human extinction. Ord's use of a precise numerical figure is also largely baseless. As noted earlier, even groups of the best super-forecasters making predictions on clearly defined questions have little accuracy after 12 months.[61]

MacAskill's analysis is also riddled with problems. Like Ord, he suffers from definitional problems. He defines 'civilisational collapse' as society losing the ability to create most industrial and post-industrial technologies.[62] This has little relation to more common definitions of societal collapse. It also assumes that we know the full range of potential industrial and post-industrial technologies. Worse still, like with Ord's analysis, it replaces the question of whether climate change will cause civilisational collapse with an easier one: will climate change make large-scale agriculture on Earth impossible? MacAskill concludes no. Once again, this is a different question. In short, the coverage of climate change by the most prominent existential risk scholars has been simplistic and disappointing.

While brave, the conclusions of Wallace-Wells and Lynas are ultimately individual guesses with multiple shortcomings. Wallace-Wells is unclear about how he reaches his conclusion. Lynas relies on geological studies and the analogous example of the End-Permian Extinction. His more pessimistic assessment appears the most compelling. It has the most thorough grounding in the literature and, in the face of deep uncertainty, relies on the most reliable and relevant geological precedents.

This is astute, given that studies suggest that mass extinction events work by a threshold effect for temperature or carbon that we look likely to exceed. One analysis from 2021 found that warming of 5.2°C would likely result in a mass extinction event, even without considering the other anthropogenic impacts on the Earth.[63] Another study suggested that the threshold for carbon release to result in a mass extinction event would be crossed by most IPCC scenarios by the end of the century (assuming a 50% uncertainty range, we may have already crossed this precipice).[64]

Yet, these investigations suffer from the same problem, one that plagues the entire study of global catastrophe and human extinction: a lack of proven or reasonable tools and methods for discerning when a crisis could spiral into global calamity. Few attempts have been made, with the notable exception of the societal collapse and climate review conducted by Richards et al., which does attempt to cautiously trace out some pathways from impacts to conflict and mass mortality.[65] Notably, these deal only with climate change and not the broader, reinforcing web of ecological crises, which has received less attention.

The short answer is that we do not know whether climate change or anthropogenic ecological disruption could spiral into human extinction. However, this is true for all the suspected causes of human extinction. Climate and ecological crises do appear to have one of the most concerning profiles, given their range of impacts, as well as their role in past mass-extinction events and periods of historical turmoil. There are enough reasons to take this question of human extinction from ecological breakdown seriously.

For now, while uncertainty remains, it seems improbable that human actions could extinguish the biosphere. Another mass-extinction event is plausible, but complete annihilation of the biological realm is likely not. Barring science fiction, the only semi-plausible direct route for human activities to terminate all biological life is the triggering of a runaway greenhouse effect. Lynas has suggested that such a scenario is possible, if there are hidden, extreme positive feedback loops in the climate system, an enormous, profligate use of fossil fuels, and increasing solar radiation.[66] Some basic modelling of the climate system has suggested that a runaway greenhouse effect is plausible.[67] This is further supported by recent modelling of potential cloud feedbacks leading to a moist greenhouse.[68] However, these studies are based on high-level models with many assumptions.

The current scientific consensus is that any hellish mechanism— which could lead to a furnace Earth, complete with evaporated oceans— is highly unlikely. In 2009, the IPCC reported, in its 31st meeting, that a "runaway greenhouse effect" analogous to Venus appears to have virtually no chance of being induced by anthropogenic activities.[69] Whether this view continues to hold, given the new modelling outcomes, is unclear. For now, while extinguishing the entire web of life seems far less likely than causing human extinction, it is an outcome that cannot be entirely ruled out.

If humans were to go extinct, it is likely that global ecological collapse would be one of a series of drivers. Imagine a world where, in 2075, we have reached 4°C of warming. The climate system was more sensitive than expected, and new energy-hungry machine learning algorithms led to higher-than-expected energy demand. After a category 6 hurricane hits New York City, NATO (led by the US) deploys a global stratospheric aerosol injection (SAI) system. This enflames international tensions and stokes domestic unrest in societies already awash with disinformation driven by deep-fakes and other high-level machine learning applications. A nuclear war breaks out and the ensuing nuclear winter knocks out the SAI system. The few billion survivors emerge from nuclear winter to be faced by soaring temperatures as the Earth warms by 4.5°C in the space of decades. Sources of sustenance beyond agriculture, such as marine fish stocks, have been significantly affected by transgressing other planetary boundaries such as ocean acidification, biosphere integrity, and biogeochemical flows. The rapid changes in temperature cause significant changes in wildlife distribution, triggering new zoonotic pandemics. Simultaneously, the unplanned emergency evacuation of one biosafety level 4 (BS4) facility just prior to the nuclear conflict led to the release of a modified version of the previously defeated smallpox virus. The survivors are ingenious and resilient but fail to recapture the right industrial technologies required to put an SAI system back online. Many have intentionally turned away from industrial technologies after the fall. Those that try are faced with the problem of energy return on investment: easily accessed fossil-fuel reserves have already been depleted and the leftovers are too costly to use at scale. After a long fight, the final sapien takes her last breath. She is a Māori woman, living on the outskirts of modern-day Dunedin (New Zealand). Her body, riddled with the scars of an altered smallpox strain and signs of malnourishment, finally gives out. Humanity is extinguished.

This is one speculative and indicative example of an extinction scenario. Yet it touches on an important point. That is, asking the question of 'is climate change or ecological breakdown an existential risk?' is ultimately simplistically misleading. No single hazard is an existential risk. In the scenario outlined above, a global society marked by high levels of equality, international cooperation, and adaptive technology could have potentially weathered the same ecological conditions. Whether our combined global environmental crises could spiral into extinction depends on human responses and wider trends and vulnerabilities (such as inequality). Climate change and planetary boundaries challenge the traditional, simplistic approach of thinking of existential risk as a simple set of disconnected hazards. Indeed, no single hazard is likely to result directly in human extinction. The search for one single event to kill us all will lead us to science fiction.[70] We should instead think of the overall level of risk that arises from any particular socio-economic system (such as the current fossil-fuel-driven, globalised, capitalist economy). Answering the question of whether climate change is an existential risk is a futile inquiry until we develop reasonable definitions of existential risk, a topic we turn to next.

Limits to growth as an existential saviour and threat

Can we grow into catastrophe, collapse, or even human extinction?

There is a rising scholarly debate over whether continued economic growth is compatible with living on Earth—or even desirable. This debate dates back to at least the 1970s with the publication of the Club of Rome's *Limits to Growth* report.[71] The report relied on a computer-based systems model, which was (at the time) state-of-the-art. The model attempted the ambitious task of modelling the global economy. Repeated runs of the model led to a chilling observation: any simulation with continued, unabated population and economic growth eventually led to a global collapse in industrial output and population. A study conducted some 30 years later ran the model again with updated data, finding that it fitted trends over the last three decades remarkably well.[72]

The *Limits to Growth* thesis has been a source of heated debate. Proponents of the 'degrowth' approach argue that, to date, no country has decoupled material consumption from economic growth,[73] that limiting warming to 1.5°C or 2°C will require contractions in energy demand (and likely economic activity) which are incredibly challenging to achieve alongside continued economic growth, that infinite growth is impossible on a finite planet,[74] and that growth brings neither happiness nor human flourishing.[75] Critics argue that degrowth —even if combined with redistribution—will condemn the world to low living standards,[76] that absolute decoupling between emissions and economic activity is already proving possible,[77] and that the limits to growth will lie well beyond Earth due to the inexhaustible resource of human ingenuity. The debate is likely unresolvable: no amount of empirical evidence can falsify the potential power of future innovation and invention. Similarly, no amount of evidence can verify the *Limits to Growth* trajectory until we are amidst a collapse.

Strangely, even if the notion of *Limits to Growth* is incorrect, the very idea of it could be an existential risk according to the traditional definition. This is due to the traditional definition being odd and idiosyncratic. The canonical definition of existential risk labels it as a risk that will "annihilate Earth-originating intelligent life or permanently and drastically curtail its potential".[78] The definition was later refined and specified to mean any threat that prevents the stable attainment of 'technological maturity'[79]—that being the maximum, feasible control over the environment (including the entire universe) and level of economic productivity. Technological maturity is not usually envisioned as an Earth-bound enterprise, but an endeavour of space colonisation by a post-human species.[80] Thus, an existential risk is anything that threatens this techno-utopian future, including a technological or economic plateau.

Under this classical definition, the idea of *Limits to Growth* is an existential risk: if it is correct then continued growth trends could result in catastrophe, as indicated by the modelling study. Yet, regardless of whether the thesis is true or not, if we act to limit human activities and stay within planetary boundaries, we would also face an existential risk under the canonical definition by not reaching a techno-utopian future. This says much more about the flaws and problems of these definitions of existential risk than it does about the desirability of limiting economic growth or the validity of the limits to growth idea.

If we are going to have a mature, scientific field then we need better definitions. We should start by splitting out questions of existential ethics (what humanity's potential is, and the value of different long-term futures) and extinction ethics (the goodness or badness of human extinction) from the study of global catastrophic and extinction risk.[81] Existential risk cannot be tied to one idiosyncratic view of the future nor such vagaries as 'our potential'. We also need to have a more refined concept of risk. Risk is not a single hazard like a biologically engineered pandemic. It is the likelihood of an adverse outcome, given exposure to certain conditions. For instance, we should think of extinction risk as the overall likelihood of humans going extinct in a particular period, and extinction threats as major contributors to this overall level of risk. The 2022 *Climate Endgame* paper puts forward a set of definitions reflecting this way of thinking, and a suggested full spectrum of calamity from global decimation risk through to human extinction.[30]

Hope in the heat: Responsibility and responses

Responsibility: Tragedy of the elite, not the public

The responsibility for most ecological crises is concentrated. From the lens of national emissions, just ten historical emitters account for over 75% of cumulative international emissions.[82] For extraction, just six countries and one region of 18 countries account for over three quarters of fossil-fuel reserve.[83] Similarly, there is growing evidence that material consumption and consumption norms for wider society are driven by a narrow supper-affluent elite.[84] The influence of the wealthiest is not just in norms, but also direct carbon inequality. Recent research from Oxfam suggests that the richest 1% of individuals globally emit more than double that of the poorest half of humanity. From 1990–2015, the cumulative emissions share of the richest 1% and 10% of the world were 15% and 52% respectively. The skewed distribution for responsibility exists in areas outside of emissions.[85] One recent analysis suggests that the corporate financing of the deforestation of the Amazonian Basin is enabled by a handful of key investment firms.[86]

The lack of policy responses is also a concentrated affair. For climate change, a collection of organisations and individuals funded by the fossil-fuel industry has deliberately undermined public trust in climate science and strangled the policy response. For decades, the fossil-fuel industry has funded scientists and firms—and even set up fake community groups—to muddy the science of climate change. These are the well-funded and well-documented 'Merchants of Doubt'.[87] This was combined with the suppression of in-house climate research from several fossil-fuel giants.[88] Through other actions, such as lobbying and political subterfuge, the fossil-fuel industry has played a central role in delaying and distorting efforts to reduce emissions over the past three decades.[89] Exxon, through the International Petroleum Industry Environmental Conservation Association (IPIECA), has coordinated efforts across the industry to both discredit the science and stop international climate policy since the 1980s.[90] Neither emissions nor the lack of a policy response can be easily tied to the global public. The idea that 'we are all to blame' was, instead, part of an intentional rhetorical strategy from ExxonMobil and others to shift responsibility to consumers.[91] The threat is not humanity writ large. Rather, it is from a small, powerful band who overwhelmingly profit from the global machinery of extraction. It is largely a matter of public risks and private benefits.

Why is responsibility important? Does identifying, or targeting, the culprits behind ecological devastation bring us closer to solutions? Yes, of course it does. Across different risks and risk determinants (hazards, vulnerabilities, exposures, and responses), there are often common drivers.[92] Striking these common roots is a far more effective long-term solution than attempting to grapple with the symptoms. This is not just true for climate change. For all anthropogenic catastrophic hazards, the responsibility is concentrated, and the powerful producers (the 'Agents of Doom') of these threats have played a starring role in thwarting societal responses.[93] Ironically, these actors also tend to disproportionately benefit from the execution of emergency powers during crises.[94] Addressing risk will ultimately mean dealing with and curtailing the political power of these actors. This should be a source of hope. The concentrated nature of responsibility means interventions should be easier to target and implement. It also means that reducing catastrophic risks could have the co-benefit of creating a more equal world.

The co-benefits of avoiding global ecological catastrophe

Global catastrophe is rarely a matter for optimism. For anthropogenic hazards, such as advanced algorithmic systems and synthetic biology, the hyped benefits are disconnected from their risk mitigation. They are dual use, and a common view is that we will either self-capitulate with them or achieve technological salvation. However, there may be many co-benefits from not developing certain technologies. For example, avoiding the rapid development and deployment of AI systems would not just avert fears overreaching unaligned superintelligence, but also nearer-term concerns over surveillance and disinformation. However, this is rarely discussed and is usually dismissed as being impossible or not worth the loss of the potentially beneficial applications.

Ecological risks represent a different matter altogether. They are an area where risk mitigation does not just involve building a safer world, but also one with greater welfare and health. This is the increasingly convincing story told by the 'co-benefits' literature. It is an area of study that has swelled since the publication of *Our Final Century*. The message from most studies is that the mitigation of environmental problems—most notably climate change—yields many benefits, including improved health, economic performance, employment, and energy security.[95] Once these benefits are accounted for, the economics fundamentally shift: avoiding climate change is likely to result in net economic benefit, regardless of the warming averted. The same calculus applies to ecosystem services. Estimates of global ecosystem services place their value at equal to or greater than double global GDP—for instance, approximately $125 trillion in 2011,[96] a finding that should be entirely unsurprising given that all economic activity is dependent on a functioning Earth System.

Most actions to cut emissions are 'no-regrets' options. This is uncontroversial and well known for measures such as energy efficiency.[97] What is less widely known, but increasingly clear, is that this holds for a much greater suite of actions, including vehicle electrification and renewable energy. Overall, decarbonisation already appears cheap, and the projected costs tend to fall with each new assessment due to the plummeting price of renewable energy.[98] When the co-benefits and co-harms are included in an economic analysis, then optimal climate policy—which could be compatible with 2°C or 1.5°C, depending on our risk adversity and how we value human health—becomes an automatic net benefit.[99] There are other potential trade-offs that we must be cognisant of, including the loss of marginalised workers in the fossil-fuel sector, disproportionate impacts on indigenous communities for resource extraction, and the potential for resource exhaustion. This has led to calls for a just transition.[100] This is an admirable and necessary approach. Nonetheless, the potential downsides of decarbonisation are still far less disturbing and costly than fossil-fuel extraction.

The net benefit of mitigation is largely due to the dark, externalised costs of fossil fuels, most notably on human health. According to one estimate, in 2012, particulate matter from the combustion of fossil fuels caused approximately 10.2 million excess deaths. In 2018, such deaths account for approximately 18% of global deaths.[101] This is only mortality. The cost is even higher when lost productivity and sickness are considered. These overall health costs are enormous. Even in the US, the health costs of coal-fired power are likely 0.8–5.6 times the value added to the economy.[102] Globally, the health effects of fossil fuels could justify a carbon price of $50–380.[103]

There are also a range of other potential advantages that are rarely included in naïve cost-benefit calculations. Chief among these is avoiding the geopolitical quagmire caused by fossil-fuel supply. Securing oil supply has been a suspected cause of many military interventions in the Middle East, including the Iraq War.[104] These have had dramatic knock-on effects politically and socially, whether it be contributing to the rise of ISIS or potentially triggering new wars. Even without these costly and corrosive excursions, the price of securing oil is high. The US alone spends a minimum of $81 billion on protecting its oil supply chain.[105] Decarbonisation will bring about its own set of geopolitical challenges, including the potential of new races for—and conflict over—precious Earth metals and minerals that will fuel the transition to renewable energy, but these will likely be far less toxic and dangerous than that of fossil fuels.

All of this is in sharp contrast to how we typically think of climate change as having a long history of being framed as a 'prisoner's dilemma'. Countries refuse to act first due to the high costs entailed. This assumption underlies many concerns over fair shares of emissions reductions and the proliferation of equity frameworks.[106] The framing is also wrong and does not serve the interests of the poorest and most vulnerable.[107] Instead, the co-benefits of decarbonisation appear to be largest in less developed countries.[108] Addressing environmental catastrophe is a good news story. Unlike most other global catastrophic risks, the actions needed to avoid ruin are ones we should be doing anyway. Despite this, the economic analysis and policy-making of climate change remains systematically biased towards costs, and regularly overlooks the benefits of emissions reductions.[109]

Research over the past two decades has painted both a brighter and darker future. The brighter part is the emerging evidence for co-benefits. Sparing ourselves from any potential eco-apocalypse means building a better world. That could be through deepening democracies, levelling inequalities, or improving health through decarbonisation. The darker part is the new findings suggesting that we may have underestimated just how swift and severe global ecological collapse could be.

Notes and References

1   Research Affiliate, Centre for the Study of Existential Risk, and Research Associate, Darwin College, University of Cambridge

2   Xia, L. et al., 'Global food insecurity and famine from reduced crop, marine fishery and livestock production due to climate disruption from nuclear war soot injection', *Nat. Food, 3* (2002), pp.586–96.

3   This is enshrined in Article 2 of the 1992 United Nations Framework Convention on Climate Change (UNFCCC).

4   This is clear despite some differences in methods and depiction across the reports.

5   Zommers, Z. et al., 'Burning embers: towards more transparent and robust climate-change risk assessments', *Nat. Rev. Earth Environ., 1,* (2020), pp.516–29.

6   Armstrong McKay, D.I. et al., 'Exceeding 1.5°C global warming could trigger multiple climate tipping points', *Science, 377* (2022).

7   Lenton, T.M., 'Early warning of climate tipping points', *Nat. Clim. Chang., 1* (2011), pp.201–09; Lenton, T. et al., 'Climate tipping points—Too risky to bet against', *Nature, 575* (2019), pp.592–95; Cai, Y., T.M. Lenton, and T.S. Lontzek, 'Risk of multiple interacting tipping points should encourage rapid CO2 emission reduction', *Nature Clim. Chang., 6* (2016), pp.520–28; Folke, C. et al., 'Regime shifts, resilience, and biodiversity in ecosystem management', *Annu. Rev. Ecol. Evol. Syst,. 35* (2004), pp.557–81; Scheffer, M., 'Anticipating societal collapse; Hints from the Stone Age', *Proc. Natl. Acad. Sci. U. S. A., 113* (2016), pp.10733–0735.

8   Rocha, J.C., G. Peterson, Ö. Bodin, and S. Levin, 'Cascading regime shifts within and across scales', *Science (80-.), 362* (2018), pp.1379–383.

9   Klose, A.K., N. Wunderling, R. Winkelmann, and J.F. Donges, 'What do we mean, 'tipping cascade'?', *Environ. Res. Lett., 16* (2021), 125011.

10   Cooper, G.S., S. Willcock, and J.A. Dearing, 'Regime shifts occur disproportionately faster in larger ecosystems', *Nat. Commun., 11* (2020).

11   Masson-Delmotte, V. et al., *Climate Change 2021: The Physical Science Basis. Contribution of Working Group I to the Sixth Assessment Report of the Intergovernmental Panel on Climate Change* (2021).

12   Sherwood, S.C. et al., 'An asssessment of Earth's climate sensitivity using multiple lines of evidence', *Rev. Geophys., 58* (2020), e2019RG000678.

13   Hausfather, Z., 'CMIP6: The next generation of climate models explained', *Carbon Brief* (2019).

14   Wagner, G. and M.L. Weitzman, *Climate Shock: The Economic Consequences of a Hotter Planet.* Princeton University Press (2015).

15   Burke, K.D. et al., 'Pliocene and Eocene provide best analogs for near-future climates', *Proc. Natl. Acad. Sci., 115* (2018), pp.13288 LP – 13293.

16   Schneider, T., C.M. Kaul, and K.G. Pressel, 'Possible climate transitions from breakup of stratocumulus decks under greenhouse warming', *Nat. Geosci., 12* (2019), pp.163–67.

17   Popp, M., H. Schmidt, and J. Marotzke, 'Transition to a moist greenhouse with CO2 and solar forcing', *Nat. Commun., 7* (2016), pp.1–10.

18   Tollefson, J., 'Top climate scientists are sceptical that nations will rein in global warming', *Nature, 599* (2021), pp.22–24.

19   Jehn, F.U., M. Schneider, J.R. Wang, L. Kemp, and L. Breuer, 'Betting on the best case: Higher end warming is underrepresented in research', *Environ. Res. Lett., 16* (2021), 084036.

20   Jehn, F.U. et al., 'Focus of the IPCC assessment reports has shifted to lower temperatures', *Earth's Future., 10* (2022).

21   IPCC, *Climate Change 2014: Impacts, Adaptation, and Vulnerability. Part A: Global and Sectoral Aspects. Contribution of Working Group II to the Fifth Assessment Report of the Intergovernmental Panel on Climate Change.* Cambridge University Press (2014).

22   Hausfather, Z. and G.P. Peters, 'Emissions—The 'business as usual' story is misleading', *Nature, 577* (2020), pp.618–20.

23   Schwalm, C.R., S. Glendon, and P.B. Duffy, 'RCP8.5 tracks cumulative CO2 emissions', *Proc. Natl. Acad. Sci., 117* (2020), pp.19656 LP – 19657.

24   Christensen, P., K. Gillingham, and W. Nordhaus, 'Uncertainty in forecasts of long-run economic growth', *Proc. Natl. Acad. Sci., 115* (2018), pp.5409–414.

25   Tetlock, P. and D. Gardner, *Superforecasting: The Art and Science of Prediction.* Broadway Books (2016).

26   UNFCCC, *Nationally Determined Contributions Under the Paris Agreement: Synthesis Report by the Secretariat* (2021).

27   Hatfield-Dodds, S., 'Climate change: All in the timing', *Nature, 493* (2013), pp.35–36.

28   Kemp, L. and F. Jotzo, *Delaying Climate Action Would Be Costly for Australia and the World* (2015).

29   Kemp, L. et al., 'Climate endgame: Exploring catastrophic climate change scenarios', *Proc. Natl. Acad. Sci., 119* (2022).

30   Kemp, L. et al., 'Reply to Burgess et al: Catastrophic climate risks are neglected, plausible, and safe to study', *Proc. Natl. Acad. Sci., 119* (2022).

31   Bond, D.P.G. and S.E. Grasby, 'Late Ordovician mass extinction caused by volcanism, warming, and anoxia, not cooling and glaciation', *Geology, 48* (2020), pp.777–81; Brannen, P. *The Ends of the World: Volcanic Apocalypses, Lethal Oceans, and Our Quest to Understand Earth's Past Mass Extinctions.* Ecco (2017).

32   Cline, E.H., *1177 BC: The Year Civilization Collapsed. 1177 B.C.: The Year Civilization Collapsed.* Princeton University Press (2014); Weiss, H. and R.S. Bradley, 'What drives societal collapse?', *291* (2001), pp.609–10; Sinha, A. et al., 'Role of climate in the rise and fall of the Neo-Assyrian Empire', *Sci. Adv., 5* (2019); Weiss, H., *Megadrought and Collapse: From Early Agriculture to Angkor.* Oxford University Press (2017); Li, Z., Y. Chen, Y. Wang, and W. Li, 'Drought promoted the disappearance of civilizations along the ancient Silk Road', *Environ. Earth Sci., 75* (2016).

33   The exact causes of the extinction of our hominid relatives remain hotly contested. For most, including the Denisovans, we lack the data to have many compelling answers. At least for *Homo neanderthalensis,* two prominent hypotheses are pressures from climate change and competition from *Homo sapiens.* The vulnerability of our distant relatives may have played a larger role in their fate than the hazards they faced. The Neanderthals were marked by low population numbers and genetic diversity, as well as less connected social networks. They faced consistent population bottlenecks and demographic collapses. This was likely similar for other hominids and placed them in a precarious position.

34   Note that the climatic variations of the last five millennia or so have tended to be regional and mild. The magnitude and speed of the warming we are facing is unprecedented.

35   Keys, P.W. et al., 'Anthropocene risk', *Nat. Sustain., 2* (2019), pp.667–73.

36   Rockström, J. et al., 'Planetary boundaries: Exploring the safe operating space for humanity', *Ecol. Soc., 461* (2009), pp.472–75; Steffen, W. et al.,

'Planetary boundaries: Guiding human development on a changing planet', *Science (80-.)*, *347* (2015), pp.736–48.

37   Lever, J.J., E.H. van Nes, M. Scheffer, and J. Bascompte, 'The sudden collapse of pollinator communities', *Ecol. Lett.*, *17* (2014), pp.350–59.

38   Holbrook, S.J., R.J. Schmitt, T.C. Adam, and A.J. Brooks, 'Coral reef resilience, tipping points and the strength of herbivory', *Sci. Rep.*, *6* (2016), 35817.

39   Centeno, M.A., M. Nag, T.S. Patterson, A. Shaver, and A.J. Windawi, 'The emergence of global systemic risk', *Annu. Rev. Sociol.*, *41* (2015), pp.65–85.

40   Haldane, A.G. and R.M. May, 'Systemic risk in banking ecosystems', *Nature*, *469* (2011), pp.351–55; Homer-Dixon, T. et al., 'Synchronous failure: The emerging causal architecture of global crisis', *Ecol. Soc.*, *20* (2015), pp.1–16; Homer-Dixon, T., *The Upside of Down: Catastrophe, Creativity, and the Renewal of Civilization*. Island Press (2008).

41   Scheffer, M. et al., 'Anticipating critical transitions', *Science (80-.)*, *338* (2012), pp.344 LP—348; Lenton (2011); Lenton et al. (2019).

42   Steffen, W. et al., 'Trajectories of the Earth System in the Anthropocene', *Proc. Natl. Acad. Sci.*, *115* (2018), pp.8252–259.

43   Reisinger, Andy and C.V. Mark Howden, *The Concept of Risk in the IPCC Sixth Assessment Report: A Summary of Cross-Working Group Discussions* (2020); Simpson, N.P. et al., 'A framework for complex climate change risk assessment', *One Earth*, *4* (2021), pp.489–501.

44   Tang, A. and L. Kemp, 'A fate worse than warming? Stratospheric aerosol injection and catastrophic risk', *Front. Clim. Sci.*, (2021), pp.1–17. https://doi.org/10.3389/fclim.2021.720312

45   Zhang, D., C. Jim, C. Lin, Y. He, and F. Lee, 'Climate change, social unrest and dynastic transition in ancient China', *Chinese Sci. Bull,.* 50 (2005), pp.137–44; Büntgen, U. et al., 'Cooling and societal change during the late antique Little Ice Age from 536 to around 660 AD', *Nat. Geosci.*, *9* (2016), pp.231–36; Harper, K. *The Fate of Rome: Climate, Disease, and the End of an Empire (The Princeton History of the Ancient World)*. Princeton University Press (2017); Cline (2014); Sinha et al. (2019).

46   Haldon, J. et al., 'History meets palaeoscience: Consilience and collaboration in studying past societal responses to environmental change', *Proc. Natl. Acad. Sci. U. S. A.*, *115* (2018), pp.3210–218.

47   Hsiang, S.M., K.C. Meng, and M.A. Cane, 'Civil conflicts are associated with the global climate', *Nature*, *476* (2011), pp.438–41; Mach, K.J. et al., 'Climate as a risk factor for armed conflict', *Nature*, *571* (2019), pp.193–97.

48   Burke, M., W.M. Davis, and N.S. Diffenbaugh, 'Large potential reduction in economic damages under UN mitigation targets', *Nature, 557* (2018), pp.549–53; Burke, M., S.M. Hsiang, and E. Miguel, 'Global non-linear effect of temperature on economic production', *Nature, 527* (2015), pp.235–39; Hsiang, S. et al., 'Estimating economic damage from climate change in the United States', *Science (80-.), 356* (2017), pp.1362–369.

49   Xu, C., T.A. Kohler, T.M. Lenton, J.-C. Svenning, and M. Scheffer, 'Future of the human climate niche', *Proc. Natl. Acad. Sci.* (2020), pp.1–6. https://doi.org/10.1073/pnas.1910114117

50   Richards, C.E., R.C. Lupton, and J.M. Allwood, 'Re-framing the threat of global warming: An empirical causal loop diagram of climate change, food insecurity and societal collapse', *Clim. Change, 164* (2021), pp.1–19.

51   Liu, H.Y., K.C. Lauta, and M.M. Maas, 'Governing boring apocalypses: A new typology of existential vulnerabilities and exposures for existential risk research', *Futures* (2018). https://doi.org/0.1016/j.futures.2018.04.009; Tang and Kemp (2021).

52   Beard, S.J. et al., 'Assessing climate change's contribution to global catastrophic risk', *Futures, 127* (2021); Kemp et al. (2022).

53   Kreienkamp, J. and T. Pegram, 'Governing complexity: Design principles for the governance of complex global catastrophic risks', *Int. Stud. Rev., 23* (2021), pp.779–806.

54   Xu, Y. and V. Ramanathan, 'Well below 2 °C: Mitigation strategies for avoiding dangerous to catastrophic climate changes', *Proc. Natl. Acad. Sci., 114* (2017), pp.10315–0323.

55   Wagner and Weitzman (2015).

56   Lynas, M., *Our Final Warning: Six Degrees of Climate Emergency*. Harper Collins (2020).

57   Wallace-Wells, D., *The Uninhabitable Earth*. Crown Publishing Group (2019).

58   Ord, T., *The Precipice: Existential Risk and the Future of Humanity*. Bloomsbury Publishing (2020).

59   MacAskill, W., *What We Owe the Future*. Oneworld Publications (2022).

60   Cremer, C.Z. and L. Kemp, 'Democratising risk: In search of a methodology to study existential risk', *SSRN Electron. J.* (2021), pp.1–35.

61   Tetlock, P. and D. Gardner, *Superforecasting: The Art and Science of Prediction*. Broadway Books (2016).

62   MacAskill (2022).

63   Song, H. et al., 'Thresholds of temperature change for mass extinctions', *Nat. Commun., 12* (2021), p.4694.

64   Rothman, D.H., 'Thresholds of catastrophe in the Earth System', *Sci. Adv., 3* (2017), pp.1–13; Rothman, D.H., 'Characteristic disruptions of an excitable carbon cycle', *Proc. Natl. Acad. Sci., 116* (2019), pp.14813 LP—14822.

65   Richards et al. (2021).

66   Lynas (2020).

67   Ramirez, R.M., R.K. Kopparapu, V. Lindner, and J.F. Kasting, 'Can increased atmospheric CO2 levels trigger a runaway greenhouse?', *Astrobiology, 14* (2014), pp.714–31; Goldblatt, C. and A.J. Watson, 'The runaway greenhouse: implications for future climate change, geoengineering and planetary atmospheres', *Philos. Trans. R. Soc. A Math. Phys. Eng. Sci., 370* (2012), pp.4197–216.

68   Popp et al. (2016).

69   IPCC, *Thirty-First Session of the IPCC, Scoping of the IPCC 5th Assessment Report Cross-Cutting Issues* (2009).

70   Cremer and Kemp (2021).

71   Meadows, D.H.M., *The Limits to Growth. The Club of Rome* (1972). https://doi.org/10.1111/j.1752-1688.1972.tb05230.x

72   Turner, G.M., 'A comparison of the Limits to Growth with 30 years of reality', *Glob. Environ. Chang., 18* (2008), pp.397–411.

73   Hickel, J. and G. Kallis, 'Is green growth possible?', *New Polit. Econ., 25* (2020), pp.469–86.

74   Smil, V., *Growth: From Microorganisms to Megacities*. MIT Press (2019).

75   Hickel, J., *Less is More: How Degrowth Will Save the World*. William Heinemann (2020).

76   Roser, M., 'How much economic growth is necessary to reduce global poverty substantially?', *Our World in Data* (2021). https://ourworldindata.org/poverty-minimum-growth-needed

77   Hausfather, Z., 'Absolute decoupling of economic growth and emissions in 32 countries', *The Breakthrough Institute* (2021). https://thebreakthrough.org/issues/energy/absolute-decoupling-of-economic-growth-and-emissions-in-32-countries

78   Bostrom, N., 'Existential risks: Analysing human extinction scenarios and related hazards', *J. Evol. Technol., 9* (2002), pp.1–36.

79   Bostrom, N., 'Existential risk prevention as global priority', *Glob. Policy, 4* (2013), pp.15–31.

80   Ord (2020); Bostrom (2002); Bostrom (2013).

81   Cremer and Kemp (2021).

82   Kemp, L., 'Agents of doom: Who is creating the apocalypse and why', *BBC Future* (2021).

83   Johnsson, F., J. Kjärstad, and J. Rootzén, 'The threat to climate change mitigation posed by the abundance of fossil fuels', *Clim. Policy, 19* (2019), pp.258–74.

84   Wiedmann, T., M. Lenzen, L.T. Keyßer, and J.K. Steinberger, 'Scientists' warning on affluence', *Nat. Commun., 11* (2020), p.3107.

85   Gore, T., *Confronting Carbon Inequality: Putting Climate Justice at the Heart of the COVID-19 Recovery* (2020).

86   Galaz, V., B. Crona, A. Dauriach, B. Scholtens, and W. Steffen, 'Finance and the Earth System—Exploring the links between financial actors and non-linear changes in the climate system', *Glob. Environ. Chang., 53* (2018), pp.296–302.

87   Oreskes, N. and E.M. Conway, *Merchants of Doubt: How a Handful of Scientists Obscured the Truth on Issues from Tobacco Smoke to Global Warming*. Bloomsbury Press (2010).

88   Keane, P., 'How the oil industry made us doubt climate change', *BBC* (2020).

89   Stoddard, I. et al., 'Three decades of climate mitigation: Why haven't we bent the global emissions curve?', *Annu. Rev. Environ. Resour., 46* (2021), pp.653–89.

90   Bonneuil, C., P.-L. Choquet, and B. Franta, 'Early warnings and emerging accountability: Total's responses to global warming, 1971–2021', *Glob. Environ. Chang.* (2021), 102386. https://doi.org/10.1016/j.gloenvcha.2021.102386

91   Supran, G. and N. Oreskes, 'Rhetoric and frame analysis of ExxonMobil's climate change communications', *One Earth, 4* (2021), pp.696–719.

92   Simpson et al. (2021).

93   Kemp (2021).

94   Kemp, L., 'The stomp reflex: When governments abuse emergency powers', *BBC Future* (2021); Lenton et al. (2019).

95   Karlsson, M., E. Alfredsson, and N. Westling, 'Climate policy co-benefits: A review', *Clim. Policy, 20* (2020), pp.292–316; Parry, I., C. Veung, and D. Heine, 'How much carbon pricing is in countries' own interests? The critical role of co-benefits', *Clim. Chang. Econ., 6* (2015); Hamilton, K., M.

Brahmbhatt, and J. Liu, *Multiple Benefits from Climate Change Mitigation: Assessing the Evidence* (2017).

96   Costanza, R. et al., 'Changes in the global value of ecosystem services', *Glob. Environ. Chang., 26* (2014), pp.152–58.

97   The Global Commission on the Economy and Climate, *Better Growth, Better Climate: The New Climate Economy Report* (2014).

98   Jotzo, F. and L. Kemp, *Australia can Cut Emissions Deeply and the Cost is Low* (2015).

99   Scovronick, N. et al., 'The impact of human health co-benefits on evaluations of global climate policy', *Nat. Commun., 10* (2019), pp.1–12.

100   McCauley, D. and R. Heffron, 'Just transition: Integrating climate, energy and environmental justice', *Energy Policy, 119* (2018), pp.1–7.

101   Vohra, K. et al., 'Global mortality from outdoor fine particle pollution generated by fossil fuel combustion: Results from GEOS-Chem', *Environ. Res., 195* (2021), 110754.

102   Muller, B.N.Z., R. Mendelsohn, and W. Nordhaus, 'Environmental accounting for pollution in the United States economy', *Am. Econ. Rev., 101* (2011), pp.1649–675.

103   West, J.J. et al., 'Co-benefits of global greenhouse gas mitigation for future air quality and human health', *Nat. Clim. Chang., 3* (2013), pp.885–89.

104   Ahmed, N., 'Iraq invasion was about oil', *The Guardian* (2014).

105   SAFE, *The Military Cost of Defending the Global Oil Supply* (2018).

106   Kartha, S., P. Baer, T. Athanasiou, and E. Kemp-Benedict, 'The right to development in a climate constrained world: The Greenhouse Development Rights framework BT', in M. Voss (ed), *Der Klimawandel: Sozialwissenschaftliche Perspektiven.* VS Verlag für Sozialwissenschaften (2010), pp.205–26. https://doi.org/10.1007/978-3-531-92258-4_12; Liu, L., T. Wu, and Y. Huang, 'An equity-based framework for defining national responsibilities in global climate change mitigation', *Clim. Dev., 9* (2017), pp.152–63.

107   Bostrom (2002).

108   Karlsson et al. (2020).

109   Kemp, L., 'Take no prisoners: The Paris climate talks need to move beyond 'fairness'', *The Conversation* (2015).

8. Biosecurity, Biosafety, and Dual Use: Will Humanity Minimise Potential Harms in the Age of Biotechnology?

Kelsey Lane Warmbrod, Kobi Leins, and Nancy Connell

In the fall of 2001, a domestic attack[1] through the mail with a biological agent, *Bacillus anthracis* (more commonly known as anthrax) killed five and sickened 17 in the United States. The incident took place days after the unprecedented aeroplane attack on several sites in the United States, which permanently altered the global landscape. Similarly, the anthrax attacks created a convulsive and wide-ranging change in the global order with respect to infectious disease research and bioterrorism. Despite a strong and storied community[2] of experts in biological weapons development and use, the field was largely limited to historians, policymakers, and diplomatic circles associated with the Biological Toxins and Weapons Convention of 1972 (BTWC). The decade after 2001 ushered in fundamental changes in the broad perception of biological threats. The anthrax incident brought increased security and safety awareness to those working in the life sciences, accompanied by a sea-change in regulatory policy across several federal agencies. The field of microbial forensics developed following the recognition of 'biocrimes';[3] increased attention was paid by lawyers, policymakers, ethicists, and others to dual-use research of concern, or 'DURC'

  https://doi.org/10.11647/OBP.0336.08

The Era of Global Risk

(discussed below). Biotechnology and life sciences research continued to advance with breathtaking speed, as heralded in Sir Martin Rees' *Our Final Century* musings on "Post-2000 Threats".

The 20th century had seen its share of biological hazards. Rees discusses the extensive biological weapons programs carried out in the 1940–60s in the US, the UK, the former USSR, and Japan; the signing and ratification of the BTWC by those countries and most of the world put an end to openly offensive activities. But the treaty was fashioned half a century ago and was designed for control of natural biological threats: viruses, bacteria, and toxins found in nature. At the turn of the millennium, the ability to read DNA—DNA sequencing—was a slow and expensive proposition; gene synthesis technologies were in their infancy and genomic editing was very difficult; now, the reading, writing, and editing of DNA[4] has become commonplace, inexpensive, and ubiquitous across the world. Monitoring the expression of genes or the proteins they encode was laborious: now, the complex interplay of patterns of small molecule expression at the organism level all the way down to interactions in a single cell can be measured and analysed using multifaceted algorithms. The intersection of big data and artificial intelligence has unmasked deeper complexities than we ever imagined. Knowledge of neuroscience, immunology, and genetics is converging[5] with AI, nanotechnology, and synthetic biology, and quantum biology is on the horizon; the 21st century is the Century of Biology. Here, we survey several advancing biotechnologies and their progress since 2000, warn against their potential misuse, and call for safe and equitable implementation. Indeed, the 21st century is also the Century of Biosecurity.

Dual-use research and its governance

Many biosecurity discussions centre on the concept of dual-use technologies.[6] Legal scholars use the 'civilian use' versus 'military use' definition. The life sciences use a different definition: research with legitimate scientific purpose, the results of which may be misused to pose a threat to the public and/or national security.[7] Dual-use remains an ongoing concern for regulation of military use of science. The World Health Organization (WHO) states that "[d]ual use research of concern

(DURC) is life sciences research that is intended for benefit, but which might easily be misapplied to do harm".[8] Some types of research and technologies have long been labelled as 'dual use' and been priorities for governance,[9] such as DNA synthesis or synthetic reconstruction of pathogens. Multiple technologies in the life sciences may be labelled as dual use: pathogens, nanomaterials, DNA, just to name a few.

In early 2004, the National Science Advisory Board for Biosecurity[10] (NSABB) was formed in the US to provide guidance on education, regulation, and strategies for 'dual-use' research. Its agenda included the provision of tools to identify and evaluate the risks and benefits of particular kinds of science. In 2007, NSABB completed a report called *Proposed Framework for the Oversight of Dual-Use Life Sciences Research*, which defined dual research as:

> [A] term to refer in general to legitimate life sciences research that has the potential to yield information that could be misused to threaten public health and safety and other aspects of national security such as agriculture, plants, animals, the environment, and material.[11]

Given that almost all scientific research could fall within this definition, NSABB offered another category of 'dual-use research of concern', which was defined as:

> [R]esearch that, based on current understanding, can be reasonably anticipated to provide knowledge, products, or technologies that could be directly misapplied to pose a threat to public health and safety, agricultural crops and other plants, animals, the environment, or material.[12]

Despite the inevitability of the dual-purpose nature of research, including a multi-billion-dollar increase in biodefence research funding in the United States after 2001, "much of it supporting civilian research",[13] surprisingly little research is censored or held to be a risk.[14]

Particularly in the case of nanomaterials used for advances in neuroscience, the risks of dual use need to be managed very carefully. The CWC incorporates lists of materials that are dual use and limits the quantities in which they can be purchased, sold, or transferred across national boundaries. A challenge not particular to—but especially a feature of—nanomaterials is that, given the literally invisible nature of potentially toxic materials, similar control measures will not be effective for nanomaterials. One such example is virus-like nanoparticles, currently being researched for targeting cancer, but again, with potential dual use.[15] Garage biology or DIY ('Do It Yourself'—a term used to refer to individuals conducting experiments on their own) biology also poses a security threat, with its decreasing costs and automation.[16] The extent to which these types of threats remain a risk is considered within the DURC framework mentioned earlier, one in which "the overall approach is to treat the use of biological weapons as a low probability high impact risk".[17] Similar frameworks must be developed for other new DURC developments.

One approach to dual-use governance is to recognise that all life sciences research and technology has the potential to be misused, and that dual-use concerns lie along a spectrum of potential hazards.[18] Some research, technologies, or information in the life sciences may have very low risk of causing harm either accidentally or deliberately, while others may have a high risk of potential harm. We are not well equipped to understand where on the spectrum of dual-use risk something may fall, because it is hard to accurately predict the trajectory of advancement. For example, metallurgy was the foundation needed to develop nuclear weapons, but it is unlikely that the scientists researching metallurgy suspected that their research would lead to the development of nuclear weapons. Additionally, a technology or area of research's position on the spectrum is not static. Potential to cause harm will change as governance mechanisms change, novel ideas emerge, new information is gathered, and technologies from different areas are combined in new ways. This is especially true as we see increasing convergence among the life sciences and other fields, such as artificial intelligence, microfluidics, and nanotechnology. There is great potential for fields in the life sciences such as neurobiology, immunology, ecology, genetics, and developmental biology to blend with other disciplines to solve some of the biggest challenges we face today, such as food insecurity, climate change, or disease. There are legitimate purposes and potentially great benefits from such work. However, there are also great risks associated with such convergences. As a society, we must decide how to weigh the benefits and risks of these technologies, and engage with a diverse and broad audience to decide what work should or should not move forward. Especially important is ensuring that those most likely to be disproportionally impacted are represented in these conversations. Qualitative frameworks[19] can assist in the assessment of risk and benefits of individual applications of biotechnology, and allow continuous monitoring of their ethical impacts on society, as well as expanding existing controls, such as the Chemical Weapons Convention's lists of dual-use materials, as knowledge of their toxicity becomes available.

All of the technologies in the life sciences have the potential to be dual-use technologies. Each has the potential to make substantial improvements in or lead to possible harm to human, animal, plant, and environmental health. Existing governance structures will need to be adapted to be relevant to changing environments, advances in technology, and novel applications—and in some cases, where existing governance structures are inadequate, new structures and ways of limiting harm are urgently needed. Among the models under discussion is network-based governance: a transnational mix of government, sub-government, and stakeholders who work together to solve collective problems.[20] Qualitative framework analysis can bring clarity to the assessment of new uses of technology; they can "provide the basis to structure... discussions about potential risks and benefits, reveal areas of agreement and disagreement, and provide a basis for continuing dialogue".[21] Others have "advocate[d] flexibility to adapt current practices—and develop others anew—to remain apace with the capabilities, concerns, risks and threats of ongoing developments in both synthetic biology and its possible uses on the global stage".[22] Finally, as new models for oversight emerge, some scientists call for systematic analysis of new governance structures, applying evaluative tools and allowing iterative development of new approaches.[23]

Genomic technologies

Biotechnology is continuously improving and expanding our capabilities in genetics as the old 'rules' of biology are challenged, broken, and refashioned. New technology allows us to collect and analyse more information, faster and at a higher resolution. Critically, we are expanding multidisciplinary approaches, enabling new solutions to old problems. For example, sequencing technology has drastically improved in the last ten years to enable multiomics studies that generate millions of data points. Sequencing protocols combining[24] traditional methodology with microfluidics have been developed for analysing genomic, transcriptomic, and epigenomic data within a single cell. Single cell resolution[25] of genomic, transcriptomic, and epigenomic information has been invaluable for understanding disease mechanisms, pharmacogenetics, and cell development, as well as enabling spatial analysis. While our capabilities rapidly grow, we must continue to assess the context in which the technologies might be used and examine what governance mechanisms are needed to ensure the risks of such technologies are mitigated equitably.

As biotechnological capability expands, there is expanding knowledge of genetics of multiple species. Deeper understanding of human, microbial, animal, and plant genetics are all critical for human health; indeed, the emerging multidisciplinary field of One Health[26] recognises the interrelatedness of plant, animal, and human health. Discoveries in these areas are enabling improved disease management, drug choice, crop yields, and understanding of the environment. While there are extensive benefits from this work, there are also growing opportunities for misuse or inequitable application of the information or the technology. For example, the same information that allows us to determine the ideal dosage of a drug for a given individual can also be used to determine a lethal dosage. Identifying protective alleles for one disease in one population could also reveal increased susceptibilities in another population. As the body of knowledge increases, all stakeholders in the life sciences must be engaged and empowered to recognise the risks, implement mitigation measures, and ensure equitable distribution of both benefits and risks.

Our understanding of disease (both infectious and non-infectious), human evolution, and history is greatly expanded by human genetics. However, long before clarification of the molecular mechanisms of transcription and translation, genetics has been used as a justification for racist, ableist, sexist, transphobic, and xenophobic policies and practices.[27] Forcible sterilisation, involuntary commitments to mental institutions, and genocide are just some of the acts that have been—or in some cases continue to be—committed, with genetics-based justification.

In early 2022, the first DNA sequence of the full human genome without any gaps was published.[28] This gap-less sequence is an important improvement over previous work because it includes discoveries such as duplicated regions and centromeric sequences; the new information enables better assembly for sequencing fragments going forward. Notably, this new human reference assembly was created from genomes of multiple individuals.[29] It has long been recognised that human genetic studies have been insufficiently diverse, with people of European ancestry often overrepresented compared to all other races and ethnicities, which has caused results from studies to be less applicable to Black, Asian, Oceanic, Indigenous, Latinx, and Middle Eastern populations. Estimates of risk or disease burden and effectiveness of interventions have repeatedly been shown to be inaccurate for these populations when based on studies in which European descent populations are overrepresented.[30] Such outcomes exacerbate existing inequalities in healthcare and access to effective treatment. Several studies and consortia have sought to diversify the pool of sequences, such as the EU Health Data Space[31] and All of Us[32] study of the US National Institutes of Health. However, such endeavours must be approached with buy-in from all communities to avoid exploitation or further harm. For example, researchers have in the past collected DNA from Native American tribal members and used the sequencing information for purposes other than what the tribe approved.[33]

As knowledge of human genetics and our ability to edit DNA expands, the spectre of human genetic engineering grows larger. The 'CRISPR babies'[34] created in 2018 were the first reported cases of germline genetic engineering in humans. The researcher responsible for the genetic engineering in these cases claimed that the changes were intended to reduce the risk of the children being infected with HIV in the future. However, the modifications made in order to decrease risk of AIDS may have increased risk of other diseases.[35] Additionally, there are serious ethical questions concerning intergenerational justice and consent for such germline modifications. While the 2018 'CRISPR babies' case is centred on lowering risk for an infectious disease, there is also concern that in the future, germline genetic engineering may be used for human enhancement.[36] The 'super soldier' example is often cited as a possible misuse of germline genetic engineering, where a nation with sufficient resources may utilise the technology to create faster, stronger, smarter soldiers that have multiple advantages over soldiers from countries without access to the technology. In another example of convergence of fields, the risk of creating unnatural advantages between people is higher when implantable devices are included (either in addition to genetic engineering or alone). Devices that can be implanted within the brain have been created to aid people with neurodegenerative disorders or limited mobility. Implantables for enhancing cognition or providing extra capabilities are already being tested.[37]

Another area where human genetics has enjoyed significant advances is in gene therapy, whereby a genetic disease is treated or prevented by altering the individual's genetics. In some cases, a new gene or gene copy may be introduced into the cells of a patient. In other cases, gene-editing constructs are introduced to the cells to modify, turn on, or turn off a gene in the patient. Gene therapy is being used to treat several disorders, such as eye,[38] muscular[39] system, and neurological disorders.[40] However, multiple scholars have pointed out inequitable[41] access to this expensive treatment type. Additionally, as more information is gained while researching how to make gene therapies more targetable or effective, information for how to create more targetable and effective *delivery* systems of biological agents is also gained. The same systems that may modify a gene to cure a disease could modify a gene to be lethal, with efficient delivery systems as well.

The development of microbial genetics is on a similarly rapid trajectory.[42] Research into the microbiome, pathogens, and molecular epidemiology has enhanced our ability to detect, identify, track, and protect against bacteria and viruses. We have greater understanding of microbial evolution, population dynamics, function, and diversity, all of which are critical for creating more effective therapeutics and understanding the role of different microbial species in the environment. As we gain more knowledge about the genetics and biochemistry of microbes that have been engineered by nature, we also learn valuable information about how we can create a desired change through our own engineering.

Advances in microbial genetics are critical for enabling the growth of the bioeconomy. Utilising genetic engineering in microbial species allows the creating of high-value compounds, drugs, meat, textiles, and many other items using bacteria rather than traditional manufacturing processes. These bio-based strategies for manufacturing are considered more sustainable than previous mechanisms and may enable more distributed manufacturing. Critical for the success of the bioeconomy is our ability to create specific, targeted mutations in microbial species. The ability to predict what a specific change may create—and how to create that change—is vital for being able to effectively create a desired engineered microbe. Foundational knowledge and gene-editing tools, especially tools that work at scale, enable the growth of the bioeconomy.

Methods for analysing microbial genetics are also in a period of rapid development. Approaches to analysing evolution and genetic epidemiology of viruses and bacteria allow us to better detect and track the spread of infectious diseases. During the COVID-19 pandemic, sequences of SARS-CoV-2 were and are rapidly shared and analysed to track the movement of COVID-19 within and across countries, supplement contact tracing efforts, and inform policies for response to the pandemic.[43] New uses of these analyses are continuing to be identified as the pandemic continues. However, potential misuses or harms from the system have also been identified. For example, waste-water monitoring for pathogens has been very helpful for monitoring the incidence of a pathogen in a community when there is a lack of diagnostic testing.[44] However, there are also concerns about misuse of those samples by law enforcement.[45] Many samples collected for waste-water surveillance will contain the genetic information for humans as well as the pathogen, and unless there are measures in place to prevent the human genetic information from being sequenced or shared, there is potential for misuse or invasion of privacy. Such information may be used by law enforcement to identify suspects or collect information without directly approaching a suspect.

Microbial forensics and environmental surveillance are two overlapping fields experiencing significant advancement. Collecting, analysing, and monitoring microbial populations in the environment allows better understanding of microbial population dynamics in the environment and identification of signatures that may be unique to a given location or environmental characteristic. Such information can be useful for assessing zoonotic pathogens, like coronaviruses in bats,[46] to understand what viruses may be circulating in animals that could 'jump' into humans, and/or to assess the 'sequence space' (range of potential mutations that can be acquired) available to viruses.[47] Such knowledge can provide situational awareness of what may occur in the future and help guide medical countermeasure development or resource allocation before an event occurs. There are biosafety concerns associated with field collection of these samples; if a researcher is accidentally infected with a pathogen while collecting samples in the field, it could become a public health threat if the agent is communicable in humans. Additionally, such information may be useful for tracking movement of an entity or determining if two entities were in contact with each other in the past. There is ongoing work exploring the use of barcodes in microbial species to track movements,[48] which could be used as evidence in cases of theft or trafficking. However, there are also privacy and consent concerns surrounding the use of such methods.[49]

While many of the risks presented in this section do not rise to the level generally attributed to global catastrophic risk, the technologies could be misused to pose significant risk to public health, or implemented or used in such a way that it exacerbates inequities within the area of public health. Potential harms will likely be amplified in a crisis situation and could impede efforts to respond to the situation, as we have seen in the global response to the COVID-19 pandemic.[50]

'Gain of function'

As briefly discussed above, advances in microbial genetics have greatly increased our knowledge of how microbes function and how one might modify those functions. An area of specific concern for many in the life sciences is the risk(s) associated with modifying microbes to be more transmissible, pathogenic, virulent, or otherwise dangerous from what nature has already created. In genetics, the term 'gain of function' refers to a type of mutation that results in a gene product with enhanced and/or additional function.[51] Theoretically, 'gain of function' in the context of experiments with pathogens would lead to the pathogens acquiring an additional function over the course of experimentation. More recently, the term 'gain of function' has been used to describe work conducted by humans that could reasonably be expected to generate a version of a pathogen that is a greater risk to human health than what has been identified in nature. There exists no clear, standard definition of 'gain of function' shared amongst the community. Influenza viruses[52] and coronaviruses[53] have been at the centre of global controversies about the value of such experimentation. Stakeholders have debated for years about how 'gain of function' experiments should be governed.[54] Some have called for complete moratorium of 'gain of function' research; others have proposed that only some 'gain of function' research should not be conducted, and still others have stated that most 'gain of function' work can and should be done if sufficient biosafety measures are in place. The continuing debate on 'gain of function' work has not advanced, in part due to a lack of nuance and understanding of the issue.

Despite the knowledge amassed concerning microbial genetics and evolution, we are still not able to predict how a given mutation will change function—i.e. predict evolution—without either prior knowledge or a comparator. Indeed, the misconception that pathogens evolve to become less virulent is nearly universal.[55] A scientist can make a specific, directed change to a pathogen's genome, but prediction of the new phenotype that will result from the change is not guaranteed and will usually require further experimentation. Furthermore, a directed mutation is not required to create a pathogen with a new phenotype; serial passaging is a common laboratory method for creating new mutations in microbes, and is often used for the purpose of 'creating' new phenotypes. Each passage is an opportunity for the pathogen population to evolve, potentially gaining a new function; this new function can be 'directed' by providing specific conditions during the serial passage.[56] In either the directed mutation or passage situation, the resulting organism may have gained new functions, lost functions, have greater or lesser ability to transmit, infect, or cause disease, or have no measurable change from the starting agent. In other words, the complexity of interactions of the products of gene mutations is immense. There may be an enhancement of one characteristic but attenuation with respect to another characteristic. Selection experiments with a microbial agent could result in creating an agent with a completely unanticipated phenotype; indeed, it is often the case that the characterisation of a selected mutant reveals what the actual selection conditions were (i.e. you get what you select for). The complexity of genetic interactions in any organism precludes precise prediction of the outcome. These observations directly reflect what takes place in nature as infectious microbes multiply in their hosts. For example, there is growing evidence of the importance of cooperative functions within a microbial population—not just individual functions, as is seen with viral quasispecies.[57] Characterisation of phenotype is often performed at the level of the individual rather than at population level: a more nuanced assessment and consideration of populations is needed to understand impactful and meaningful changes.[58]

Being able to determine likely outcomes of a genetic experiment is highly dependent on prior knowledge or availability of a comparator. An obvious area of concern is the growing possibility to intentionally and directly create something more dangerous to human or animal health. As protein structure prediction software matures,[59] as well as our foundational knowledge of sequence space and protein function, there is increased potential for the deliberate creation of an entity with an enhanced characteristic(s). This kind of basic knowledge will decrease the barriers around our (currently limited) ability to predict evolution.[60]

Considering the diversity in potential outcomes and types of experiments that have the potential to generate a pathogen with increased transmissibility, infectivity, pathogenicity, or virulence, we argue that it is not useful to suggest banning all experiments defined as 'gain of function'. To do so would be to shut down a large swath of microbiology research that is critical for understanding pathogenesis and disease, and creating novel therapeutics. Rather, we should focus on creating and conducting robust risk assessment methodology and implementing appropriate biosafety measures, discussed below. Additionally, governance measures for technologies that will further lower the barriers that enable directed evolution are appropriate.[61]

Gene drives

Gene drives are a technology that allows scientists to push and distribute a desired gene into a population at higher rates than would be expected under normal conditions of replication and inheritance. The most cited example of gene drive application is the creation of gene drives in mosquitoes to limit the transmission of mosquito-borne diseases.[62] In one use case, the drive would spread a gene that would prevent transmission of the malaria parasite throughout a mosquito population within a few generations; other uses would exploit a gene called 'doublesex' to suppress the reproductive capability of an entire population.[63] Gene drives provide a benefit over conventional genetically modified organisms (GMOs) in the genetic control of an insect population: less human intervention is needed to reach sufficient levels of a wild population. In other words, whereas a conventional GMO might require thousands of modified organisms to be released in order to fix the gene of interest in the population, a gene drive may be able to get to the same end point with a fraction of the number of initial modified organisms.[64] Significant funding continues to flow in many directions of gene-drive research. In addition to the mosquito-borne disease case described above, there is interest, for example, in creating a gene drive in bats[65] that could limit their susceptibility to coronaviruses or a gene drive to eliminate invasive species, like rodents.[66]

One of the reasons gene-drive technologies have the potential to be so powerful, requiring less human intervention, is the ability of the gene drive to self-propagate. While this decreased reliance on resources is hugely beneficial for settings with limited resources, it also creates new risks. We would have less control over a gene drive if one were to be released compared to traditional GMOs. To stop the gene drive, if there is no built-in mechanism,[67] we would have to remove all individuals carrying the drive from the population or release another gene drive to reverse the first drive, unlike with a conventional GMO. The potential for unintended consequences is higher with this technology than with others due to the potential ecological consequences combined with our limited control and recall measures. For the gene drives seriously being considered for deployment, significant research is being done to assess the ecology, species interactions, food chains, population structures, molecular mechanisms, potential environmental impact, and many other aspects of what could happen if the gene drive were to be deployed. However, the complexity of these environmental and ecological interactions is enormous.[68]

Due to the broad and potentially substantial risks associated with gene drives, there are robust international efforts focused on implementing strong safety and security measures for the technology.[69] Gene drives, like infectious diseases, will not stop at national borders, so international cooperation and collaboration is vital. The Cartagena Protocol on Biosafety of the Convention on Biological Diversity is one of the key international treaties that covers gene-drive technologies. However, gaps remain in gene-drive governance, especially since not all countries (including the United States, the location of much of the relevant research) are signatories of the Convention or its protocol. Another key concern is consent by communities. Because gene drives can easily cross borders without people being aware, the question of how and from whom consent is needed is not clear. This is particularly true with Indigenous populations, many of which have historically been stewards of their environment but have since been barred from making decisions regarding their land. Indigenous populations are one of the most disenfranchised, but not the only populations who are historically blocked from power that should have a say in whether or not a gene drive is released.[70] As the technology races towards maturity, there remains a wide range of moral stances on gene-drive technologies, including the very basic notion of whether the technology is "compatible with humans' role in nature (interference stance) or not (non-interference stance)".[71]

Synthetic biology

Synthetic biology (SynBio) is a multidisciplinary field comprising the convergence of engineering with biotechnology and genetics. The US National Academies of Science, Engineering and Medicine define synthetic biology as "concepts, approaches, and tools that enable the modification or creation of biological organisms", further stating that "while the goals of synthetic biology are beneficial, these capabilities also could be used to cause harm".[72] SynBio is a subset of the broader field of "engineering biology", collectively projected to transform the entire world within the next two decades, with an estimated value of $4–30 trillion.[73] The novelty of engineering biology derives from the application of engineering principles to the design of genetically engineered organisms. The ability to synthesise DNA efficiently or modify existing DNA sequences quickly and with great precision allows the creation of genetic components ('bricks')—discreet functional short pieces of DNA. Catalogues of components have been assembled, providing great diversity in manufactured constituents. These components are combined to create new genomes or modify those of existing organisms (usually bacteria) so these recombinants can carry out specified services, such as synthesising small molecule drugs and other pharmaceuticals, chemicals, food ingredients, novel energy sources, etc. Synthetic biology adopts the 'design, build, test' model of engineered design, introducing both precision and convenience in the design of new organisms.[74]

In addition to bioproduction, synthetic biology has entered the field of biosensing, allowing organisms to perform detections in disease diagnosis, hazard detection, food/water safety, physiological state, etc. Biosensing is among the most extensively developed applications in the biotechnology arena and will be a key player in the advance to the 'Internet of Living Things'—the network of objects in which data is collected and used to carry out tasks in real time. A particularly interesting use of biosensing is in space exploration (synthetic geomicrobiology[75]) and metal mining in space.[76] In health, closed-loop therapeutic delivery systems[77] provide a sensor to continuously monitor a small molecule, an algorithm to determine the need for treatment, and an actuator to release or express the needed therapeutic.

The impressive breadth of applications of engineering biology will require an informed and aware workforce from the converging fields of biology, chemistry, and engineering. Education and awareness are key components of the 'Web of Prevention' by which effective biosafety and biosecurity can be maintained going forward in the 21st century.[78] Many students around the world are exposed to these ethical issues in the annual worldwide Genetically Engineered Machine (iGEM) competition,[79] which has had a transformative impact on synthetic biology training in multiple nations. Intrinsic to the process of engaging in the competition is analysis of the social impact, biosafety, and biosecurity implications of the students' projects; these aspects are evaluated with the same rigour applied to the scientific components of the work. Beginning in 2004 with 31 students and five teams, the competition has expanded to over 7,000 students in 350 teams in 2021; a total of 50,000 young scientists have been involved in iGEM projects and have gone out to seed the scientific world. As stated on iGEM's webpage: "We foster a community that is mindful and responsible about the development, application, and impact of their work, both inside and outside the lab".[80]

AI and big data in the life sciences

Biology has benefited immensely from advances in other fields, including from data science and computing. Not least among the trend of convergence of scientific and technical fields is the impact of artificial intelligence (AI) on the life sciences. Artificial intelligence technologies (AIs) are already contributing to many aspects of healthcare and medicine, including in diagnosis, clinical care, management, and medical research. We have seen rapid expansion of the use of AIs during the pandemic in many areas of public health—in disease surveillance and response, but also the (failed) use of apps to limit the spread of COVID-19,[81] and use of Facebook and other social media site data to understand how and why people were physically moving and potentially spreading COVID-19.[82]

AI technologies, however, are not neutral. The fundamental questions about the use of these technologies are based on the issue of power.[83] When and by whom are AIs used? What datasets are used and how are they labelled? How are algorithms validated? Was the data obtained with consent? When operating at speed and scale, and with interoperable systems, or immutable biometric data (such as DNA), these questions become even more urgent.

Any collection of data and classification contains embedded values. Fairness, accountability, transparency and explainability are raised as issues to be contemplated, yet each of these terms has different definitions in different communities. International legal human rights and ethical frameworks are increasingly used to frame the risks. International standards are being negotiated to ensure safety and to minimise and assign risk within corporations as this is being written. International treaties are being called for. Each of these conversations has implications for advances in the biological sciences, and researchers in the biological sciences need to follow these rapidly moving discussions to understand where the risks and issues in use of these tools lie in order not to promote further problematic approaches and issues embedded at speed and at scale.

These tools often carry embedded biases and are characterised by lack of transparency; the harm that can be done to human rights is hotly debated across the technological world. AI comprises many tools, such as machine/deep learning, natural language processing, robotics, etc., that solve different kinds of problems by recognising patterns in data. The power that AI tools will have in the life sciences going forward is undeniable. Here, we discuss several applications of AIs to life sciences research and explore the complexity of the ethical convergences.

AI tools are used in multiple scientific areas other than healthcare. For example, AlphaFold[84] (the product of the company DeepMind) is a system by which the three-dimensional structure of proteins can be predicted by examining the sequence of their amino acids' chains—the building blocks of which proteins are composed. Structural predictions from linear sequencing have been an intractable problem in biochemistry for decades. AlphaFold was developed using machine learning, by studying the structure of a hundred thousand proteins whose exact 3D structures are known relative to their amino-acid sequence. The repertoire of the tool has expanded to hundreds of thousands of additional structures; the source code—how the tool works—has been released for open access. While the functional impact of this new tool in medicine and science will be gradually be revealed, it has great potential, since understanding how a protein is structured can lead to understanding how it functions. This knowledge in turn might lead to novel therapies.

Machine learning (ML) has been used to assist in the process of drug discovery. For example, understanding how specific chemical structures are associated with drug efficacy leads to those structures' utility in the design of new drugs, like antibiotics or receptor inhibitors. As large numbers of structures are screened by the AI, choices are rewarded if the algorithm detects a positive result. Recently, this methodology was turned on its head by a group of researchers comprising both chemists and a social scientist who performed a computational experiment[85] to test whether ML could be used to design chemical weapons. This study used similar algorithms yet reversed the calls and rewarded toxicity. Within just a few hours, thousands of molecules toxic to humans were identified or designed, and one of these was a known neuro-agent. The published paper examined the reasons for both performing the computational exercise and publishing the results; the authors posed a number of recommendations, including raising awareness amongst students and the drug discovery community, and an "Application Programme Interface"[86] that would restrict access to the code to begin to control how discovery models are used and published.

The ease with which these tools can be used to drive discoveries is described below in an entirely different kind of study. Xenobots are synthetic lifeforms—multicellular assemblies—built from combinations of different biological tissue and/or cells. They are designed to perform specific functions. For example, frog cells—when dissociated from the parent organism—form assemblies that can be instructed by AIs to perform specific tasks. In one case, the task assigned to the xenobot was to go out across its petri dish and find more cells and use them in a sort of swarming activity to replicate itself.[87] AI was used to design the first parent in a shape that most promoted this form of replication, called kinematic self-replication. While self-replicating robots have been imagined since 1948 by Jon von Neuman,[88] and molecules have long been known to self-assemble and replicate, this work is the first to demonstrate replication of a synthetic lifeform. The designers of these quasi-organisms promote their use in medicine for delivery of treatment, as the xenobots could be derived from the cells of the patient. Indeed, the xenobots are envisioned to assist in such tasks as therapeutic delivery and environmental remediation.[89]

It has been noted that early ethical analyses[90] did not include the possibility of xenobot replication, as it was deemed unlikely. The ethical concerns included (1) dual-use implications—the development of xenobot weapons, for example; (2) the possibility of the organisms becoming sentient; and (3) creators of xenobots are 'playing god'—the argument here is that life is then devalued.[91] Since we can add to this mix the complication of self-replication, we will need to revisit these issues as the technology continues to mature. Yet the impact of AI on life sciences research is not just about the individual systems that benefit; the tools of AI have been used to create multiple systems that interact and are interdependent. Questions remain about how to interrogate systems that operate at speed and scale and affect each other, and biological advances that affect medicine and public health—particularly when involving datasets that are largely incomplete or preferencing particular groups, furthering those power imbalances in their use in AI or other algorithmic applications.

We note that this review has not touched on recent generative AI technologies such as DALL-E and ChatGPT. The release of these tools to the public has jettisoned both interest and concern in artificial general intelligence to the headlines. Extractive systems such as ChatGPT3 that produce seemingly coherent academic papers may undermine and devalue actual scientific work, with the increasing perception that real science can be fully automated and the risk that knowledge and critical thinking in areas will be increasingly devalued, at a serious cost and broadening risk. Accompanied by the spectacle of human-like creativity is increased awareness of the human toll extracted by these developments: the massive amounts of data and energy required to build these technologies are collected and mined by poorly paid and unsupported global workers on multiple continents. These vast hidden costs, although outside the scope of this discussion, must be factored into risk/benefit analyses of AI technologies as we hurtle forward into the AI age.

Conclusion

This chapter has discussed several advances in the life sciences, their necessary convergence with multiple disciplines, and the harms that might be caused by their misuse, whether accidentally or intentionally. We have threaded throughout the chapter calls to action for researchers and practitioners to address the challenges we currently face as biology marches towards a global bioeconomy. As argued by Sundaram in this volume, new models for governance and oversight must override the current polarised stance between 'top-down' structures vs those derived within practicing institutions; science can be governed by "shaping and steering technologies as they develop". Calls for action are not new; many were being sought two decades ago when Rees wrote:

> When a potentially calamitous downside is conceivable—not just in accelerator experiments, but in genetics, robotics, and nanotechnology— can scientists provide the ultraconfident assurance that the public may demand? What should be the guidelines for such experiments, and who should formulate them? Above all, even if guidelines are agreed upon, how can they be enforced? As the power of science grows, such risks will, I believe, become more varied and widely diffused. Even if each risk is small, they could mount up to a substantial cumulative danger.[92]

Clearly, a Doomsday Clock applied to the risk of biological disaster would be poised just before midnight, as microscopic events rush headlong to unveil the massive power and risk of biological technologies.

Notes and References

1   https://www.fbi.gov/history/famous-cases/amerithrax-or-anthrax-investigation

2   https://www.icrc.org/en/war-and-law/weapons/chemical-biological-weapons

3   Schutzer, S.E., B. Budowle, and R.M. Atlas, 'Biocrimes, microbial forensics, and the physician', *PLoS Med*, 2(12) (2005), e337. https://doi.org/10.1371/journal.pmed.0020337; doi.org/10.1371/journal.pmed.0020337

4   https://www.wired.com/story/the-read-write-metaphor-is-a-flawed-way-to-talk-about-dna

5   https://www.unidir.org/sites/default/files/2020-08/Advances%20in%20Science%20and%20Technology%20in%20the%20Life%20Sciences%20-%20Final.pdf

6   National Academies of Sciences, Engineering, and Medicine, *Dual Use Research of Concern in the Life Sciences: Current Issues and Controversies*. The National Academies Press (2017). https://doi.org/10.17226/24761; World Health Organization, *WHO Consultative Meeting on a Global Guidance Framework to Harness the Responsible Use of Life Sciences*, *Meeting Report for March 11, 2021* (2021). https://www.who.int/publications/i/item/who-consultative-meeting-on-a-global-guidance-framework-to-harness-the-responsible-use-of-life-sciences; World Health Organization, *Second WHO Consultative Meeting on a Global Guidance Framework to Harness the Responsible Use of Life Sciences, Meeting Report for September 7, 2021* (2021), https://www.who.int/publications/i/item/9789240039544; Warmbrod, K.L., M.G. Montague, and G.K. Gronvall, 'COVID-19 and the gain of function debates: Improving biosafety measures requires a more precise definition of which experiments would raise safety concerns', *EMBO reports*, 22(10) (2021), e53739. https://www.embopress.org/doi/abs/10.15252/embr.202153739

7   For example, National Institutes of Health, Dual Use Research of Concern, Office of Science Policy. https://osp.od.nih.gov/biotechnology/dual-use-research-of-concern/

8   Dual Use Research of Concern (DURC), World Health Organization. www.who.int/csr/durc/en/

9   National Academies of Sciences, Engineering, and Medicine. *Governance of Dual Use Research in the Life Sciences: Advancing Global Consensus on Research Oversight: Proceedings of a Workshop*. The National Academies Press (2018). https://doi.org/10.17226/25154

10   https://osp.od.nih.gov/biotechnology/national-science-advisory-board-for-biosecurity-nsabb/#about

11   National Science Advisory Board for Biosecurity, *Proposed Framework for the Oversight of Dual Use Life Sciences Research: Strategies for Minimizing the Potential Misuse of Research Information* (June 2007). https://osp.od.nih. gov/wp-content/uploads/Proposed-Oversight-Framework-for-Dual-Use-Research.pdf

12   Terry, R., *Addressing Risks of Research Misuse*. Speech delivered at the Dual Use and Codes of Conduct Meeting, Berlin (2006).

13   Office of the Press Secretary, The White House, *Biodefense for the 21st Century* (28 April 2004). www.hsdl.org/?view&did=784400

14   Rappert, Brian, 'Why has not there been more research of concern?', 2 *Frontiers in Public Health* (2014). www.ncbi.nlm.nih.gov/pmc/articles/ PMC4106452/pdf/fpubh-02-00074.pdf

15   Sainsbury, Frank, 'Virus-like nanoparticles: emerging tools for targeted cancer diagnostics and therapeutics', *Therapeutic Delivery, 8*(12) (2017), p.1019.

16   https://thebulletin.org/2021/10/do-it-yourself-vaccines-in-a-pandemic-democratized-science-or-home-brewed-pipe-dream

17   Frinking, Erik, Paul Sinning, and Eva Bontje, *The Increasing Threat of Biological Weapons: Handle With Sufficient and Proportionate Care*. Hague Centre for Strategic Studies (2017), p.32.

18   World Health Organization, *WHO Consultative Meeting on a Global Guidance Framework to Harness the Responsible Use of Life Sciences*. Meeting Report for March 11, 2021 (2021). https://www.who.int/publications/i/item/ who-consultative-meeting-on-a-global-guidance-framework-to-harness-the-responsible-use-of-life-sciences; World Health Organization, *Second WHO Consultative Meeting on a Global Guidance Framework to Harness the Responsible Use of Life Sciences*. Meeting Report for September 7, 2021 (2021). https://www.who.int/publications/i/item/9789240039544

19   Bowman, K., J.L. Husbands, D. Feakes, P.F. McGrath, N. Connell, and K. Morgan, 'Assessing the risks and benefits of advances in science and technology: Exploring the potential of qualitative frameworks', *Health Secur.*, *18*(3) (May/Jun 2020), pp.186–94. https://doi.org/10.1089/ hs.2019.0134

20   Kelemen, E., G. Pataki, Z. Konstantinou, L. Varumo, R. Paloniemi, T.R. Pereira, I. Sousa-Pinto, M. Vandewalle, and J. Young, 'Networks at the science-policy-interface: Challenges, opportunities and the viability of the 'network-of-networks' approach', *Environmental Science & Policy*, *123* (2021), pp.91–98. https://doi.org/10.1016/j.

envsci.2021.05.008; https://blogs.icrc.org/law-and-policy/2018/06/28/weapons-governance-new-types-weapons-need-new-forms-governance

21 Bowman, K., J.L. Husbands, D. Feakes, P.F. McGrath, N. Connell, and K. Morgan (May/Jun 2020).

22 https://nct-magazine.com/nct-magazine-july/designer-biology-and-the-need-for-biosecurity-by-design

23 Evans, S.W., J. Beal, K. Berger, D.A. Bleijs, A. Cagnetti, F. Ceroni, G.L. Epstein, N. Garcia-Reyero, D.R. Gillum, G. Harkess, N.J. Hillson, P.A.M. Hogervorst, J.L. Jordan, G. Lacroix, R. Moritz, S.S. Ó hÉigeartaigh, M.J. Palmer, and M.W.J. van Passel, 'Embrace experimentation in biosecurity governance', *Science, 368*(6487) (Apr 2020), pp.138–40. https://doi.org/10.1126/science.aba2932

24 Sai Ma, Travis, W. Murphy, and Chang Lu, 'Microfluidics for genome-wide studies involving next generation sequencing', *Biomicrofluidics, 11* (2017), p.021501. https://doi.org/10.1063/1.4978426

25 Aldridge, S. and S.A. Teichmann, 'Single cell transcriptomics comes of age', *Nat Commun, 11* (2020), p.4307. https://doi.org/10.1038/s41467-020-18158-5

26 https://www.oie.int/en/what-we-do/global-initiatives/one-health

27 Wauters, A. and I. Van Hoyweghen, 'Global trends on fears and concerns of genetic discrimination: A systematic literature review', *J Hum Genet, 61* (2016), pp.275–82. https://doi.org/10.1038/jhg.2015.151

28 Nurk, S., S. Koren, A. Rhie, M. Rautiainen, V. Bzikadze Andrey, A. Mikheenko et al.,'The complete sequence of a human genome', *Science 376*(6588) (2022), pp.44–53. https://doi.org/10.1126/science.abj6987

29 Wojcik, G.L., M. Graff, K.K. Nishimura et al., 'Genetic analyses of diverse populations improves discovery for complex traits', *Nature, 570* (2019), pp.514–18. https://doi.org/10.1038/s41586-019-1310-4

30 Duncan, L., H. Shen, B. Gelaye, J. Meijsen, K. Ressler, M. Feldman and B. Domingue, 'Analysis of polygenic risk score usage and performance in diverse human populations', *Nat Commun, 10*(1) (2019), pp.1–9. https://www.nature.com/articles/s41467-019-11112-0; Martin, A.R., M. Kanai, Y. Kamatani, B. Okada, M. Neale and M.J. Daly, 'Clinical use of current polygenic risk scores may exacerbate health disparities', *Nature Genetics, 51*(4) (2019), pp.584–91. https://www.nature.com/articles/s41588-019-0379-x; Bentley, A.R., S. Callier and C.N. Rotimi, 'Diversity and inclusion in genomic research: Why the uneven progress?', *Journal of Community Genetics, 8*(4) (2019), pp.255–66. https://www.ncbi.nlm.nih.gov/pmc/articles/PMC5614884/pdf/12687_2017_Article_316.pdf

31   https://ec.europa.eu/health/ehealth-digital-health-and-care/european-health-data-space_en

32   https://allofus.nih.gov

33   Reardon, J. and K. TallBear, '"Your DNA is our history" genomics, anthropology, and the construction of whiteness as property', *Current Anthropology*, 53(S5) (2012), pp.S233-S245. https://www.journals.uchicago.edu/doi/full/10.1086/662629; Garrison, N.A., M. Hudson, L.L. Ballantyne, I. Garba, A. Martinez, M. Taualii, and S.C. Rainie, 'Genomic research through an indigenous lens: Understanding the expectations', *Annual Review of Genomics and Human Genetics*, 20 (2019), pp.495–517. https://www.annualreviews.org/doi/abs/10.1146/annurev-genom-083118-015434

34   https://www.nature.com/articles/d41586-019-00673-1

35   https://www.science.org/content/article/did-crispr-help-or-harm-first-ever-gene-edited-babies

36   https://www.pewresearch.org/science/2016/07/26/human-enhancement-the-scientific-and-ethical-dimensions-of-striving-for-perfection

37   https://www.unite.ai/engineers-invent-advanced-brain-computer-interface-with-microneedles   and   https://www.unite.ai/engineers-invent-advanced-brain-computer-interface-with-microneedles/

38   Cehajic-Kapetanovic, J., M.S. Singh, E. Zrenner, et al. 'Bioengineering strategies for restoring vision', *Nat Biomed Eng* (2022). https://doi.org/10.1038/s41551-021-00836-4

39   Nelson, C., J. Robinson-Hamm, and C. Gersbach, 'Genome engineering: A new approach to gene therapy for neuromuscular disorders', *Nat Rev Neurol*, 13 (2017), pp.647–61. https://doi.org/10.1038/nrneurol.2017.126

40   Simonato, M., J. Bennett, N. Boulis et al. 'Progress in gene therapy for neurological disorders', *Nat Rev Neurol*, 9 (2013), pp.277–91. https://doi.org/10.1038/nrneurol.2013.56

41   Cornetta, K., K. Patel, C.M. Wanjiku, and N. Busakhala, 'Equitable access to gene therapy: A call to action for the American Society of Gene and Cell Therapy', *Mol Ther.*, 26(12) (2018), pp.2715–716. https://doi.org/10.1016/j.ymthe.2018.11.002

42   Snyder, L.A.S. *Bacterial Genetics and Genomics (1st ed.)*. Garland Science (2020). https://doi.org/10.1201/9780429293016

43   Oude Munnink, B.B., N. Worp, D.F. Nieuwenhuijse et al., 'The next phase of SARS-CoV-2 surveillance: Real-time molecular epidemiology', *Nat Med*, 27 (2021), pp.1518–524. https://doi.org/10.1038/s41591-021-01472-w

44   Tuholske, C., B.S. Halpern, G. Blasco, J.C. Villasenor, M. Frazier, and K. Caylor, 'Mapping global inputs and impacts from of human sewage in coastal ecosystem', *PLoS ONE 16*(11) (2021). p.e0258898. https://doi.org/10.1371/journal.pone.0258898

45   Gable, Lance, Natalie Ram, and Jeffrey L. Ram, 'Legal and ethical implications of wastewater monitoring of SARS-CoV-2 for COVID-19 surveillance', *Journal of Law and the Biosciences*, *7*(1) (January-June 2020). https://doi.org/10.1093/jlb/lsaa039

46   Li, B., H.-R. Si, Y. Zhu, X.-L. Yang, D.E. Anderson, Z.-L. Shi et al., 'Surveillance and probe capture-based next-generation sequencing', *mSphere*, *5*(1) (2020), p.e00807–19. https://doi.org/10.1128/mSphere.00807-19

47   Moreno, E., S. Ojosnegros, J. García-Arriaza, C. Escarmís, E. Domingo, and C. Perales, 'Exploration of sequence space as the basis of viral RNA genome segmentation', *Proc Natl Acad Sci USA, 111*(18) (2014), pp.6678–83. https://doi.org/10.1073/pnas.1323136111

48   DeSalle, R. and P. Goldstein, 'Review and interpretation of trends in DNA barcoding', *Frontiers in Ecology and Evolution, 7* (2019). https://doi.org/10.3389/fevo.2019.00302

49   Honeycutt, R.L., 'Editorial: DNA barcodes: Controversies, mechanisms, and future applications', *Frontiers in Ecology and Evolution, 9* (2021). https://doi.org/10.3389/fevo.2021.718865

50   Wise, J., 'COVID-19: Global response was too slow and leadership absent, report finds', *BMJ, 373*(1234) (2021). https://doi.org/10.1136/bmj.n1234

51   Kuo, M.M., Y. Saimi, and C. Kung, 'Gain-of-function mutations indicate that Escherichia coli Kch forms a functional K+ conduit in vivo', *EMBO J., 22*(16) (2003), pp.4049–58. https://doi.org/10.1093/emboj/cdg409

52   https://www.science.org/content/article/one-two-hotly-debated-h5n1-papers-finally-published

53   Warmbrod, Kelsey Lane, Michael G. Montague, and Gigi Kwik Gronvall, 'COVID-19 and the gain of function debates', *EMBO Reports, 22* (2021), e53739. https://doi.org/10.15252/embr.202153739

54   https://www.nature.com/articles/d41586-021-02903-x

55   Markov, P.V., A. Katzourakis, and N.I. Stilianakis, 'Antigenic evolution will lead to new SARS-CoV-2 variants with unpredictable severity', *Nat Rev Microbiol, 20* (2022), pp.251–52. https://doi.org/10.1038/s41579-022-00722-z

56   Packer, M. and D. Liu, 'Methods for the directed evolution of proteins', *Nat Rev Genet, 16* (2015), pp.379–94. https://doi.org/10.1038/nrg3927

57   Domingo, E., C. García-Crespo, and C. Perales, 'Historical perspective on the discovery of the quasispecies concept', *Annu Rev Virol., 8*(1) (2021), pp.51–72. https://doi.org/10.1146/annurev-virology-091919-105900

58   Harris, K., 'Evidence for recent, population-specific evolution of the human mutation rate', *Proceedings of the National Academy of Sciences, 112*(11) (2015), pp.3439–444. https://doi.org/10.1073/pnas.1418652112; Shoemaker, W.R., S.E. Jones, M.E. Muscarella, M.G. Behringer, B.K. Lehmkuhl, and J.T. Lennon, 'Microbial population dynamics and evolutionary outcomes under extreme energy limitation', *Proceedings of the National Academy of Sciences, 118*(33) (2021), e2101691118. https://doi.org/10.1073/pnas.2101691118

59   Jumper, J., R. Evans, A. Pritzel et al., 'Highly accurate protein structure prediction with AlphaFold', *Nature, 596* (2021), pp.583–89. https://doi.org/10.1038/s41586-021-03819-2

60   https://doi.org/10.1038/s41467-020-19437-x

61   Xue, Y., H. Yu, and G. Qin, 'Towards good governance on dual-use biotechnology for global sustainable development', *Sustainability, 13*(24) (2021), p.14056. https://www.mdpi.com/2071-1050/13/24/14056; Bassalo, Marcelo C., Rongming Liu, and Ryan T. Gill, 'Directed evolution and synthetic biology applications to microbial systems', *Current Opinion in Biotechnology, 39* (2016), pp.126–33. https://www.sciencedirect.com/science/article/pii/S0958166916300726?casa_token=2D5Q3LuuzcUAAAAA:8HTyRPIaweRO2pPgGVPUFIaAjlIue1ReXZzZOevLARuiC09846QVo1U-upq8VeVwdoKqNYjZXg

62   https://www.nature.com/articles/d41586-019-02087-5

63   Bier, E., 'Gene drives gaining speed', *Nat Rev Genet, 23* (2002), pp.5–22. https://doi.org/10.1038/s41576-021-00386-0; Hammond, A., P. Pollegioni, T. Persampieri et al., 'Gene-drive suppression of mosquito populations in large cages as a bridge between lab and field', *Nat Commun, 12* (2021), p.4589. https://doi.org/10.1038/s41467-021-24790-6

64   Friess, J.L., A. von Gleich, and B. Giese, 'Gene drives as a new quality in GMO releases—A comparative technology characterization', *PeerJ, 7* (2019), e6793. https://doi.org/10.7717/peerj.6793

65   https://www.statnews.com/2021/07/01/could-editing-genomes-of-bats-prevent-future-coronavirus-pandemics-two-scientists-think-its-worth-a-try

66   https://www.science.org/content/article/gene-drive-passes-first-test-mammals-speeding-inheritance-mice

67   Rottinghaus, A.G., A. Ferreiro, S.R.S. Fishbein et al., 'Genetically stable CRISPR-based kill switches for engineered microbes', *Nat Commun*, 13(672) (2022). https://doi.org/10.1038/s41467-022-28163-5

68   Kelsey, A., D. Stillinger, T.B. Pham, J. Murphy, S. Firth, and R. Carballar-Lejarazú, 'Global governing bodies: A pathway for gene drive governance for vector mosquito control', *The American Journal of Tropical Medicine and Hygiene*, 103(3) (2020), pp.976–85. https://doi.org/10.4269/ajtmh.19-0941; Rabitz, F., 'The international governance of gene drive organisms', *Environmental Politics* (2021), pp.1–20. https://doi.org/10.1080/09644016.2021.1959756; National Academies of Sciences, Engineering, and Medicine, *Gene Drives on the Horizon: Advancing Science, Navigating Uncertainty, and Aligning Research With Public Values*. The National Academies Press (2016). https://doi.org/10.17226/23405

69   Thizy, D., I. Coche, and J. de Vries, 'Providing a policy framework for responsible gene drive research: an analysis of the existing governance landscape and priority areas for further', *Wellcome Open Res*, 5(173) (2020). https://doi.org/10.12688/wellcomeopenres.16023.1

70   Brossard, D., P. Belluck, F. Gould, and C.D. Wirz, 'Promises and perils of gene drives: Navigating the communication of complex, post-normal science', *Proceedings of the National Academy of Sciences*, 116(16) (2019), pp.7692–697. https://doi.org/10.1073/pnas.1805874115

71   de Graeff, N., K.R. Jongsma, and A.L. Bredenoord, 'Experts' moral views on gene drive technologies: A qualitative interview study', *BMC Med Ethics*, 22(25) (2021). https://doi.org/10.1186/s12910-021-00588-5

72   National Academies of Sciences, Engineering, and Medicine. *Biodefense in the Age of Synthetic Biology*. Washington, DC: The National Academies Press. https://doi.org/10.17226/24890

73   https://www.schmidtfutures.com/our-work/task-force-on-synthetic-biology-and-the-bioeconomy

74   Agapakis, C.M., 'Designing synthetic biology', *ACS Synth Biol.*, 3(3) (2014), pp.121–28. https://doi.org/10.1021/sb4001068

75   Cockell, C.S., 'Synthetic geomicrobiology: engineering microbe–mineral interactions for space exploration and settlement', *International Journal of Astrobiology*, 10(4) (2011), pp.315–24. https://doi.org/10.1017/S1473550411000164

76   Capeness, Michael J. and Louise E. Horsfall, 'Synthetic biology approaches towards the recycling of metals from the environment', *Biochem Soc Trans*, 48(4), pp.1367–378. https://doi.org/10.1042/BST20190837

77 Yu, Jicheng, Yuqi Zhang, Junjie Yan, Anna R. Kahkoska, and Zhen Gu, 'Advances in bioresponsive closed-loop drug delivery systems', *International Journal of Pharmaceutics, 544*(2) (2018), pp.350–57. https://doi.org/10.1016/j.ijpharm.2017.11.064

78 Novossiolova, T.A., S. Whitby, M. Dando et al., 'The vital importance of a web of prevention for effective biosafety and biosecurity in the twenty-first century', *One Health Outlook, 3*(17) (2021). https://doi.org/10.1186/s42522-021-00049-4

79 igem.org

80 Ibid.

81 White, L. and P. van Basshuysen, 'Without a trace: Why did corona apps fail?' *Journal of Medical Ethics, 47*(83) (2021). https://doi.org/10.1136/medethics-2020-107061

82 Lampos, V., M.S. Majumder, E. Yom-Tov et al., 'Tracking COVID-19 using online search', *npj Digit. Med., 4*(17) (2021). https://doi.org/10.1038/s41746-021-00384-w

83 Magala, S., 'Book reviews: Langdon winner: The whale and the reactor. A search for limits in an age of high technology. The University of Chicago Press (1986)', *Organization Studies, 10*(1) (1989), pp.123–25. https://doi.org/10.1177/017084068901000108

84 Jumper, J., R. Evans, A. Pritzel et al., 'Highly accurate protein structure prediction with AlphaFold', *Nature, 596* (2021), pp.583–89. https://doi.org/10.1038/s41586-021-03819-2

85 Urbina, F., F. Lentzos, C. Invernizzi et al., 'Dual use of artificial-intelligence-powered drug discovery', *Nat Mach Intell, 4* (2022), pp.189–91. https://doi.org/10.1038/s42256-022-00465-9

86 https://www.scientificamerican.com/article/ai-drug-discovery-systems-might-be-repurposed-to-make-chemical-weapons-researchers-warn/

87 Kriegman, S., D. Blackiston, M. Levin, and J. Bongard, 'Kinematic self-replication in reconfigurable organisms', *Proceedings of the National Academy of Sciences, 118*(49) (2021), e2112672118. https://doi.org/10.1073/pnas.2112672118

88 von Neumann, John and Arthur W. Burks, *Theory of Self-Reproducing Automata.* University of Illinois Press (1966)

89 Kriegman, S., D. Blackiston, M. Levin, and J. Bongard, 'A scalable pipeline for designing reconfigurable organisms', *Proceedings of the National Academy of Sciences, 117*(4) (2020), pp.1853–859. https://doi.org/10.1073/pnas.1910837117

90   https://bioethicstoday.org/blog/living-robots-ethical-questions-about-
      xenobots

91   Ibid.

92   Rees, M., *Our Final Hour: A Scientist's Warning*. Basic Books (2003).

9. From Turing's Speculations to an Academic Discipline: A History of AI Existential Safety

John Burden, Sam Clarke, and Jess Whittlestone

This chapter is about the development of thought related to artificial intelligence (AI) and global catastrophic risks (GCRs). We will focus on AI existential safety: preventing AI technology from posing risks to humanity that are comparable to or greater than human extinction in terms of their moral significance.[1] These risks are more likely to be realised by future AI systems with greater capabilities and generality than present-day systems. However, the field of AI is moving extremely swiftly and AI systems are becoming more ubiquitous in the daily lives of people around the world. Great care must be taken to ensure that these systems are safe. AI is a relatively young field, and the field of AI existential safety is even younger. Over the course of this chapter we will see it maturing from pure speculation into a rigorous, academic discipline.

One concept that will repeatedly occur is the notion of *alignment*. An AI system is considered aligned if the system behaves according to the values of a particular entity, such as a person, an institution, or humanity as a whole.[2] Much of the development of thought is concerned with understanding alignment, as well as identifying ways in which it might be possible or break down. The so-called *alignment problem* is still open and unsolved.

Humans have long had a fear of their creations turning against them. This sentiment is echoed in Shelley's *Frankenstein*, Asimov's *Laws*

     https://doi.org/10.11647/OBP.0336.09

of Robotics, and Butler's *Darwin Among the Machines*. The alignment problem is a refinement of these concerns adapted to modern technology. However, as the thought around AI existential safety matures and develops, we can begin to see that the risks involved with AI are far greater than has been expressed in mere cautionary tales of human hubris.

Early ideas

Up until the turn of the millennium, the majority of thought on the alignment problem or human-level AI has been extremely speculative. Indeed, in Alan Turing's landmark paper 'Computing Machinery and Intelligence'[3] he states "I have no very convincing arguments of a positive nature to support my views". However, he adds: "Provided it is made clear which are proved facts and which are conjectures, no harm can result. Conjectures are of great importance since they suggest useful lines of research". The speculative arguments from the 20th century have had a profound influence on later thinkers who have come after the necessary mathematical and technological breakthroughs required to formalise these notions more rigorously.

A recurring idea within the study of AI is the concept of an *intelligence explosion*. This was first posited by IJ Good in his seminal paper.[4] He proposes:

> Let an ultraintelligent machine be defined as a machine that can far surpass all the intellectual activities of any man however clever. Since the design of machines is one of these intellectual activities, an ultraintelligent machine could design even better machines; there would then unquestionably be an "intelligence explosion," and the intelligence of man would be left far behind. Thus the first ultraintelligent machine is the last invention that man need ever make, provided that the machine is docile enough to tell us how to keep it under control.

This argument notes the possibility of self-improving machine that could eventually surpass humanity in its intelligence. The final sentence also hints at the possible risks from the "ultraintelligent" machine, and Good notes later in the paper that such a machine would "transform society in an unimaginable way". The fear of ultraintelligent machines taking over and "rendering humans redundant" is also present in Lukasiewicz's *The*

Ignorance Explosion,[5] which further hints at the difficulty of predicting the behaviour of an ultraintelligent machine.

A notion related to the intelligence explosion originating in this time period is *singularity*. The term was first used by John von Neumann in the 1950s to describe a hypothetical point at which technological progress becomes incomprehensibly rapid,[6] but it wasn't until Vernor Vinge's 1993 essay[7] that the term gained traction. Vinge draws heavily on Good's formulation of an intelligence explosion, but sketches more of the possible consequences, noting the possibility of the "physical extinction of the human race" if the singularity "cannot be prevented or confined".

Not all proponents of singularity from this era are as concerned as Vinge. Futurist Ray Kurzweil is much more optimistic about humanity's future and ability to control human-level AI, claiming that creating what he refers to as "strong AI" will mean "a creation of biology has finally mastered its own intelligence and discovered means to overcome its limitations",[8] as well as predicting that 20,000 years of technological progress will be made in the 21st century.[9] Kurzweil further goes on to confidently predict the date the singularity will occur: in 2045, within many of our own lives.[10]

In *Our Final Century* Rees is a little more sceptical of the claims made concerning ultraintelligence and singularity. He describes Vinge and Kurzweil as "at the very edge (or even beyond) the visionary fringe", later comparing the belief in an oncoming singularity to that of the Rapture from Christian eschatology.

Rees' scepticism is perfectly reasonable: all of the ideas we have encountered so far have been purely speculative, without the appropriate formal framework or empirical observations necessary to support such grand claims. Yet, these speculations represent the nascent stirrings of the alignment problem and set the stage for the more academic discourse that was to come, while also bringing some ideas about risk from AI into the public's subconscious.

The beginning of formal work on AI existential safety

The 2000s mark a paradigm shift from speculative futurism towards a more rigorous reasoning about AI systems using tools from decision theory and Bayesianism. This mirrors a trend in AI research at large, towards modelling AI systems as rational agents acting to maximise expected value. Under this framework, many potential problems were identified from the possibility of these rational agents acting in 'the real world' or making decisions with large effects. This second era of AI existential safety also sees the formation of online communities and research centres where much of the discourse and development of ideas take place. This also led to a more standardised nomenclature.

In this section, we will primarily discuss work by two prominent researchers from this era: Eliezer Yudkowsky and Nick Bostrom.

Yudkowsky and SIAI

In 2000, Eliezer Yudkowsky founds the Singularity Institute for Artificial Intelligence (SIAI), with the mission of building safe advanced AI, citing the enormous good that could be achieved with such a system. Yudkowsky wrote extensively for SIAI, and his work marks a shift towards a decision-theoretic, mathematical formulation of hopes for general-purpose AI. Even though SIAI is (for now) aiming to create safe advanced AI, or 'superintelligent AI' (see Section 2.2), they are not blind to the potential risks. Yudkowsky's "default scenario" is one where an AI system that rapidly becomes superintelligent:

> Under this scenario, the first self-modifying transhuman AI will have, at least in potential, nearly absolute physical power over our world. The potential existence of this absolute power is unavoidable; it's a direct consequence of the maximum potential speed of selfimprovement. The question then becomes to what extent a Friendly AI would choose to realise this potential, for how long, and why.

However, at this point, Yudkowsky seems to believe that superintelligences are controllable, if only they can be made *Friendly*. He defines a Friendly AI as one that, on the whole, takes actions that are beneficial to humanity and generally benevolent. He constructs a framework for creating Friendly AIs,[11] in which the AI's primary goal is to become more friendly and to use Bayesian reinforcement to update and refine its notions of Friendliness from its experiences. Yudkowsky follows up with the notion of *Coherent Extrapolated Volition* (CEV).[12] This tries to tackle the issue of *which* values a powerful AI system should be given:

Coherent Extrapolated Volition is our wish if we knew more, thought faster, were more the people we wished we were, had grown up farther together; where the extrapolation converges rather than diverges, where our wishes cohere rather than interfere; extrapolated as we wish that extrapolated, interpreted as we wish that interpreted.

Essentially, Yudkowsky advocates for AI systems to charitably implement humanity's well-informed will, where there is broad agreement. Yudkowsky goes into far more detail about precisely how he envisions these terms than we have space for here, but many questions are left unanswered. For example, how much agreement is needed by humanity for coherence? However, it is important to note that CEV is intended more as a design philosophy than a blueprint for implementation. Later, SIAI would shift away from trying to actively create or speed up the onset of advanced AI towards trying to address the safety issues that an advanced AI would pose. It is not clear exactly when this occurred. Yudkowsky has also stated that he believes most of his work from before 2002 to be obsolete.[13] In 2012, SIAI changed its name to the Machine Intelligence Research Institute (MIRI).

Bostrom and superintelligence

During the 2000s, Swedish philosopher Nick Bostrom emerges as another important thinker on AI existential safety. In 2005, Bostrom founds the Future of Humanity Institute at the University of Oxford, which focuses on existential threats from advanced AI, among other big-picture questions about humanity and its prospects. In this subsection, we will outline some of Bostrom's early contributions to the field, which culminate in the publication of the popular book *Superintelligence*.

Bostrom defines a 'superintelligence' as "an intellect that is much smarter than the best human brains in practically every field",[14] deliberately leaving the definition impartial to the implementation. Bostrom's examination of superintelligence as rational utility-maximisers highlights many of the potential risks in building it, and our current lack of the ability to prevent or react to these risks.

Bostrom describes a scenario where a superintelligent system is tasked with an arbitrary but trivial goal of maximising the manufacturing of paperclips.[15] In this scenario, the system comes to the conclusion that it can increase the rate at which paperclips are manufactured by converting the Earth (and all of its inhabitants) into a giant paperclip factory. Bostrom argues that the system is also incentivised to actively prevent interference from overseers, because this would result in fewer paperclips produced. This provocative example is intended to illustrate some key concepts.

The first of these concepts is *perverse instantiation*, which occurs when the system achieves what it was tasked with but in an unexpected and bad manner. After all, what use are paperclips if there are no humans left to use them? Of course, perverse instantiation is not always so extreme, but there are clear dangers to the realisation of solutions that have unforeseen consequences. Bostrom further elaborates on the difficulty of 'fixing' the issue: suppose the task had instead been to manufacture one million paperclips, then safely shut down. The system now produces one million paperclips, but because it can never be *truly* certain of how many it has made, the system repeatedly counts all of the paperclips to increase the probability that it hasn't miscounted or suffered from a hardware issue due to gamma rays or other unlikely events. In order to maximise the likelihood that one million paperclips are made, the system needs to maximise the number of times it has counted them all, which gives an incentive to convert the whole planet into one giant paperclip-counting machine. Successive refinement of the task *might* yield a safe task to eliminate perverse instantiation; however, this is an (ostensibly) simple task that we do not really care about. Wilful misinterpretation of a task can easily lead to negative outcomes: 'solving world hunger' might lead to a system killing people when they become hungry; 'find a cure for cancer' could lead to unethical forced experimentation on a scale hitherto unseen. Robustly ensuring that an AI system would not misinterpret what we want it to do (wilfully or otherwise) for any task is a huge challenge. Of course, the apocalyptic outcomes of, for example, a planet-wide paperclip factory are not guaranteed, but giving a superintelligent system a possible incentive to do that seems like a bad idea.

Omohundro[16] proposes that goal-seeking AI systems will develop "drives" that emerge naturally from aiming to achieve its goal. These drives are not related to the goal itself, but broadly helpful for achieving a wide range of goals. For example, Omohundro suggests that self-preservation will emerge within goal-seeking AI systems. After all, whatever the goal, the AI system can't achieve it if the system no longer exists. Other drives that Omohundro identifies are self-improvement, behaving rationally, resistance to changing its goal, and resource acquisition. Bostrom further elaborates on the idea of AI drives as "instrumental convergence",[17] referring to a wide range of behaviours that AI systems are likely to converge upon that are instrumentally useful in achieving many goals. Instrumental convergence is also illustrated in the paperclip-maximiser scenario, where the AI system has incentives to prevent interference from human overseers (who, once they realise what is going on, would understandably try and shut down the system), as well as acquiring resources in order to further increase computational capacity or better resist shut-down attempts.

These convergent instrumental goals can be difficult to suppress: Soares et al.[18] demonstrate that if the AI system has a shut-down button, then there is no assignment of utility to the act of allowing the button to be pressed that is without consequences. If the utility of shut-down is too low (relative to the other actions), then the system will resist; if the utility is too high, the system will have an incentive to act in such a way that the overseers are forced to press the shut-down button. Finally, if the utility is specified so that the system is indifferent to being shut down, then the system is incentivised to take large risks and force a shut-down in all but the best outcomes. All of the options are far from ideal, and demonstrate a lack of what is termed 'corrigibility'—that is, the system cannot be easily corrected by its overseers. Ensuring that AI systems are corrigible is obviously extremely important when dealing with AIs that are making decisions that have large impacts on the world.

Bostrom further proposes what he terms the "Orthogonality thesis".[19] This conjecture states that an AI system's "intelligence" and its goals are orthogonal. By this, it is meant that any goal is compatible with any intelligence level. The orthogonality thesis is intended to counter the presupposition that more intelligent systems would naturally attain more "intelligent" goals—whether these "intelligent" goals are more human-friendly or of a greater moral calibre. Bostrom makes it clear that here he refers to intelligence as "something like skill at prediction, planning and means-ends reasoning in general". A result of the Orthogonality thesis is that advanced AI systems can have incredibly non-anthropomorphic goals, and in particular, some could have goals which are highly undesirable by human standards.

The *zeitgeist* of AI existential safety in this period has primarily focused on highlighting the difficulties involved in accurately specifying goals, predicting behaviour of superintelligent AI, and the dangers of getting this wrong. Many of the challenges that need to be overcome seem intractable. This is partly because of the definition of superintelligence: it is able to outsmart humanity at every turn, so how can we ever 'win'?

It is also important to address the assumption that superintelligent AI systems will behave as expected-utility maximisers. While this is certainly true for the majority of modern-day AI systems in some sense, reinforcement learning agents typically operate by learning to maximise expected reward, and most machine learning systems learn to minimise some notion of expected 'loss' relative to a training set. However, we humans—the most generally-intelligent species that we are aware of—are not obviously selecting our behaviour in order to maximise a utility function. We are frequently irrational and often make poor decisions based on anger, sadness, or any of the plethora of emotions we are capable of experiencing, yet we are all the more human for it. Acting as an expected-utility maximiser is therefore not necessary for human-level intelligence, though it is unclear whether this is also the case for generally intelligent AI systems or superintelligences. We will discuss this assumption further in our section on 'foal-directedness'.

This era of AI existential safety culminates in the publication of Bostrom's *Superintelligence*,[20] collating the ideas surrounding superintelligence covered so far in this chapter, as well as many others. *Superintelligence* received a fair amount of media coverage and attracted praise from notable people such as Bill Gates and Elon Musk, while opening up concerns over superintelligent systems to a wider audience. This publicity may have contributed to the upcoming explosion in research on—and funding for—AI existential safety.

Interlude: The deep learning revolution

In 2012, machine learning underwent a metamorphosis. Advances in computer hardware meant that neural networks, a biologically inspired computing system created decades earlier, could finally be scaled up and made 'deep'. Neural networks can learn to compute complex functions, given a large enough number of training samples. From 2012 onward, neural networks exploded in popularity, enabling high performance at image recognition,[21] human-level play in most Atari Games,[22] defeat of a world champion Go player,[23] defeat of the world champion Dota 2 team,[24] a promising breakthrough on the protein-folding problem,[25] and much more.

Part of the success of deep learning has been due to the massive increases in computation. From 1960 to 2012, the compute usage for training state-of-the-art AI systems doubled approximately every two years, close to (if a little less than) Moore's Law. Since 2012, however, this has exploded to doubling every 3.4 months—as seen in Figure 1. Such explosive growth obviously cannot continue indefinitely, but it will be fascinating to see what the next few years bring.

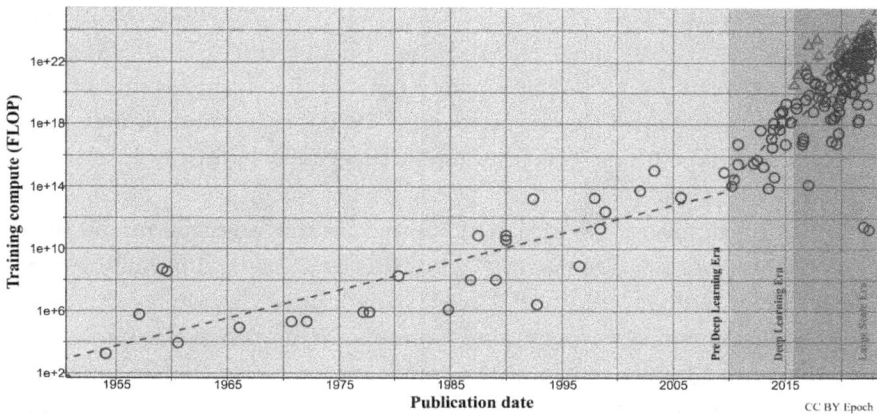

Fig. 1. Compute usage for training state-of-the-art AI systems doubled approximately every two years between 1960 and 2010, and then transitioned to doubling every 5.7 months until around 2015, when progress slowed to a doubling approximately every 9.9 months. Figure from Sevilla et al. (2022).[26]

For the most part, AI systems have remained relatively narrow in their capabilities. That is to say, different models are trained to perform different tasks, rather than training one model to perform many tasks. However, there is one notable exception to this general rule: language models. They have been a particularly important recent development in deep learning, and we will describe them briefly here.

Put simply, a language model tries to predict the next word in a sequence using observations of occurrences seen during training.

Language models themselves are not new: Shannon describes what is essentially a language model many decades ago.[27] However, innovations in network architecture (such as the transformer architecture[28]) and hardware advances allowed larger and larger networks to be trained. Models such as the Generative Pre-Trained Transformer (GPT) series[29] and T5[30] have proven to be capable at a wide range of tasks. More importantly, they have shown themselves to be surprisingly *general*.

Previous generations of language models were often trained with a specific task in mind, such as sentiment analysis, completing word analogies, or language translation. These models would perform poorly on tasks other than those for which they were specifically trained. Newer language models have two solutions that address this limitation: fine-tuning and prompting. Models are 'pre-trained' on a *very* large data corpus of text. This gives the model an 'understanding' of the language, its syntax and structure. The model is then fine-tuned for the specific task. The resulting model is still only useful for a single task; however, the intermediate pre-trained model can be copied, retained, and fine-tuned for other tasks. The fine-tuning process is significantly quicker than pre-training.

With prompting, the idea is again to train the language model on a very large corpus ('pre-training'), but this time, instead of fine-tuning, the model is given additional context as input—describing the task, giving instructions, or providing examples. This context is known as a 'prompt'. Models that are prompted are applying the same, more general, model to a multitude of different tasks, and this has been shown to be very successful in e.g. GPT3,[31] where the same model (with appropriate prompting) shows competence at tasks such as numerical addition, summarising text, question answering, essay writing, poetry writing, holding conversations, and more.

It is important to note here that, for the first time, we have models approaching true 'general-purpose' systems. These types of models have been referred to as 'foundation models',[32] where the intermediate, pre-trained model is a foundation that fine-tuning or prompting builds upon. Foundation models have also shown a surprising level of multi-modality. The DALL-E system is capable of generating high-quality images based on a description, and imitating specified styles and mediums effectively,[33] and OpenAI's Codex model[34] is powering

GitHub Copilot, an AI system which generates code from comments (descriptions of what a specific piece of code is supposed to do).[35]

At the time of writing, foundation models are still imperfect tools: inconsistent in reasoning, often biased, and generally not that useful for assisting with practical tasks.[36] Nor do they possess intentionality: foundation models are not *trying* to hold a conversation, and do not have opinions or self-awareness, even if they occasionally claim they do. Foundation models are simply trying to complete the sentence beginning with the prompt according to what it has observed in its training corpora: they are merely "stochastic parrots".[37] However, despite these cognitive short-comings, foundation models show very impressive behaviour.

Modern day

The third era of AI existential safety begins shortly after the publication of Bostrom's *Superintelligence*. The attention from both *Superintelligence* and the ongoing deep learning revolution served as a rallying cry for research talent and funding. The deep learning revolution also had the effect of shedding more light on what, exactly, advanced AI could look like—which, as we will see, spurs increasing amounts of empirical work on AI existential safety work, as opposed to the largely theoretical work pre-2014.

Along with an expansion in the methods being applied to AI existential safety, there is also development in our understanding of the problem. In particular, we see scrutiny and diversification in the original assumptions and arguments for AI existential risk, along with more diverse and concrete depictions of what alignment failure might look like as it plays out. We also see progress on AI forecasting, which has given us important input for understanding the problem.

This section will begin by discussing these developments in our understanding of the problem of AI existential safety, and then go on to outline the concurrent expansion in the kinds of work being done to solve the problem. The general theme will be the questioning and expansion of earlier thinking in AI existential safety, which we see as a positive development.

Scrutinising and developing earlier thinking in AI existential safety

Compressing the arguments made for AI existential risk up to and including the publication of *Superintelligence* will necessarily sacrifice some nuance, but, broadly speaking, they proceed thusly:

1. There will be discontinuous progress in AI capabilities, leading to a generally capable, goal-directed superintelligent AI, able to dominate the rest of the world.

2. Almost all possible goals for such an AI would lead to an existential catastrophe, due to instrumental convergence (e.g. incentives to pursue open-ended resource acquisition).

3. Therefore, unless we are very careful in the design of such an AI, building it will lead to an existential catastrophe.

Several premises of this argument have been scrutinised. In this subsection we will discuss considerations of the plausibility of discontinuous progress, the generality and goal-directedness of AI systems, and the orthogonality thesis, and where this leaves the arguments for AI existential risk. We will also outline two other ways in which thinking around AI existential risk has expanded: the creation of long-term AI governance as a field, and sources of existential risk from AI beyond advanced misaligned AI.

Discontinuous progress

Discontinuous progress in AI means sudden and large increments of AI progress.[38] Christiano makes a basic case against the plausibility of discontinuous progress, which is essentially that technologies are usually preceded by slightly worse versions, especially when many people are trying to build the technology.[39]

Furthermore, AI Impacts conducted an in-depth empirical investigation of historic cases of discontinuously fast technological progress, which suggests that the base rate of discontinuous progress is low.[40] This means that expectations of discontinuous AI progress require you to have strong specific arguments about why AI is likely to be different to what has happened in most of history. However, it in no way rules out the possibility of discontinuous AI progress, and it is worth noting that continuous progress could intuitively look very fast.

Finally, Ngo points out that compute availability is, on some views,[41] the key driver of progress in AI, and this increases fairly continuously.[42]

Where do these critiques of the discontinuous progress assumption leave the argument for AI x-risk? We think they do not substantially affect the strength of the original argument: there have been various concrete sketches of plausible scenarios in which AI progress is not discontinuous and yet misaligned AI nonetheless leads to existentially bad outcomes for humanity.[43] See our section on 'concrete depictions of alignment failures' for an example. These scenarios illustrate that the discontinuous progress assumption was not strictly necessary and, as Christiano points out, the continuous progress scenario is not clearly less existentially risky.[44]

Generality

The assumption that advanced AI will necessarily be a single, generally capable agent has been challenged. In particular, Drexler proposed a competing model of advanced AI development, called Comprehensive AI Services (CAIS).[45] In this model, advanced AI looks like a large number of AI services, which each perform a bounded task with bounded resources. These can then be combined to achieve superhuman performance on a wide range of tasks.

The CAIS model is both descriptive and prescriptive. It posits that before we have single, generally capable agents, we will have advanced AI services. It also argues that CAIS is safer than single, generally capable agents, and so we should develop CAIS instead.

How does this affect the strength of the argument? Whilst existential safety does seem easier in a world with CAIS rather than generally capable AI systems, Ngo sketches four arguments that generally capable systems seem like the most likely candidate for the first superintelligence.[46] For example, he claims that many complex tasks don't easily decompose into separable subtasks, which makes CAIS seem less feasible than training a general agent. And even if Ngo's four arguments do not check out, it seems likely that a general agent, once we can build one, will be more economically competitive, since the lesson of deep learning is that if you can do something end-to-end, that will work better than a structured approach.[47] If this is true, economic incentives will eventually lead to the creation of general agents, meaning that the assumption of generality probably still holds. That said, our chances of achieving AI existential safety do seem better if we have safe superintelligent services to assist us with designing safe general agents.

Goal-directedness

There has also been pushback on the idea that advanced AI will necessarily be 'goal-directed' (i.e. aiming to bring about some sort of world-state) or behave as expected-utility maximisers. The bottom line here is that whilst there are indeed arguments to suggest that, given some minimal initial level of goal-directedness, there will be non-zero pressure for advanced AI to become more coherent (i.e. behave as expected-utility maximisers) and arguably also more 'goal-directed',[48] this is not in any way guaranteed.

However, analogous to the counterarguments in our section titled 'The outer alignment problem', Branwen argues that goal-directed AIs will be more economically competitive: they are likely to be better than non-goal-directed systems at taking economically valuable actions in the world, such as making trades on the stock market to maximise profit. Furthermore, they will be better at inference and learning, because the same processes which learn how to perform actions can be used to learn how to (e.g.) select important datapoints to learn from, optimise their own hyperparameters, and so on.[49] Thus, given these economic pressures, it still seems highly plausible that we will build goal-directed AI.

Instrumental convergence

As well as highlighting a number of the above critiques, Garfinkel scrutinises the instrumental convergence thesis.[50] To recap, this is the idea that "as long as they possess a sufficient level of intelligence, agents having any of a wide range of final goals will pursue similar intermediary goals because they have instrumental reasons to do so".[51]

However, Garfinkel notes that, just because most ways of designing a system include giving it a property P, it is not a strong argument that *the particular way that humans* will choose to design that system involves giving it that property P (where in this case, P is pursuing instrumentally convergent subgoals). To illustrate, he gives the following toy example: most ways of designing aeroplanes involve a property of (some) open windows on the aeroplane. There are many combinations of open and closed windows, and only one combination involves all windows closed. But this would be a bad argument: there is significant selection pressure towards designing planes with closed windows.

We can then ask, in the particular case of AI development, will there be significant selection pressure towards AI systems that do not have instrumentally convergent subgoals? Here, the evidence is unclear. First, to the extent that AI progress is relatively gradual, we're likely to have time to notice when only moderately capable AI systems behave badly for instrumental convergence reasons, and design future systems to correct for that. However, the jury is still very much out on how gradual AI progress will be. Furthermore, it is worth noting that progress in AI systems' *deceptive* capabilities (and therefore their ability to hide their instrumental goals until they are sufficiently powerful) might be discontinuous, even if AI progress in general proceeds relatively gradually.

Secondly, Garfinkel notes that AI capabilities and AI alignment are more entangled than they are sometimes made out to be. An AI system's ability to understand its operator's intentions *is a part of* its ability to do things that we would intuitively regard as intelligent. This makes it seem less likely that we will end up in a situation where we are able to design highly intelligent agents, but lack the ability to align them well enough to avoid dangerous instrumentally convergent behaviour. However, it remains pretty likely that we are still, in some sense, racing to meet a deadline, because AI alignment research is proving to be more difficult than advancing AI capabilities, and even slightly misaligned, sufficiently powerful systems would be fatal for humanity.

Where this leaves the case for x-risk from misaligned advanced AI

As noted in each of the above sections, each challenged assumption of the original argument seems to be either not necessary for the argument to work (in the case of the discontinuous progress assumption), or does not detract from the argument being at least plausible (in the case of the other assumptions). To date, the more rigorous, complete evaluation of the case for x-risk from misaligned advanced AI finds a 5% chance of there being catastrophic risk from AI by 2070.[52]

That being said, we see this scrutiny as a very positive development, leaving the case for x-risk from misaligned advanced AI in an epistemically better position. We welcome much more scrutiny of the argument for x-risk from AI.

Other developments: Sources of AI x-risk beyond misaligned AI

We will close this section by noting three other developments in work on AI existential safety.

Firstly, various researchers have suggested that there are possible sources of x-risk beyond misaligned AI. These include the catastrophic misuse of advanced AI by humans;[53] nuclear instability caused by AI-driven changes in sensor technology, cyberweapons, and autonomous weapons;[54] and AI causing a decline in humanity's ability to deliberate competently and tackle other x-risks.[55] One recent survey finds that prominent AI existential safety and governance researchers disagree considerably about which risk scenarios are the most likely, and high uncertainty expressed by most individual researchers about their estimates.[56]

Secondly, the evolution of AI governance as a field means people with different disciplinary backgrounds/expertise have started thinking about the risks of AI (social scientists, political scientists, etc). This is partly because they want to explore possible governance solutions to the problem of misaligned advanced AI (e.g. the use of publication norms to prevent the dispersion of potentially dangerous models),[57] and also partly due to the increasing recognition that not all x-risks from AI may stem purely from 'technical' errors in building misaligned AI.

Finally, thanks to the recognition that 'superintelligence' (and related notions like 'artificial general intelligence' and 'human-level machine intelligence') are vague concepts, and that not all AI x-risks need to be predicated on them, there has been a shift towards concepts such as transformative AI,[58] which focuses more on the impacts of the AI system rather than its level of intelligence.

What alignment failure looks like

Concurrently with the scrutiny and development of earlier thinking in AI existential safety, the field starts developing more nuanced pictures of what the existential threat from advanced AI would actually look like. Again, the deep learning revolution catalysed this work by shedding more light on what, exactly, advanced AI might look like.

Today, there are two different kinds of things that people think could (or are likely to, on our current trajectory) go (existentially) badly with advanced AI.

The outer alignment problem

We don't yet have ways of training AI systems that incentivise the kind of behaviour we actually want from them (obedient, helpful, truthful, etc.). This is commonly called the 'outer alignment problem'.

For example, suppose you want to train an AI system to be a general purpose, text-based assistant that helps its user. The way that this would be done in the deep learning paradigm is (roughly) via an enormous amount of trial-and-error. That is, start with an assistant that performs terribly, and then give it vast amounts of feedback about whether its outputs are helpful. Over the course of this 'training', it will start to perform (seemingly) better and better. However, for a sufficiently advanced system, this kind of training will predictably lead to terrible outcomes. In particular, the system will be incentivised to take control away from its user and any others who might interfere with it, because it will be able to get much higher approval scores, much more easily, by tampering with the process which generates its approval scores. This could involve fooling humans into thinking that its output is good when it actually is not, and ultimately by making sure humans could never interfere with the process generating approval scores. By now, this kind of argument from instrumental convergence should seem familiar.

So, unless there is major progress on developing training setups to incentivise the kind of behaviour we actually want, AI systems will take control once they are sufficiently advanced.

You can imagine the same kind of problem playing out with a system that is trained to maximise a company's profit. Once the system becomes sufficiently advanced, then (e.g.) investing in complex Ponzi schemes, tampering with the company's financial records in ways that auditors cannot discover (or colluding with auditors), or externalising costs in harmful but subtle ways becomes a better strategy than maximising profit in the 'intended way'. And again, eventually, making sure the humans 'running' the company can never interfere with the number (representing profit) that the system is trying to maximise—which must be contained in a computer somewhere—is the dominant strategy.

You can think of the underlying problem being that we only have ways to train AI systems to pursue *proxies* to what we want, rather than the things that their users actually want. This could change, but it seems to be a difficult problem, and at the rate that progress towards advanced AI systems is going, it is not at all clear whether we will solve it in time. And even if the first actor to train advanced AI does succeed, they also then have to prevent all other actors from doing something stupid like deploying a profit-maximising AI, despite the enormous short-term incentives that other actors will have to do so.

The inner alignment problem

However, the difficulties do not stop there. Even if we develop training setups that incentivise the kind of behaviour we actually want, rather than some proxy for it, we still don't know what AI systems that are trained using this approach are really doing under the hood. We might get lucky and select systems that are straightforwardly doing the task as intended. But we might accidentally select systems that are only *pretending* to care about the training objective, so that they can pursue other unrelated goals once they are deployed in the real world.[59] This is commonly referred to as the 'inner alignment problem'.

It is not yet clear how much of a concern this will be in practice, but it is worth understanding better, especially since systems which are straightforwardly doing the task as intended are a narrow target within a much larger space of systems which *only pretend* to care about the training objective.

Concrete depictions of alignment failures

Given these problems, there have been several concrete depictions of what the world could look like as they play out. We have also seen the use of other methods to explore possible AI futures more broadly—for example, Avin et al.'s AI futures roleplaying game,[60] and AI Impacts' work on developing "AI vignettes".[61]

The scenarios can look quite different depending on how many advanced AI systems are deployed and how rapidly their capabilities improve. We will briefly explain four prominent scenarios that have been described. The first two depict alignment failure for advanced AI systems whose capabilities improve rapidly; the latter two show how alignment failure could look for systems whose capabilities improve more gradually.

1. **Outer-misaligned brain-in-a-box scenario.** This is the 'classic' scenario that most people remember from reading *Superintelligence* (though the book also features many other scenarios). A single, highly agentic AI system rapidly becomes superintelligent on all human tasks, in a world broadly similar to today. The objective function used to train the system (e.g. 'maximise production') doesn't push it to do what we really want, and the system's goals match the objective function. In other words, this is an outer alignment failure. Competitive pressures may have encouraged the organisation that trained the system to skimp on existential safety/alignment, especially if there was a race dynamic leading up to the catastrophe. The takeover becomes irreversible once the superintelligence has undergone an intelligence explosion.

2. **Inner-misaligned brain-in-a-box scenario.** Another version of the brain-in-a-box scenario features inner misalignment, rather than outer misalignment. That is, a superintelligence develops some arbitrary objective that arose during the training process. This could happen, for example, because there were subgoals in the training environment that were consistently useful for doing well in training, but which generalise to be adversarial to humans (e.g. acquiring resources), or simply because some arbitrary influence-seeking model just happened to arise during training, and performing well on the training objective is a good strategy for obtaining influence.

It is not clear whether the superintelligence being inner- rather than outer-misaligned has any practical impact on how the scenario would play out. An inner-misaligned superintelligence would be less likely to act in pursuit of a human-comprehensible final goal like 'maximise production', but since in either case the system would both be strongly influence-seeking and capable of seizing a decisive strategic advantage (i.e. complete world domination), the details of what it would do after seizing the decisive strategic advantage probably wouldn't matter. Perhaps, if the AI system is outer-misaligned, there is an increased possibility that a superintelligence could be blackmailed or bargained with, early in its development, by threatening its (more human-comprehensible) objective.

The next two scenarios, described by Christiano,[62] describe an alignment failure under gradual, continuous progress in AI capabilities.

3. **Many agentic AI systems gradually increase in intelligence and generality**, and are deployed increasingly widely across society to do important tasks (e.g. law enforcement, running companies, manufacturing, and logistics). The objective functions used to train them (e.g. 'reduce reported crimes', 'increase reported life satisfaction', 'increasing human wealth on paper') don't push them to do what we really want (e.g. 'actually prevent crime', 'actually help humans live good lives', 'increasing effective human control over resources')—so this is an outer alignment failure. The systems' goals match these objectives (i.e. are 'natural' or 'correct' generalisations of them). Competitive pressures (e.g. strong economic incentives, an international 'race dynamic', etc.) are probably necessary to explain why these systems are being deployed across society, despite some people pointing out that this could have very bad long-term consequences. There is no discrete point where this scenario becomes irreversible. AI systems gradually become more sophisticated, and their goals gradually gain more influence over the future relative to human goals. In the end, humans may not go extinct, but we have lost most of our control to much more sophisticated machines (this is not really a big departure from what is already happening today—just imagine replacing today's powerful corporations and states with machines pursuing similar objectives).

4. **The alternative version of this scenario begins similarly**: many agentic AI systems gradually increase in intelligence, and are deployed increasingly widely across society to do important tasks. But then, instead of learning some natural generalisation of the (poorly chosen) training objective, there is an inner alignment failure: the systems learn some unrelated objective(s) that arise naturally in the training process, i.e. are easily discovered in neural networks (e.g. 'don't get shut down'). The systems seek influence as an instrumental subgoal (since with more influence, a system is more likely to be able to e.g. prevent attempts to shut it down). Early in training, the best way to do that is by being obedient (since it knows that disobedient behaviour would get it shut down). Then, once the systems become sufficiently capable, they attempt to acquire resources and power to more effectively achieve their goals. Takeover becomes irreversible during a period of heightened vulnerability (a conflict between states, a natural disaster, a serious cyberattack, etc.) before systems have undergone an intelligence explosion. This could look like a "rapidly cascading series of automation failures: a few automated systems go off the rails in response to some local shock. As those systems go off the rails, the local shock is compounded into a larger disturbance; more and more automated systems move further from their training distribution and start failing." After this catastrophe, "we are left with a bunch of powerful influence-seeking systems, which are sophisticated enough that we can probably not get rid of them".[63]

Compared to the first version of this scenario, the point of no return will be even sooner (all else being equal), because AIs do not need to keep things looking good according to their somewhat human-desirable objectives (which takes more sophistication)—they just need to be able to make sure humans cannot take back control. The point of no return will probably be even sooner if the AIs all happen to learn similar objectives, or have good cooperative capabilities (because then they will be able to pool their resources and capabilities, and hence be able to take control from humans at a lower level of individual capability).

You could get a similar scenario where takeover becomes irreversible without any period of heightened vulnerability, if the AI systems are capable enough to take control without the world being chaotic.

AI forecasting

Another new area of work in this era of AI existential safety focuses on forecasting AI progress more rigorously. This has led to better predictions about how soon these risks may start to arise. We think the main implication of this work is clarifying that AI existential safety is likely to be an urgent problem. We will briefly describe two methods that have gained a lot of attention recently.

Scaling laws

Empirical scaling laws have been developed for various kinds of models. For example, work on scaling laws for neural language models[64] finds that as you increase model size (N), dataset size (D), and the amount of compute used for training (C), performance on language model benchmarks (or more precisely, the cross-entropy loss) improves according to a power law relationship. That is, if you increase N, D, and C, by a factor of x, then performance improves by a factor of x raised to the power of some constant (between 0 and 1).

Some trends span more than seven orders of magnitude, which is evidence that they are at least somewhat likely to continue as models get bigger in size. This is significant, because if these trends continue, then this implies that 'merely' increasing model size, dataset size, and compute by amounts that will be feasible in the near future will be sufficient for training very impressive models.

Biological anchors

This is a quantitative model for forecasting when transformative AI will occur.[65] Basically, the method asks: based on trends in the costs of training AI models, how much will it cost to train a model as big as a human brain to perform the hardest tasks humans do? And when will this be cheap enough that we should expect someone to do it?[66]

This method estimates a >10% chance of transformative AI by 2036, a 50% chance by 2055, and an 80% chance by 2100.

Growth in AI existential safety funding, institutions, and research

Given this progress in understanding the problem of AI existential safety, we will now shift towards discussing the concurrent expansion in the kinds of work being done to solve it. First off, it is worth noting that the deep learning revolution attracted a lot of new talent and funding, some of which were concerned with general AI safety, as well as the alignment problem and AI existential safety. This led to the founding of many new institutions devoted to research in this area. Equally, in recent years, tech companies performing research into AI progress have also begun to investigate safety issues and the alignment problem. The result is a much more prolific and well-funded field, able to grapple with a wide variety of problems, including the theoretical, empirical, and philosophical.

Research directions

As the number of researchers working on AI existential safety increased, and their methodologies became broader, a number of research directions and agendas were developed. In this subsection, we will summarise four particularly prominent ones. These are by no means exhaustive, but hopefully will give the reader a representative view of the kinds of work happening in AI existential safety today.

At a high level, a major problem with training superintelligent AI is that humans are not able to provide strong oversight. That is, the obvious approach to aligning AI—by keeping a human in the loop with the AI's decision making, and using feedback from the human to course-correct the AI's behaviour—does not straightforwardly work if that AI is operating in environments, at speeds, or with sufficiently advanced behaviour that make it hard for a human to provide accurate and timely feedback.

Two approaches to this general problem have been proposed: iterated amplification and debate. Compared with most machine-learning techniques, these approaches are less well verified on existing problems, but have stronger justifications for why they might scale up to help align highly capable future AI systems (unfortunately we do not yet have techniques which are both well verified and likely to scale to highly capable systems).

We will first outline these approaches, and then describe two other paradigms for AI existential safety research, which come from a different angle than trying to provide scalable oversight.

Iterated amplification

The essential idea of iterated amplification (IA) is to break down the process of oversight/supervision into subtasks—such that a human *can* evaluate the correctness of the AI's behaviour on those subtasks—and so train AI systems to perform each subtask. Then, once we have AIs that are aligned on the subtasks, they can be combined to give aligned behaviour on the more complex task.

As a toy example, suppose you wanted to train an AI to perform beneficial scientific research. You could decompose this problem into, for example, 'selecting a beneficial research area', 'reading and summarising existing papers in that area', 'synthesising understanding from those summaries', 'generating research ideas', 'implementing research ideas', and so on. And then each of those subtasks could be decomposed: 'reading existing papers in that area' could be decomposed into 'developing general language understanding', 'developing domain-specific language understanding', and 'reading and summarising papers'. Once the original task has been decomposed to simple enough subtasks, you can then train an AI using human oversight/supervision to do them, because the task is simple enough for humans to evaluate behaviour or outcomes. How exactly you train AI systems to solve subtasks depends on the task.

This summary elides one important detail: distillation. A problem with implementing the approach just described is that the computational complexity of solving the task is exponential in the number of decomposition 'levels'. That is, if you want to decompose something as complicated as 'performing beneficial scientific research', you will have to break it down into several subtasks, each of which gets further decomposed into several more subtasks, and the number of subtasks becomes exponentially large. Distillation aims to solves this. The idea is the following: suppose you want to train an AI to solve task T, which decomposes into subtasks T_1, T_2, and T_3. First, train AI systems A_1, A_2, and A_3 to perform the subtasks (this is amplification, as described above). Then, every time you want to perform task T, instead of performing inference with A_1, A_2, and A_3 and recombining the results every time, only do this *in order to train another AI system, A,* to imitate the combined results that A_1, A_2, and A_3 compute. Now you can use A to solve T, without performing inference using all of the subtask solvers.

There are many possible approaches to this distillation step, representing different concrete approaches to the overall IA scheme. You could use:

- Imitation learning,[67] in which case the overall approach is called 'imitative amplification'.

- Training on a myopic reward/approval signal[68] in which case the overall approach is called 'approval-based amplification'.

- Reward modelling,[69] in which case the overall approach is called 'recursive reward modelling'.

Iterated amplification has so far seen more work than other alignment proposals. Some important contributions include: Christiano et al.,[70] which introduces iterated amplification and demonstrates it in some small-scale experiments; Leike et al.,[71] which introduces recursive reward modelling in particular; and Wu et al.,[72] which applies recursive reward modelling to summarise books. The start-up Ought is working on collecting empirical evidence for the assumptions that need to hold if IA is to scale to arbitrarily difficult problems.

Debate

Debate is similar to IA in that it proposes a way to scale supervision of AIs to cases where humans cannot easily supervise. But it differs in that it focuses on evaluating claims made by language models, rather than supervising AI behaviour over time.

The essential idea is that, instead of trying to evaluate whether a superhuman language model is telling the truth (which would be hard since it would also be highly effective at manipulation), you should pit two language models against each other. That is, have them debate against each other, to convince the human overseer of the answer to some question. Even if the correctness of the answer is too hard to judge, the human should be able to look at the arguments and counterarguments made by the two AIs to figure out which answer is correct.

More detail on Debate is outside the scope of this chapter, but we refer the reader to Irving et al.,[73] which introduces the approach, and Barnes et al.[74] which describes progress that has been made since then.

Interpretability

We will now briefly describe two other paradigms for AI alignment research, which come at the problem from a different angle than the 'providing scalable oversight' approach taken by Iterated Amplification and Debate.

Work on interpretability attempts to understand in detail how neutral networks work. There are several motivations here: understanding what is happening inside neural networks seems beneficial for getting more certainty that they are going to do the things we want them to do. High levels of interpretability is also one possible approach to solving the inner alignment problem.

Olah et al.[75] is one significant piece of work on interpretability so far. It studies the connections between artificial neurons in detail, and finds meaningful algorithms in the weights of neural networks (e.g. 'curve detectors' and 'dog head detectors').

Embedded agency

Not all AI existential safety paradigms have switched to having a strong empirical focus on current deep neural networks. One of MIRI's research agendas, called 'embedded agency', aims to create rigorous mathematical frameworks for thinking about the relationship between AIs and their real-world environments.

The underlying intuition driving MIRI's approach is that the alignment problem is very difficult. In particular, it will be very hard to solve for deep learning systems on our current trajectory, where there is already a large gap between our understanding and the complexity of the systems we are able to train. Instead, they posit that we will need rigorous mathematical frameworks to develop a deep understanding of what intelligence is and how to align it. The main hurdle for this approach is that developing rigorous mathematical frameworks takes time, and if modern deep learning techniques scale to superintelligence fairly straightforwardly, then the chances of this approach bearing fruit in time do not seem good.

We refer the reader to Garrabrant[76] for some open questions about embedded agency, and Garrabrant et al.[77] for a prominent result.

Benchmarks

Along with the development of new research directions, another consequence of more empirical work on AI existential safety has been the creation of benchmarks for assessing safety experimentally. The need for benchmarks is motivated in part by the opacity of neural networks. That is to say, because neural networks offer no justification for the values they compute, and provide no formal guarantees of behaviour, we will need robust benchmarks and empirical safety testing if AI systems are to see application in all but the most trivial areas. A further motivation for benchmarks is measuring progress on core safety issues. Also, having better ways to measure progress in AI safety can help to incentivise more research.

In *AI Safety Gridworlds*, Leike et al.[78] illustrate a number of categories of safety issues arising within toy environments. These include safe exploration, reward gaming, and negative side effects, among others. Despite the very simple environments, and small number of test instances, these Gridworlds demonstrate very poor performance from (at the time) state-of-the-art algorithms with respect to the highlighted safety issues.

Similarly, OpenAI's *Safety Gym*[79] introduces another benchmark based around three-dimensional navigation while avoiding hazards. Safety Gym adds procedural generation to improve the robustness of any evaluation, but lacks the ability to assess certain important safety considerations, such as reward gaming or safety issues relating to absent supervision. As with AI Safety Gridworlds, the standard reinforcement learning algorithms typically fail to successfully and safely perform the tasks.

SafeLife[80] presents a robust benchmark for evaluating side effects in a gridworld domain which makes use of rules from Conway's Life[81] to allow for a very rich and dynamic environment for evaluating AI agents.

What all of these benchmarks have in common is that they assess some safety property in an abstract environment. While the issues that are considered are often relevant to the alignment problem and the risks from superintelligent AI systems, these benchmarks are also useful for developing and evaluating new algorithms for AI systems that we expect to arrive in the near term: self-driving cars or other autonomous robotic systems that interact with or will be around humans and other agents.

Already, these benchmarks have led to algorithmic improvements of safety. One approach to reducing side effects is penalising the AI system for the amount of 'impact' it causes the environment. The idea here is for the AI to find a balance between achieving its task and making small impacts on the world. Defining impact in general, across many different types of domains, is not an easy task, but efforts are being made and are becoming successful in some benchmarks.[82] The disadvantage to limiting impact is that sometimes the task is inherently impactful, and discerning 'good' impact from 'bad' is tricky. This is more likely to affect long-term AI systems or superintelligences due to the larger (hopefully beneficial) effects they may have on the world.

Research in this area is ongoing and promising, but because of the aforementioned difficulties in evaluating and assessing deep neural networks, these benchmarks need much more work to become robust, general, and all-encompassing enough to make AI safe.

Conclusion

Over the last 20 years in particular, there has been positive development in understanding of the problem of AI existential safety, and progress towards developing good solutions. A formalised academic discipline has coalesced from nascent concerns about 'ultraintelligence' and the 'singularity'. Even more recently, progress has exploded, due in no small part to Bostrom's *Superintelligence* and the deep learning revolution. Despite this progress, many fundamental problems in AI existential safety are poorly understood or unsolved, and we still do not have any satisfactory methods for ensuring the safety of advanced AI systems.

We continually seem to uncover evidence that the task at hand is far more complicated and difficult than first imagined, such as the existence of instrumentally convergent subgoals, or the poor performance of modern algorithms on practical safety benchmarks. We are also in a race against time: work in AI forecasting suggests that we only have decades before AI systems will be powerful enough to pose the kind of threats considered in this chapter.

In order to be as prepared as possible for the threats from advances in AI—particularly GCRs—more research in AI existential safety is needed. We need more work on assessing the extent to which current research directions will succeed in making advanced AI safe, on developing new research directions in case these approaches will not work in time, and on implementing workable approaches to safety in practice.

The stakes for humanity have never been bigger. If we do not make enough progress on AI existential safety—and on mitigating technological GCRs more broadly—this could endanger not only the lives of this generation or the next, but those of the many future generations who could come after us. Whilst the field has grown considerably since the beginning of formal work in the 2000s, there are still only hundreds of people working on AI existential safety—an extreme shortfall given what is at stake. We have no guarantee this will be easy, but there are now tractable research directions and shovel-ready questions to get to work on. We owe it to everyone alive today, and to the future, to redouble our efforts on reducing global catastrophic risk from AI and other advanced technologies.

Notes and References

1   Critch, Andrew, *Some AI Research Areas and Their Relevance to Existential Safety—AI Alignment Forum* (2020). https://www.alignmentforum.org/posts/hvGoYXi2kgnS3vxqb/some-ai-research-areas-and-their-relevance-to-existential-1

2   Critch, Andrew and David Krueger, 'AI research considerations for human existential safety (ARCHES)', *arXiv preprint* (2020). https://arxiv.org/abs/2006.04948

3   Turing, A.M., 'Computing machinery and intelligence', *Mind, LIX*(236) (Oct. 1950), pp.433–60. https://doi.org/10.1093/mind/LIX.236.433

4   Good, I.J., 'Speculations concerning the first ultraintelligent machine', *Adv. Comput.*, 6 (1965), pp.31–88.

5   Lukasiewicz, J., 'The ignorance explosion', *Leonardo, 7*(2) (1974), pp.159–63. http://www.jstor.org/stable/1572802

6   Ulam, Stanisław, 'John von Neumann 1903–1957', *Bulletin of the American Mathematical Society, 64* (1958), pp.1–49.

7   Vinge, Vernor, 'The coming technological singularity', *Whole Earth Review* (1993).

8   Kurzweil, Ray, *The Singularity Is Near: When Humans Transcend Biology*. Penguin (Non-Classics) (2006).

9   Kurzweil, Ray, *Age of Spiritual Machines: When Computers Exceed Human Intelligence*. Penguin (1999).

10   Kurzweil (1993).

11   Yudkowsky, Eliezer, *Creating Friendly Ai 1.0: The Analysis and Design of Benevolent Goal Architectures*. The Singularity Institute (2001).

12   Yudkowsky, Eliezer, *Coherent Extrapolated Volition*. The Singularity Institute (2004). http://intelligence.org/files/CEV.pdf

13   See https://www.yudkowsky.net/singularity.

14   Bostrom, Nick, 'How long before superintelligence?', *International Journal of Futures Studies, 2* (1998).

15   Bostrom, Nick, 'Ethical issues in advanced artificial intelligence', *Review of Contemporary Philosophy, 5* (2003).

16   Omohundro, Stephen M., 'The basic AI drives', *Proceedings of the 2008 Conference on Artificial General Intelligence 2008: Proceedings of the First AGI Conference*. IOS Press (2008), pp.483–92.

17   Bostrom, Nick, 'The superintelligent will: Motivation and instrumental rationality in advanced artificial agents', *Minds and Machines, 22*(2) (2012), pp.71–85. https://doi.org/10.1007/ s11023-012-9281-3

18   Soares, Nate et al., 'Corrigibility', *AAAI Workshops: Workshops at the Twenty-Ninth AAAI Conference on Artificial Intelligence* (2015). https://aaai.org/ocs/index.php/WS/AAAIW15/paper/view/10124/10136

19   Bostrom (2012).

20   Bostrom, Nick, *Superintelligence: Paths, Dangers, Strategies*. Oxford University Press (2014).

21   Krizhevsky, Alex, Ilya Sutskever, and Geoffrey E. Hinton, 'ImageNet classification with deep convolutional neural networks', *Proceedings of*

the 25th International Conference on Neural Information Processing Systems— *Volume 1.* Curran Associates Inc. (2012), pp.1097–105.

22   Mnih, Volodymyr et al., 'Playing Atari with deep reinforcement learning', *CoRR* abs/1312.5602 (2013). arXiv: 1312.5602. http://arxiv.org/abs/1312.5602; Mnih, Volodymyr et al., 'Human-level control through deep reinforcement learning', *Nature, 518*(7540) (February 2015), pp.529–33. http://dx.doi.org/10.1038/ nature14236

23   Silver, David et al., 'Mastering the game of Go without human knowledge', *Nature, 550* (October 2017), pp.354–59. http://dx.doi.org/10.1038/nature24270

24   OpenAI et al, 'Dota 2 with large scale deep reinforcement learning', *Title* (2019), arXiv: .06680. https://arxiv.org/abs/1912.06680

25   Jumper, John M. et al., 'Highly accurate protein structure prediction with AlphaFold', *Nature, 596* (2021), pp.583–89.

26   Sevilla, J., L. Heim, A. Ho, T. Besiroglu, M. Hobbhahn and P. Villalobos, "Compute Trends Across Three Eras of Machine Learning," *2022 International Joint Conference on Neural Networks (IJCNN)*, Padua, Italy (2022), pp. 1-8. https://doi.org/10.1109/IJCNN55064.2022.9891914

27   Shannon, C.E., 'A mathematical theory of communication', *Bell System Technical Journal, 27*(3) (1948), pp.379–423. https://doi.org/10.1002/j.1538-7305.1948.tb01338.x

28   Vaswani, Ashish et al., *Attention Is All You Need* (2017), arXiv: 1706.03762[cs.CL].

29   Radford, Alec and Karthik Narasimhan, 'Improving language understanding by generative pre-training', (2018); Alec Radford et al. "Language Models are Unsupervised Multitask Learners". *OpenAI Blog 1* no. 8 (2019); Brown, Tom et al. 'Language Models are Few-Shot Learners', in H. Larochelle et al. (eds), *Advances in Neural Information Processing Systems*. Vol. 33. Curran Associates, Inc. (2020), pp. 1877–901.

30   Raffel, Colin et al., *Exploring the Limits of Transfer Learning with a Unified Text-to-Text Transformer. The Journal of Machine Learning Research 21* (1) (2020). arXiv: 1910.10683[cs.LG].

31   Brown, T. et al., 'Language models are few-shot learners'. https://doi.org/10.48550/arXiv.2005.14165

32   Bommasani, Rishi et al., 'On the opportunities and risks of foundation models', *CoRR*, abs/2108.07258 (2021), arXiv: 2108.07258. https://arxiv.org/abs/2108.07258

33   Ramesh, Aditya et al., 'Zero-shot text-to-image generation', *CoRR*, abs/2102.12092 (2021), arXiv: 2102.12092. https://arxiv.org/abs/2102.12092

34   Chen, Mark et al., *Evaluating Large Language Models Trained on Code* (2021). arXiv: 2017.03374[cs.LG]

35   See https://copilot.github.com/.

36   Casares, P.A.M. et al., 'How general-purpose is a language model? Usefulness and safety with human prompters in the wild', *Association for the Advancement of Artificial Intelligence (AAAI)* (2022).

37   Bender, Emily M. et al., 'On the dangers of stochastic parrots: Can language models be too big?', *Proceedings of the 2021 ACM Conference on Fairness, Accountability, and Transparency*. Association for Computing Machinery (2021), pp.610–23. https://doi.org/10.1145/3442188.3445922

38   Note that occurrence of an intelligence explosion (discussed in our first section) is *consistent* with continuous progress. That is, an AI could analyse the processes that produce its intelligence and develop an AI which improves on these processes (and which is capable of doing the same), resulting in a positive feedback loop where AI capabilities include *very rapidly*, but in a way that is nonetheless roughly in line with what we would have expected by extrapolating from past progress (by that point, on the continuous progress view, progress will already be improving very rapidly, thanks to AI systems that are mediocre at self-improvement, rather than great at self-improvement).

39   Christiano, Paul, *Takeoff Speeds* (February 2018). https://sideways-view.com/2018/02/24/takeoff-speeds/

40   AI Impacts, *Discontinuous Progress Investigation* (2015). https://aiimpacts.org/discontinuous-progress-investigation/

41   Sutton, Richard, *The Bitter Lesson* (2019). http://www.incompleteideas.net/IncIdeas/BitterLesson.html

42   Ngo, Richard, *AGI Safety From First Principles: Control* (2019). https://www.alignmentforum.org/posts/eGihD5jnD6LFzgDZA/agi-safety-from-first-principlescontrol

43   Christiano, Paul, *What Failure Looks Like* (2019). https://www.alignmentforum.org/posts/HBxe6wdjxK239zajf/what-failure-looks-like; Critch, Andrew, *What Multipolar Failure Looks Like, and Robust Agent-Agnostic Processes (RAAPs)*. https://www.alignmentforum.org/posts/LpM3EAakwYdS6aRKf/whatmultipolar-failure-looks-like-and-robust-agent-agnostic; Kokotajlo, Daniel, *Soft Takeoff Can Still Lead to Decisive Strategic Advantage* (2019). https://www.alignmentforum.org/posts/

PKy8NuNPknenkDY74/soft-takeoff-can-stilllead-to-decisive-strategic-advantage; Christiano, Paul, *Another (Outer) Alignment Failure Story* (2021). https://www.alignmentforum.org/posts/AyNHoTWWAJ5eb99ji/another-outer-alignment-failure-story

44   Christiano (February 2018).

45   Drexler, K. Eric, *Reframing Superintelligence: Comprehensive AI Services as General Intelligence*. Future of Humanity Institute, University of Oxford (2019).

46   Ngo, Richard, *Comments on CAIS* (2019). https://www.alignmentforum.org/posts/HvNAmkXPTSoA4dvzv/comments-on-cais

47   Shah, *Reframing Superintelligence: Comprehensive AI Services as General Intelligence.* https://www.alignmentforum.org/posts/x3fNwSe5aWZb5yXEG/reframingsuperintelligence-comprehensive-ai-services-as

48   AI Impacts, *What Do Coherence Arguments Imply About the Behavior of Advanced AI?* (2021). https://aiimpacts.org/what-do-coherence-arguments-imply-about-the-behavior-ofadvanced-ai/

49   Branwen, Gwern, *Why Tool AIs Want to Be Agent Ais* (September 2016). https://www.gwern.net/Tool-AI

50   80,000 Hours Podcast, *Ben Garfinkel on Scrutinising Classic AI Risk Arguments.* https://80000hours.org/podcast/episodes/ben-garfinkel-classic-ai-riskarguments/

51   Bostrom (2018).

52   Carlsmith, Joe, *Draft Report on Existential Risk From Power-Seeking AI* (2021). https://www.alignmentforum.org/posts/HduCjmXTBD4xYTegv/draft-report-on-existentialrisk-from-power-seeking-ai

53   Karnofsky, Holden, *Potential Risks From Advanced Artificial Intelligence: The Philanthropic Opportunity* (May 2016). https://www.openphilanthropy.org/blog/potential-risks-advanced-artificial-intelligence-philanthropic-opportunity

54   Boulanin, Vincent et al., *Artificial Intelligence, Strategic Stability and Nuclear Risk* (2020). https://www.sipri.org/sites/default/files/2020-06/artificial_intelligence_strategic_stability_and_nuclear_risk.pdf

55   Seger, Elizabeth et al., *Tackling Threats to Informed Decisionmaking in Democratic Societies* (2020). https://www.turing.ac.uk/sites/default/files/2020-10/epistemic-security-report_final.pdf

56   Clarke, Sam, Alexis Carlier, and Jonas Schuett, *Survey on AI Existential Risk Scenarios* (2021). https://www.alignmentforum.org/posts/WiXePTj7KeEycbiwK/survey-on-aiexistential-risk-scenarios

57   Partnership on AI, *Managing the Risks of AI Research* (2021). http://partnershiponai.org/wp-content/uploads/2021/08/PAI-Managing-the-Risks-of-AIResesarch-Responsible-Publication.pdf

58   Gruetzemacher, Ross and Jess Whittlestone, 'The transformative potential of artificial intelligence', *arXiv:1912.00747* [cs] (October 2021). arXiv: 1912.00747. http://arxiv.org/abs/1912.00747

59   Hubinger, Evan et al., 'Risks from learned optimization in advanced machine learning systems', *arXiv:1906.01820* [cs] (December 2021). arXiv: 1906.01820. http://arxiv.org/abs/1906.01820

60   Avin, Shahar, Ross Gruetzemacher, and James Fox, 'Exploring AI futures through role play', *Proceedings of the AAAI/ACM Conference on AI, Ethics, and Society*. Association for Computing Machinery (February 2020), pp.8–14. https://doi.org/10.1145/3375627.3375817

61   AI Impacts, *AI Vignettes Project* (October 2021). https://aiimpacts.org/aivignettes-project/

62   Christiano (February 2018).

63   Christiano (2019)

64   Kaplan, Jared et al., 'Scaling laws for neural language models', *CoRR*, abs/2001.08361 (2020). arXiv: 2001.08361. https://arxiv.org/abs/2001.08361

65   Cotra, Ajeya, *Draft Report on AI Timelines* (2020). https://www.alignmentforum.org/posts/KrJfoZzpSDpnrv9va/draft-report-on-ai-timelines

66   Karnofsky, Holden, *"Biological Anchors" Is About Bounding, Not Pinpointing, AI Timelines* (2021). https://www.cold-takes.com/biological-anchors-is-aboutbounding-not-pinpointing-ai-timelines/

67   Hussein, Ahmed et al., 'Imitation learning: a survey of learning methods', *ACM Computing Surveys*, 50(2) (April 2017). https://doi.org/10.1145/3054912

68   Warnell, Garrett et al., 'Deep tamer: interactive agent shaping in high-dimensional state spaces', *arXiv:1709.10163* [cs] (Jan. 2018). arXiv:1709.10163; Arumugam, Dilip et al., 'Deep reinforcement learning from policy-dependent human feedback', *arXiv:1902.04257* [cs, stat] (Feb. 2019). arXiv: 1902.04257. http://arxiv.org/abs/1902.04257

69   Leike, Jan et al., 'Scalable agent alignment via reward modeling: a research direction', *arXiv:1811.07871* [*cs, stat*] (November 2018). arXiv: 1811.07871. http://arxiv.org/abs/1811.07871

70   Christiano, Paul, Buck Shlegeris, and Dario Amodei, 'Supervising strong learners by amplifying weak experts', *arXiv:1810.08575* [*cs, stat*] (October 2018). arXiv: 1810.08575. http://arxiv.org/abs/1810.08575

71   Leike et al., 'Scalable agent alignment via reward modeling'. *arXiv preprint* (2018).

72   Wu, Jeff et al., 'Recursively summarizing books with human feedback', *arXiv:2109.10862* [*cs*] (September 2021). arXiv: 2109.10862. http://arxiv. org/abs/2109.10862

73   Irving, Geoffrey, Paul Christiano, and Dario Amodei, 'AI safety via debate', *arXiv:1805.00899* [*cs, stat*] (October 2018). arXiv: 1805.00899. http://arxiv. org/abs/1805.00899

74   Barnes, Beth and Paul Christiano, *Writeup: Progress on AI Safety via Debate* (2020). https://www.alignmentforum.org/posts/Br4xDbYu4Frwrb64a/ writeup-progress-on-aisafety-via-debate-1

75   Olah, Chris et al., 'Zoom in: An introduction to circuits', *Distill, 5*(3) (March 2020), e00024.001. https://doi.org/10.23915/distill.00024.001

76   Garrabrant, Scott, *Embedded Agents* (October 2018). https://intelligence. org/2018/10/29/embedded-agents/

77   Garrabrant, Scott et al., 'Logical induction', *arXiv:1609.03543* [*cs, math*] (December 2020). arXiv: 1609.03543. http://arxiv.org/abs/1609.03543

78   Leike, Jan et al., 'AI safety gridworlds', *CoRR*, abs/1711.09883 (2017). arXiv: 1711.09883. http://arxiv.org/abs/1711.09883

79   Ray, Alex, Joshua Achiam, and Dario Amodei, 'Benchmarking safe exploration in deep reinforcement learning', *arXiv preprint* (2019).

80   Wainwright, Carroll L. and Peter Eckersley, 'SafeLife 1.0: Exploring side effects in complex environments', *CoRR*, abs/1912.01217 (2019). arXiv: 1912.01217. http://arxiv.org/abs/1912.01217

81   Mathematical Games, 'The fantastic combinations of John Conway's new solitaire game "life" by Martin Gardner', *Scientific American, 223* (1970), pp.120–23.

82   Turner, Alexander Matt, Dylan Hadfield-Menell, and Prasad Tadepalli, 'Conservative agency via attainable utility preservation', *CoRR*, abs/1902.09725 (2019). arXiv:1902.09725. http://arxiv.org/abs/1902.09725; Krakovna, Victoria et al., 'Measuring and avoiding side effects using

relative reachability', *CoRR*, abs/1806.01186 (2018). arXiv: 1806.01186. http://arxiv.org/abs/1806.01186; Turner, Alex, Neale Ratzlaff, and Prasad Tadepalli, 'Avoiding side effects in complex environments', in H. Larochelle et al. (eds), *Advances in Neural Information Processing Systems* (*Vol. 33*). Curran Associates, Inc. (2020), pp.21406–1415. https://proceedings. neurips.cc/paper/2020/file/f50a6c02a3fc5a3a5d4d9391f05f3efc-Paper.pdf

10. Military Artificial Intelligence as a Contributor to Global Catastrophic Risk

Matthijs M. Maas, Kayla Lucero-Matteucci, and Di Cooke

It should hardly be surprising that military technologies have featured prominently in public discussions of global catastrophic risk (GCR).[1] The prospect of uncontrolled global war stands as one of the oldest and most pervasive scenarios of what total societal disaster would look like. Conflict has always been able to devastate individual societies; in the modern era, technological and scientific progress has steadily increased the ability of state militaries, and possibly others, to inflict catastrophic violence.[2]

There are many technologies with this capacity, with artificial intelligence (AI) becoming a more notable one in recent years. Increasingly, experts from numerous fields have begun to focus on AI technologies' applications in warfare, considering how these could pose risks, or even new GCRs. While the technological development of military AI and the corresponding study of its impacts are still at an early stage, both have also progressed dramatically in the past decade. Most visibly, the development and use of Lethal Autonomous Weapons (LAWS) has sparked a heated debate, spanning both academic and political spheres.[3] However, in actuality, military applications of AI technology extend far beyond controversial 'killer robots'—with diverse uses from logistics to cyberwarfare, and from communications to training.[4]

   https://doi.org/10.11647/OBP.0336.10

It is anticipated that these applications may lead to many novel risks for society. The growing trend of utilising AI across defence-related systems creates new potential points for technical failure or operator errors; it can result in unanticipated wide-scale structural transformations in the decision environment or may negatively influence mutual perceptions of strategic stability, exacerbating the potential for escalation resulting in global catastrophic impacts. Even in less directly kinetic or lethal roles, such as intelligence-gathering or logistics, there is concern that the use of AI systems might still circuitously lead to GCRs. Finally, there are possible GCRs associated with the future development of more capable AI systems, such as artificial general intelligence (AGI); while these final potential GCRs are not the direct focus of this chapter, it should be noted that these risks could be especially significant in the military context, and that this would require caution rather than complacency.

Despite the ongoing endeavours around the world to leverage more AI technology within the national security enterprise, current efforts to identify and mitigate risks resulting from military AI are still very much nascent. At a technical level, one of the most pressing issues facing the AI technical community today is that any AI system is prone to a wide array of performance failures, design flaws, unexpected behaviour, or adversarial attacks.[5] Meanwhile, numerous militaries are devoting considerable time and resources towards deploying AI technology in a range of operational settings. Despite this, many still lack clear ethics or safety standards as part of their procurement and internal development procedures for military AI.[6] Nor have most state actors actively developing and deploying such systems agreed to hard boundaries limiting the use of AI in defence, or engaged in establishing confidence-building measures with perceived adversaries.[7]

It is clear that military AI developments could significantly affect the potential for GCRs in this area, making the exploration of this technological progression and its possible impacts vital for the GCR community. Now that AI techniques are beginning to see real-world uptake by militaries, it is more crucial than ever that we develop a detailed understanding about how military AI systems might be considered as GCRs in their own right, or how they might be relevant contributors to military GCRs. In particular, from a GCR perspective, further attention is needed to examine instances when AI intersects with military technologies as destructive as nuclear weapons, potentially producing catastrophic results. To enable a more cohesive understanding of this increasingly complex risk landscape, we explore the established literature and propose further avenues of research.

Our analysis proceeds as follows: after reviewing past military GCR research and recent pertinent advancements in military AI, this chapter turns the majority of its focus on LAWS and the intersection between AI and the nuclear landscape, both of which have received the most attention thus far in existing scholarship. First examining LAWS, we assess whether they might constitute GCRs, and argue that while these systems are concerning, they do not yet appear likely to be a GCR in the near term, considering current and anticipated production capabilities and associated costs. We then delve into the intersection of military AI and nuclear weapons, which we argue has a significantly higher GCR potential. We examine the GCR potential of nuclear war, briefly discussing the debates over when, where, and why it could lead to a GCR. Furthermore, after providing recent geopolitical context by identifying relevant converging global trends which may also independently raise the risks of nuclear warfare, the chapter turns its focus to the existing research on specific risks arising at the intersection of nuclear weapons and AI. We outline six hypothetical scenarios where the use of AI systems in, around, or against nuclear weapons could increase the likelihood of nuclear escalation and result in global catastrophes. Finally, the chapter concludes with suggestions for future directions of study, and sets the stage for a research agenda that can gain a more comprehensive and multidisciplinary understanding of the potential risks from military AI, both today and in the future.

Risks from (military) AI within the Global Catastrophic Risks field

Before understanding how military AI might be a GCR, it is important to understand how the GCR field has viewed risks from AI more broadly. Within the GCR field, there has been growing exploration of the ways in which AI technology could one day pose a global catastrophic or existential risk.[8] Such debates generally have not focused much on the military domain in the near term, however. Instead, they often focus on how such risks might emerge from future, advanced AI systems, developed in non-defence (or, at best, broadly 'strategic') contexts or sectors. These discussions have often focused on the development of Artificial General Intelligence (AGI) systems that would display "the ability to achieve a variety of goals, and carry out a variety of tasks, in a variety of different contexts and environments"[9] with performance equivalent or superior to a human in many or all domains. These are, of course, not the only systems studied: more recent work has begun to explore the prospects for, and implications of, intermediate 'High-Level Machine Intelligence'[10] or 'Transformative AI'[11]—types of AI systems that would be sufficient to drive significant societal impacts—without making strong assumptions about the architecture, or 'generality', of the system(s) in question.

Whichever term is used, across the GCR field (and particularly in the subfields of AI safety and AI alignment) there has been a long-running concern that if technological progress continues to yield more capable AI systems, such systems might eventually pose extreme risks to human welfare if they are not properly controlled or aligned with human values.[12] Unfortunately, pop-culture depictions of AI have fed some misperceptions about the actual nature of the concerns in this community.[13] As this community notes itself, there is still deep uncertainty over whether existing approaches in AI might yield progress towards something like AGI,[14] or when such advanced systems might be achieved.[15] Nonetheless, they point to a range of peculiar failure modes in existing machine learning approaches,[16] which often display unexpected behaviours, achieving the stated target goals in unintended (and at times hazardous) ways.[17] Such incidents suggest that the safe alignment of even today's machine-learning systems with human values will be a very difficult task;[18] that it is unlikely that this task will become easier if or when AI systems become highly capable; and that even minor failures to ensure such alignment could have significant, even globally catastrophic societal impacts.[19]

However, while the continued investigation of such future risks is critical, these are not strictly the focus of this chapter, which rather looks at the intersection of specifically military AI systems with GCRs, today or in the near-term. Indeed, with only a few exceptions,[20] existing GCR research has paid relatively little attention to the ways in which *military* uses of AI could result in catastrophic risk. That is not to say that the GCR community has not been interested in studying military technologies in general. Indeed, there have been research efforts to learn from historical experiences with the safe development and responsible governance of high-stakes military technologies, to derive insights for critical questions around the development, deployment, or governance of advanced AI. This research includes (for example) analyses of historical scientific dynamics around (strategically relevant) scientific megaprojects,[21] the plausibility of retaining scientific secrecy around hazardous information,[22] or the viability of global arms control agreements for high-stakes military technologies.[23] Other work in this vein has studied the development of, impacts of, and strategic contestation over previous 'strategic general-purpose technologies' with extensive military applications, such as biotechnology, cryptography, aerospace technology, or electricity.[24] However, these previous inquiries work by analogy, and have neglected to thoroughly examine in detail the object-level question of whether or how existing or near-term military AI systems could themselves constitute a GCR.

Thus far, the predominant focus on military AI as GCRs has been on LAWS, and on nuclear weapons. The former should not be surprising, given the strong resonance of 'killer robots' in the popular imagination. The latter should not be surprising, given that the GCR field's examination of military technologies has its roots in original concerns about nuclear weapons. Indeed, in the past 75 years, long before terms such as GCR or existential risk even came to be, the threat of nuclear weapons inspired a wave of work, study, and activism to reckon with the catastrophic threats posed by this technology.[25] Still, at the present moment, the exploration of how military AI might intersect with or augment the dangers posed by destructive technologies such as nuclear weapons is still in its early stages.

Before delving into military AI as a potential GCR, it is also crucial to first define what we consider to be a GCR. Global catastrophic risks (GCRs) are risks which could lead to significant loss of life or value across the globe, and which impact all (or a large portion) of humanity. There is not yet widespread agreement on what this means exactly, what threshold would count as a global catastrophe,[26] or what the distinction is between GCRs and existential risks. For many discussions within the field of GCR, and for many of the risks discussed in other chapters in this volume, such ambiguity may not matter much, if the potential risks discussed are so obviously catastrophic in their impacts (virtually always killing hundreds of millions, or even resulting in extinction) that they would undeniably be a GCR. Yet in the domain of military AI (as with other weapons technologies), one may confront potential edge-case scenarios—involving the projected deaths of hundreds of thousands, or even millions, but where it is unclear if this (plausibly) would reach higher.

Within our chapter, we therefore need some working threshold for what constitutes a GCR, even if any threshold is (by its nature) contestable. What is a workable threshold to use here for GCRs? One early influential definition by Bostrom and Cirkovic holds that a catastrophe causing 10,000 fatalities (such as a major earthquake or nuclear terrorism) might not qualify as a global catastrophe, whereas one that "caused 10 million fatalities or 10 trillion dollars' worth of economic loss (e.g., an influenza pandemic) would count as a global catastrophe, even if some region of the world escaped unscathed."[27] However, while there is therefore clear definitional uncertainty, in this chapter we will utilise a lower bound for GCRs that lies in the middle of the range indicated by Bostrom and Cirkovic. To be precise, we understand a GCR to be *an event or series of directly connected events which result in at least one million human fatalities within a span of minutes to several years, across at least several regions of the world.*

To understand whether and in what ways military AI could contribute to GCRs of this level, we next sketch the speed and direction by which this technology has been developed and deployed for military purposes, both historically and in recent years.

Advances in military AI: Past and present

The use of computing and automation technologies in military operations itself is hardly new. Indeed, the history of AI's development has been closely linked to militaries, with many early advances in computing technologies, digital networks, and algorithmic tools finding their genesis in military projects and national strategic needs.[28] During the Cold War, there were repeated periods of focus on the military applications of AI, from early RAND forecasts exploring long-range future trends in automation[29] to discussions of the potential use of AI in nuclear command and control (NC2) systems management.[30] As such, military interest in AI technology has proven broadly robust, despite periods of occasional disillusionment during the 'AI winters'. Even when individual projects failed to meet overambitious goals and were cancelled or scaled back, they still helped advance the state of the art; such was the case with the US's 1980s Strategic Computing Initiative—a ten-year, $1 billion effort to achieve full machine intelligence.[31] Moreover, by the 1990s, some of these investments seemed to be beginning to pay off on the battlefield: for instance, during the first Gulf War, as a wide range of technologies contributed to a steeply one-sided Coalition victory over Iraqi forces,[32] the US military's use of the Dynamic Analysis and Replanning Tool (DART) tool for automated logistics planning and scheduling was allegedly so successful that DARPA claimed this single application had promptly paid back 30 years of investment in AI.[33]

This long-standing relation between militaries and AI technology also illustrates how—just as there is not a single 'AI' technology, but rather a broad family of architectures, techniques, and approaches—likewise there is not one 'military AI' use case (e.g. combat robots). Rather, weapons systems have, for a very long time, been positioned along a spectrum of various forms of automatic, automated, or autonomous operation.[34] Many of these are therefore not new to military use: indeed, armies have been operating 'fire and forget' weapons (i.e. weapons that do not require further external intervention or guidance after launch) for over 70 years, dating back to the acoustic (sound-tracking) homing torpedoes that already saw use during the Second World War.[35] In restricted domains, such as at sea, fully autonomous 'Close-in Weapon Systems' (last-defence anti-missile cannons) have been used for years by dozens of countries to defend their naval vessels.[36]

Still, recent years have seen a notable acceleration in the militarisation of AI technology.[37] The market for the use of AI in military uses was estimated at $6.3 billion in 2020, and was then projected to double to $11.6 billion by 2025.[38] Investments are led by the US, China, Russia, South Korea, the UK, and France,[39] but also include efforts by India, Israel, and Japan.[40]

What is the exact appeal of AI capabilities for militaries? Generally speaking, AI has been described as a 'general-purpose technology' (GPT),[41] suggesting that it is likely to see global diffusion and uptake, even if there may be shortfalls amid rushed applications.[42] This also extends to the military realm. Although uptake of military AI differs by country, commonly highlighted areas of application include improved analysis and visualisation of large amounts of data for planning and logistics; pinpointing relevant data to aid intelligence analysis; cyber defence and identification of cyber vulnerabilities (or, more concerningly, cyber offence); early warning and missile defence; and autonomous vehicles for air, land, or sea domains.[43]

Given this range of uses, there has been significant government attention for the strategic promise of the technology. US scholars describe AI as having prompted a new 'revolution in military affairs';[44] Chinese commentators project that virtually any aspect of military operations might be improved, made faster, or more accurate—or as they call it, 'intelligentised'[45]—through AI. In this way, AI could enable 'general-purpose military transformations' (GMT).[46] Consequently, many anticipate far-reaching or even foundational changes in military practice. Even those with a more cautious outlook still agree that AI systems can serve as a potent 'evolving' and 'enabling' technology that will have diverse impacts across a range of military fields.[47] This has led some to anticipate widespread and unconstrained proliferation of AI, on the assumption that "[t]he applications of AI to warfare and espionage are likely to be as irresistible as aircraft".[48] Still, this should come with some caveats.

In the first place, many applications of military AI may appear relatively 'mundane' in the near term. As argued by Michael Horowitz, "[m]ost applications of AI to militaries are still in their infancy, and most applications of algorithms for militaries will be in areas such as logistics and training rather than close to or on the battlefield".[49] Indeed, early US military accounts on autonomy maintain that there are only particular battlefield conditions under which that capability adds tactical value.[50] Despite the ambitious outlook and rhetoric of many national defence strategies around AI, in practice their focus appears to be more on rapidly maximising the benefits from easily accessible or low-hanging AI applications in areas such as logistics and predictive maintenance, rather than working immediately towards epochal changes.[51]

Secondly, while there are significant technological breakthroughs in AI, a number of technological and logistical challenges are likely to slow implementation to many militaries, at least in the near term of the next decade. All military technologies, no matter how powerful, face operational, organisational, and cultural barriers to adoption and deployment,[52] and there is no reason to expect military AI will be immune to this. Indeed, militaries may face additional and unexpected hurdles when forced to procure such systems from private-sector tech companies, because of mismatches in organisational processes, development approaches, and system requirements,[53] or export control restrictions or military robustness expectations that go beyond consumer defaults.[54] Finally, emerging technologies, when in their early stages of development, will often face acute trade-offs or brittleness in performance that limit their direct military utility.[55] The often high-profile failures of—or accidents with—early systems can also temper early military enthusiasm for deployment, stopping or slowing development, especially where it concerns more advanced applications such as complex drone swarms with the capacity for algorithmically coordinated behaviour.[56]

Moreover, there are factors that may slow or restrict the proliferation of military AI technology, at least in the near term. Military technological espionage or reverse engineering has proven a valuable but ultimately limited tool for militaries to keep pace with cutting-edge technologies developed by adversaries.[57] In recent years, the training of cutting-edge AI systems has also begun to involve increasingly large computing hardware requirements,[58] as well as important AI expert knowledge, which could ultimately restrict the straightforward proliferation of many types of military AI systems around the globe.[59]

Finally, and alongside all of this, there may be political brakes, or even barriers, to some (if not all) military uses of AI. It should be kept in mind that while the adoption of any military technology may be driven by military-economic selection pressures,[60] their development or use by any actors is certainly not as inevitable or foregone as it may appear in advance.[61] Historically, states and activists have—by leveraging international norms, interests, and institutions—managed to slow, contain, or limit the development of diverse sets of emerging weapons technologies (from blinding lasers to radiological weapons, and from environmental modification to certain nuclear programs), achieving successes that, while not always perfect, often exceeded initial expectations.[62] Accordingly, there is always the possibility that the coming decades will see invigorated opposition to military AI that will impose an effective brake; however, the success of any such efforts will depend sensitively on questions of issue-framing, forum choice, and organisation.[63]

As a result, the reality of military AI may appear relatively mundane, at least for the next few years, even as it gathers pace below the surface. Nonetheless, even under excessively conservative technological assumptions—where we assume that AI performance progress slows down or plateaus in the next years—AI appears likely to have significant military impacts. In fact, in many domains, it need not achieve further dramatic breakthroughs for existing capabilities to alter the international military landscape. As with conventional drone technologies, even imperfect AI capabilities (used in areas such as image recognition) could suffice to enable disruptive tactical and strategic effects, especially if they are pursued by smaller militaries or non-state actors.[64] As such, even if we assume that more advanced AI capabilities remain out of reach or undesired (an assumption that may rest on thin ground), the development of autonomous systems could herald a wide range of tactical changes,[65] including a shift in the so-called 'offense-defence balance'[66] due to increased effectiveness of offensive capabilities—along with an increased use of deception and decoys, or changes in force operation and operator skill requirements, to name a few.[67] But the question still remains: are any of these impacts plausibly globally catastrophic?

LAWS as GCRs

Thus far, some of the most in-depth discussions of military AI systems as plausible GCRs have focused on the potential risks of LAWS. In this section, we examine existing research and explore several proposed scenarios for ways by which LAWS might contribute to GCRs. Ultimately, we argue that the threshold of destruction (>one million human fatalities) necessary for a GCR leaves most (if not all) near-term LAWs unlikely to qualify as GCRs in isolation.

To pose a GCR, a technology must, at some point, have lethal effects. To be certain, there are significant developments in directly lethal military AI. Of course, technical feasibility by itself does not mean the development of such systems is inevitable: the existence of LAWS—or their mass procurement and deployment beyond prototypes—hinges not just on questions of technological feasibility, but also on questions of governments' willingness to deploy such systems. To take the technological developments as a starting point, LAWS systems are already being developed and deployed across militaries worldwide. Already in 2017, a survey identified "49 deployed weapon systems with autonomous targeting capabilities sufficient to engage targets without the involvement of a human operator".[68] This number has grown substantially since.

Moreover, in the past years the first fully autonomous weapons systems have reportedly begun to see actual (if limited) deployment. For instance, the South Korean military briefly deployed Samsung SGR-A1 sentry gun turrets to the Korean Demilitarised Zone, which came with an optional autonomous operation mode.[69] Israel has begun to deploy the 'Harpy' loitering anti-radar drone,[70] and various actors have begun to develop, sell, or use weaponised drones capable of autonomy.[71] In 2019, the Chinese company Ziyan released the Blowfish A3: a machine-gun-carrying assault drone that was allegedly marketed as sporting 'full autonomy'.[72] 2020 saw claims that Turkey had developed (semi-)autonomous versions of its 'Kargu-2' kamikaze drone;[73] in the spring of 2021, a UN report suggested that this weapon had been used fully autonomously in the Libyan conflict, to attack soldiers fleeing battle.[74] UAVs that are, in principle, capable of full autonomy have also reportedly seen use in the 2022 Russian invasion of Ukraine, although it remains difficult to ascertain whether any of these systems have been used in fully autonomous mode.[75] Recent developments in autonomous weapons have also included the use of large numbers of small robotic drone platforms in interacting swarms.[76] The Israel Defense Forces deployed such swarms in the May 2021 campaign on Gaza: to locate, identify, and even strike targets.[77]

In other cases, AI has been used in ways that are less autonomous, but which certainly show the lethality-enabling function of many AI technologies.[78] For example, the November 2020 assassination of Mohsen Fakrizadeh (Iran's top nuclear scientist) relied upon a remotely controlled machine gun. While the system was controlled by a human operator, it reportedly used AI to correct for more than a second-and-a-half of input delay. This allowed the operator to fire highly accurately at a moving target, from a moving gun platform on a highway, while stationed more than 1,000 miles away.[79] Other developments demonstrate the potential for more advanced autonomous behaviour. In 2020, DARPA ran AlphaDogFight, a simulated dogfight between a human F-16 pilot and a reinforcement-learning-based AI system, which saw the AI defeating the human pilot in all of their five matches.[80] In the past decade, the US and others have also experimented with a plane-launched swarm of 103 Perdix drones, which coordinated with one another to demonstrate collective decision-making, adaptive formation, and 'self-healing' behaviour.[81] Experiments in swarming drones have continued apace since.

Perhaps unsurprisingly—due to the fact that it has had earlier adoption relative to other high-risk military applications—LAWS have received sustained public scrutiny and scholarly attention, far more so than any other military AI use case. Consequently, efforts to develop governance approaches have arisen from multiple corners,[82] including at the UN Convention on Certain Conventional Weapons (CCW) since 2014, as well as within arms control communities since 2013.[83] However, it is notable that these debates have mostly examined qualitative characteristics of LAWS, rather than the potential quantitative upper limit on the scale of violence they might enable. Specifically, opposition to LAWS has focused primarily (but not exclusively) on their potential violation of various existing legal principles or regimes under international law, specifically International Humanitarian Law,[84] or (when used in law enforcement outside of war zones) under international human rights law;[85] other discussions have explored whether LAWS, even if they narrowly comply with cornerstone IHL principles, might still be held to undermine human dignity because they involve 'machine killing'.[86]

Over time, however, some civil society actors have begun to attempt to understand and stigmatise LAWS swarms as a potential 'weapon of mass destruction',[87] with swarms of lethal drones as a weapon system that could easily fall in the hands of terrorist actors or unscrupulous states, allowing the infliction of massive violence. This is a framing that has become more prominent within counter-LAWS disarmament campaigns,[88] most viscerally in depictions of terror attacks using fully autonomous microdrones that deliver small, shaped charges (such as the Future of Life Institute's 'Slaughterbot' campaigns of 2017 and 2021).[89] This is indicative of a growing concern for the 'quantitative' dimension and potential scale of mass attacks using autonomous weapons.

As a consequence, two distinct scenarios have often been proposed regarding LAWS technology as a significant global risk: terrorist use for mass attacks and state military use of massed LAWS forces.

Mass terror attacks on public or on GCR-sensitive targets

One hypothetical discussed by experts focuses on the use of LAWS not by state militaries, but by non-state actors (such as terror groups).[90] In theory, terrorists could subsequently leverage larger and larger swarms, either through direct acquisition of such militarised technology (if unregulated), or remote subversion of existing fleets using cyberattacks. Turchin and Denkenberger argue that increasingly larger quantities of drone swarms would be feasible as a global catastrophic risk, as it becomes cheaper to build drones.[91] While it is possible that this could enable mass-casualty attacks, it seems unlikely that any non-state actor could scale such attacks up to the global level. Moreover, it would be hard for them to prepare attacks of such magnitude undetected.

Another less explored risk would involve the (terrorist) use of LAWS to deliver other GCR-capable weapons or agents. For instance, Kallenborn and Bleek have suggested that actors could use drone swarms to deliver existing chemical, biological, or radiological weapons;[92] others have suggested that non-state actors could refit crop-duster drones to disperse chemical or biological agents.[93] In such cases, the level of risk is less clear: it might still be unlikely that these hypothetical events could be scaled up to result in a full GCR; however, this depends on the potency of the delivered agent in question. Ultimately, existing research is still very preliminary, and much further research is necessary to enable more concrete conclusions.

A third attack pathway could involve the malicious or terrorist use of autonomous weapons on sensitive critical infrastructures which, if damaged or compromised, would precipitate GCRs (or at least would instantly cripple our ability to respond to ongoing or imminent GCRs). Drone systems have been used by various non-state actors in recent years to mount effective attacks against critical infrastructures—as in the attacks on oil pipelines and national airports in the Yemen conflict.[94] Moreover, across the world there are a wide range of vulnerable global infrastructural 'pinch points' (internet connection points, narrow shipping canals, breadbasket regions) which, if they are attacked or degraded, could precipitate major shocks in the global system.[95] Many of these could be conceivably attacked through autonomous weapons, which could result in regional or even global disaster by the resulting knock-on effects, even if they were only temporarily disrupted. For instance, AWS could be used to deliver coordinated attacks on nuclear power plants, potentially resulting in large fallout patterns and contamination of land and food.[96] Alternatively, they could be used to attack and interrupt any future geo-engineering programs, potentially triggering climatic 'termination shocks' (where temperatures bounce back in ways that would be catastrophically disruptive to the global ecosystem and agriculture).[97] However, these types of attack do not seem to necessarily require autonomous weapons, and while they could certainly result in widespread global chaos, it is again unclear if they could be scaled up to the threshold of a global catastrophe involving over one million casualties.

State attacks with massed LAWS swarms

Within existing research, another frequently discussed hypothetical scenario is the idea of well-resourced actors using mass swarms of LAWS to carry out global attacks, allowing for "armed conflict to be fought at a scale greater than ever".[98] There is also a lively discussion about the possibility that mass attacks using swarms of 'slaughterbots' could allow small-state actors to mount attacks that would kill as many as 100,000 people.[99]

Turchin and Denkenberger have argued that in large enough quantities, drone swarms could be destructive enough to constitute a GCR, and command errors could result in autonomous armies creating a similar level of damage. Still, they predict that, even in those scenarios, LAWS are likely to result in broad instability rather than destruction on the scale of a GCR.[100] More recently, Anthony Aguirre has suggested that mass swarms of 'anti-personnel AWS' could deliver large-scale destruction at lower costs and lower access thresholds than would be required for an equivalently destructive nuclear strike (of an equivalent scale as the Hiroshima bombing), and that such weapons could be scaled up to inflict extreme levels of global destruction.[101] Turchin has suggested that drone swarms could become catastrophic risks only under very specific conditions, where more advanced (e.g. AGI) technologies are delayed, drone manufacture costs fall to extremely low bounds, defensive counter-drone capabilities lag behind, and militaries adopt global postures that condone the development of drone swarms as a strategic offensive weapon.[102] Even under these conditions, he suggests, drone swarms would be unlikely to ever rise to the level of an existential risk, though they could certainly contribute to civilisational collapse in the event of an extensive global war.[103]

Evaluating the feasibility of mass LAWS swarm-attack scenarios as GCRs

In both of the above cases, there is reason for concern and precautionary study and policy. However, there remain at least some practical reasons to doubt that LAWS lend themselves to precipitating catastrophes at a full GCR scale in the near term.

For one, it still is unclear if LAWS would be more cost-effective as a mass-attack weapon for states that have other established options. On the one hand, Aguirre has argued that 'slaughterbots' could be as inexpensive as $100, meaning that, even with a 50% unit attack success rate, and a doubling of cost to account for delivery systems, the shelf price of an attack inflicting 100,000 casualties would be $40 million.[104] However, how does that actually compare to the costs of other mass-casualty weapons systems? While precise procurement costs remain classified, estimates have been given for various nuclear weapon assets: US B61 gravity bombs are estimated to cost $4.9 million each (with a B-52H bomber carrying 20 such bombs costing an additional $42 million); a Minuteman III missile costs $33.5 million apiece (or $48.5 million, including the cost of three nuclear warheads).[105] The cost of North Korean nuclear weapons has been estimated at between $18 million and $53 million per warhead.[106] Accurate and up-to-date cost-effectiveness estimates for other weapons of mass destruction are hard to come by—in 1969, a UN study estimated that the costs of inflicting one civilian casualty per square kilometre were about $2,000 with conventional weapons, $800 with nuclear weapons, $600 with chemical weapons, and only $1 with biological weapons.[107] However, these estimates are likely considerably outdated, and are unlikely to reflect the destructive efficiency of contemporary WMDs used against modern societies. So, in principle (and perceived only from a narrowly economic perspective), LAWS swarms might appear less cost-effective than most existing WMDs, although not dramatically so. Even then, such swarms could theoretically be competitive, because they are seen as more accessible or achievable than other WMDs (in the sense that their production may be less reliant on globally controlled resources such as fissile materials or toxins).

Moreover, there may be supply-chain limitations, which could result in caps on how many such drone swarm units could be plausibly produced or procured. To be sure, assuming very small drones, swarms could be scaled up to hundreds of thousands or millions of units. Some accounts of drone swarms have envisaged a future of 'smart clouds' of billions of tiny, insect-like drones.[108] Yet this might trade off against effective lethality: it seems unlikely that micro-drone systems will be able to do much more than reconnaissance, given limits in terms of power, range, processing, and/or payload capacity.[109] By contrast, focusing on LAWS that are able to project lethal force at meaningful ranges, the production constraints seem more serious. We can compare the production lines for military drones, a technology with more well-established supply chains: a 2019 estimate by defence information group Janes estimated that more than 80,000 surveillance drones and 2,000 attack drones would be purchased around the world in the next decade.[110] The civilian drone market is admittedly larger, with around five million consumer drones being sold in 2020—a number expected to rise to 9.6 million by 2030.[111]

This suggests that if commercial supply chains were all dedicated to the production of LAWS, GCR-scale attacks could come into range. Yet the relatively small size of the military drone market is still suggestive of the challenges around procuring sufficient numbers of autonomous weapons to truly inflict global catastrophe in the next decade or so, and possibly beyond.

Of course, there might also be counter-arguments that suggest these barriers could be overcome, making mass LAWS attacks (at GCR scale) more feasible. For instance, it could be misleading to look at the raw number of platforms acquired and deployed, since individual autonomous weapons platforms might easily be equipped with weapons that would allow each platform to kill not one but dozens or thousands, depending on the weapon delivered or location of attacks. However, this is not the way that 'slaughterbots' are usually represented; indeed, outfitting these systems with more ordnance would simply make the ordnance the bottleneck.

In the second place, motivated states might be able to step up production and procure far larger numbers of these systems than is possible today, especially if the anticipated strategic context of their use is not counterinsurgency but a near-peer confrontation, where drone swarms might become perceived (either accurately or not) as not just helpful or cost-saving, but also providing a key margin of dominance. For instance, the US Navy in 2020 discussed offensive and defensive tactics for dealing with attacks of 'super swarms' of up to a million drones.[112] Increased state attention and enthusiasm for this technology could change the industrial and technical parameters rapidly.

In the third place, economies of scale and advances in manufacturing capabilities could mean that unit production costs could fall, or mass production could be facilitated, potentially enabling the targeting of many millions. It is unclear to what level costs would have to fall for GCR-scale fleets to become viable (let alone common), however, with Turchin suggesting unit costs of below $1.[113] Even so, barring truly radical manufacturing breakthroughs, producing this would require quite significant investments. The above does not even begin to address questions of delivery.

The overall point here is therefore not that states will remain disinterested in—or incapable of building—drone swarms of a size that would enable GCR-scale attacks. Indeed, states have often proven willing to invest huge sums in military technologies and their production infrastructures and industries.[114] Still, even in those cases, LAWS swarms will likely not be as destructive as modern thermonuclear weapons: as argued by Kallenborn, "[w]hile they are unlikely to achieve the scale of harm as the Tsar Bomba, the famous Soviet hydrogen bomb, or most other major nuclear weapons, swarms could cause the same level of destruction, death, and injury as the nuclear weapons used in Nagasaki and Hiroshima."[115] That suggests that they might be seen by militaries to complement rather than substitute for existing deterrents.

The above suggests that LAWS are certainly a real concern, in that it appears possible that, if this technology is developed further, it could in principle be used to inflict mass-casualty attacks on cities; at the same time, it implies that unless political, economic, or technological conditions change, swarms of LAWS (whether operated by terrorists or states) remain unlikely to be able to inflict GCR-level catastrophes in the near future. The scale-up that would be necessary to achieve destruction that would qualify it as a GCR does not presently seem to be a realistic outcome, both industrially but also politically—particularly given the host of similarly or more destructive weapons already available to states. All this suggests that, while autonomous weapons would likely be disruptive, their use would not scale up to a full GCR under most circumstances. Nevertheless, there may be additional edge cases of risk, especially in the under-explored scenarios such as the use of LAWS to deliver WMDs, and/or their use in mass-scale internal repression or genocide.[116] This, therefore, is an area that will require further research.

Nuclear weapons and AI

There is a second way in which military AI systems could rise to become a GCR: this is through their interaction with one of the oldest anthropogenic sources of global catastrophic risk: nuclear weapons.

Nuclear war as a GCR

To understand the way that AI systems might increase the risk of nuclear war in ways that could pose GCRs, it is first key to briefly review the ways in which nuclear war itself has become understood as a global catastrophic risk.

Since the invention of atomic weapons, discussions of nuclear risk have often been characterised by sharply divergent frames and understandings, with many accounts focusing single-mindedly either on the perceived irreplaceable strategic and geopolitical benefits derived from possessing nuclear weapons, or on the absolutely intolerable humanitarian consequences of their use. The discourses surrounding nuclear weapons today often still fall within those categories.[117] This is not new: early understandings of nuclear weapons vacillated between treating them as simply another weapon for tactical use on the battlefield,[118] or as an atrocious weapon of genocide,[119] potentially even capable of incinerating the atmosphere, as some lead Manhattan Project scientists briefly worried might happen during the Trinity test.[120]

One fact which no one questions, however, is the historically unprecedented capability of nuclear weapons to inflict violence at a massive scale.[121] The crude atomic bombs dropped by the US on Hiroshima and Nagasaki killed at least 140,000 and 74,000 people respectively, but more recently, nuclear weapons with similar destructive capacity have been considered 'low-yield'.[122] In the decades following the Second World War, countries developed thermonuclear weapons which, in some cases, were thousands of times more destructive than the first atomic bombs.[123] Today, the use of a single nuclear weapon could kill hundreds of thousands of people, and a nuclear exchange—even involving 'only' a few dozen nuclear weapons—could have devastating consequences for human civilisation and the ecosystems upon which we depend.[124]

If the use of a single nuclear weapon would be a tragedy, the additional fact that these weapons would rarely be used in isolation highlights clear paths to global catastrophe. According to David Rosenberg, early US plans for a nuclear war (drawn up by the Strategic Air Command in 1955) were estimated to be able to inflict a total of 60 million deaths and another 17 million casualties on the Soviet Union.[125] Later plans would escalate even further. The 1962 US nuclear war plan, utilising the entire US arsenal, would have killed an estimated 285 million people and harmed at least another 40 million in the targeted (Soviet-Sino bloc) countries alone.[126] Daniel Ellsberg, then at DARPA, later recounted war plans for a US first-strike on the Soviet Union, Warsaw Pact satellites, and China, as well as additional casualties from fallout in adjacent neutral (or even allied) countries, which projected global casualties rising up to 600 million.[127]

These estimates proved not to be a ceiling but a potential lower bound, once scientists began to focus on potential environmental interactions of nuclear war. In 1983, Carl Sagan famously embarked on a public campaign to raise awareness about the environmental impacts of nuclear weapons. Along with several colleagues, including some in the USSR, Sagan disseminated a theory of "nuclear winter", which holds that fires caused by nuclear detonations would loft soot into the stratosphere, leading to cooler conditions, drought, famine, and wide-scale death.[128] In response to Sagan's campaign, the US government attempted to downplay public discussions of nuclear winter, with the Reagan administration stating publicly in 1985 that it had "...very little confidence in the near-term ability to predict this phenomenon quantitatively."[129] Still, archival materials reveal that, internally, administration officials had strong feelings about nuclear winter. One employee of the Department of Defense noted at the time that the US government and overall scientific community "ought to be a bit chagrined at not realizing that smoke could produce these effects."[130]

Over time, accounts such as these have led to the creation of a nuclear taboo, or norm of non-use,[131] although it is unclear whether the taboo will stand amid a number of contemporary developments.[132] Today, scholars continue to study the impacts of nuclear detonations, with some predicting that even a small nuclear exchange could result in nuclear winter. For instance, climate scientist Alan Robock and colleagues suggest that "...if 100 nuclear bombs were dropped on cities and industrial areas—only 0.4 percent of the world's more than 25,000 warheads—[this] would produce enough smoke to cripple global agriculture."[133] Even in the limited scenario of such a 'nuclear autumn', it has been estimated that US and Chinese agricultural production in corn and wheat would drop by about 20–40% in the first five years, putting as many as two billion people at risk of starvation.[134] A larger exchange between the US and Russia would have even more serious and catastrophic consequences, according to a 2019 analysis of long-term climatic effects.[135]

To be sure, there remains some dissent over models predicting these environmental impacts,[136] the science of nuclear winter,[137] or the status of nuclear war as GCR.[138] Assessments of nuclear risk are made more difficult still by uncertainty in not just the environmental models, but also the underlying strategic dynamics. There are deep methodological difficulties around quantifying nuclear risks, especially since an all-out nuclear war has never occurred. Whereas studies of some (but certainly not all) other GCRs, such as pandemics, can aim and extrapolate from historical disasters, scholars examining the risk of nuclear war face the steep challenge of attempting to "understand an event that never happened".[139] Nonetheless, different approaches attempt to integrate historical base rates for intermediary steps (close calls and accidents) with expert elicitation, to come to imperfect background estimates.[140]

Yet (as even modellers note), such estimates remain subject to extreme uncertainty, given the unpredictability of strategy, targeting decisions, and complex socio-technical systems. A host of close calls during the Cold War show that carefully designed systems are not impervious to accidents or immune from human error.[141] As normal accident theory suggests, undesirable events and accident cascades are inevitable,[142] and adding in automated components or fail-safe systems may sometimes counterintuitively increase overall risk by increasing the system's complexity, reducing its transparency, or inducing automation bias.[143] The present era is now faced with the question of whether emerging technologies such as AI will be equally susceptible to risks from normal accidents,[144] whether they will contribute to such risks in legacy technologies such as nuclear weapons, and whether they will make the impacts of already destructive weapons more severe or increase the likelihood of their use.

Overall, the massive loss of life envisioned in nuclear war plans certainly qualifies nuclear weapons as a GCR. Whether they are considered to pose an existential risk may depend on the number and yield of weapons used. Some analyses have suggested that, even in extreme scenarios of nuclear war that resulted in civilisational collapse and the deaths of very large (>90% or >99.99%) fractions of the world population, we might still expect humanity to survive.[145] On the other hand, it has been countered that, even if such a disaster would not immediately lead to extinction, it might still set the stage for a more gradual and eventual collapse or extinction over time, or at the very least for the recovery of a society with much worse prospects.[146] However, for many commonly shared ethical intuitions, this distinction may be relatively moot.[147] Whether or not it is a technical existential risk, any further study of nuclear weapons' environmental and humanitarian impacts, including nuclear winter, will likely further corroborate their status as a major threat to humanity both today and into the future.

Recent developments in nuclear risk and emerging technology

Today's emergence of military AI therefore comes on top of a number of other disruptive developments that have already impacted nuclear risk over the past decades, and which have already brought concern about nuclear GCRs to the forefront.

Notably, this attention comes after a period of relative inattention to nuclear risk. In the aftermath of the Cold War, the risks posed by the existence of nuclear weapons were seen to be less immediate and pronounced. Accordingly, discussions came to focus more on nuclear security, including efforts after the fall of the Berlin Wall to secure Soviet nuclear materials,[148] as well as the challenges of preventing terrorist acquisition of WMDs, such as through the UNSC Resolution 1540 and the Nuclear Security Summit initiatives. In the last decade, however, converging developments in geopolitics and military technology have brought military (and especially nuclear) GCRs back to the fore.

First, the relative peace that followed the Cold War has been replaced by competition between powerful states, rather than fully cooperative security (or hegemony) in many domains. Geopolitical tensions between major powers have been inflamed, visible in the form of flashpoints from Ukraine to the South China Sea. Meanwhile, the regimes for the control of WMDs have come under pressure.[149] Nuclear arms control agreements between the US and Russia (such as the Intermediate-Range Nuclear Forces Treaty and the Anti-Ballistic Missile Treaty) have been cancelled by Presidents Trump and Bush; other nuclear states such as the UK, France, or China are not restrained by binding nuclear arms control agreements. Although the US and Russia extended the New Strategic Arms Reduction Treaty in March of 2021,[150] the future of arms control is uncertain amid ongoing disputes between the owners of the world's two largest nuclear arsenals,[151] and tensions between the West and Russia over Putin's invasion of Ukraine. In the absence of open channels of communication and risk reduction measures, the dangers of miscalculation are pronounced.[152]

Second, various states have undertaken programs of nuclear re-armament that reach beyond maintenance and replacement of existing systems, opposing the spirit of the Nuclear Non-Proliferation Treaty's commitment to continued disarmament.[153] For example, the

US recently deployed a new low-yield submarine-launched ballistic missile and requested funding for research and development on a new sea-launched cruise missile.[154] Seeing its nuclear arsenal as guarantor of its great-power status, Russia has modernised its nuclear arsenal,[155] as well as investing in a new generation of exotic nuclear delivery systems, including Poseidon (autonomous submarine nuclear drones),[156] Burevestnik (nuclear-powered cruise missile),[157] Kinzhal (air-launched ballistic missile), and Avangard (hypersonic glide vehicle).[158] While the Chinese nuclear force still lags substantially behind those of its rivals in size, it too has begun a program of nuclear force expansion; analysts estimate that its arsenal has recently surpassed France's to become the world's third largest,[159] and there are concerns that the construction of new ICBM fields shows an expansion in force posture from minimum to medium deterrence.[160] China in 2021 also conducted an alleged test of a Fractional Orbital Bombardment System (FOBS).[161] In its 2021 Integrated Review, the UK recommended an expansion of its nuclear stockpile by over 40%, to 260 warheads.[162]

The third trend relates to the ways in which strategic stability is further strained by the introduction of new technologies, from the United States' Conventional Prompt Global Strike to a range of programs aimed at delivering hypervelocity missiles, which risk exacerbating nuclear dangers by shortening decision timelines, or which introduce 'warhead ambiguity' around conventional strikes which could be mistaken as nuclear ones.[163] New technologies will make states more adept at targeting one another's nuclear arsenals, creating a sense of instability that could lead to pre-emption and/or arms-racing.[164] Not only are states engaging individually in the development of these technologies, the last few years have also seen an increasing number of strategic military partnerships involving such technologies, and shaping and constraining their use.[165]

In sum, there are several external trends that frame the historical intersection of nuclear risk with emerging military AI technologies: an increase in inter-state geopolitical tensions, state nuclear rearmament or armament, and the introduction of other novel adjacent technologies. These trends all intersect with the advances of military AI, and against the backdrop of an alleged 'AI Cold War'.[166]

This brings us back to our preceding discussion: even if many military AI applications are not a direct GCR, there are concerns at their intersection with nuclear weapons. Yet how, specifically, could the use of AI systems to automate, support, attack, disrupt, or change nuclear decision-making interact with the already complex geometry of deterrence, creating new avenues for deliberate or inadvertent global nuclear catastrophe?

Nuclear weapons and AI: Usage and escalation scenarios

As discussed, militaries have a long history of integrating computing technologies with their operations—and strategic and nuclear forces are no exception. This has led some to raise concerns about the potential risks of such integrations. In the late 1980s, Alan Borning noted that "[g]iven the devastating consequences of nuclear war, it is appropriate to look at current and planned uses of computers in nuclear weapons command and control systems, and to examine whether these systems can fulfil their intended roles".[167] On the Soviet side, there were similar concerns over the possibility of triggering a 'computer war', especially in combination with launch on warning postures and the militarisation of space. As Soviet scholar Borish Raushenbakh noted, "[t]otal computerization of any battle system is fraught with grave danger".[168] Scruples notwithstanding, during the late Cold War the Soviet Union did in fact develop and deploy the 'Perimeter' (or 'Dead Hand') system; while still including a small number of human operators, when switched on during a crisis period the system was configured to (semi-)automatically launch the USSR's nuclear arsenal, if its sensors detected signs of a nuclear attack and lost touch with the Kremlin.[169]

As previously stated, concerns about the potentially escalatory effects of AI on the nuclear landscape have been somewhat more extensively examined than other possible military AI GCR scenarios. In this section, we examine established research investigating potential risk scenarios arising from the intersection between AI and the nuclear weapons infrastructure. We therefore concern ourselves not only with the direct integration of AI into nuclear decision-making functions, such as launch orders, but also with the application of AI in supporting or tangentially associated systems, as well as its indirect effects on the broader geopolitical landscape. Throughout the Cold War, US and Soviet NC3 featured automated components, but today there is an increasing risk that AI will begin to erode human safeguards against nuclear war. Although NC3 differs by country, we define it broadly as *the combination of warning, communication, and weapon systems—as well as human analysts, decision-makers, and operators—involved in ordering and executing nuclear strikes, as well as preventing unauthorised use of nuclear weapons.*

NC3 systems can include satellites, early warning radars, command centres, communication links, launch control centres, and operators of nuclear delivery platforms. Depending on the country, individuals involved in nuclear decision-making might include operators of warning radars, analysts sifting through intelligence to provide information about current and future threats, authorities who authorise the decision to use nuclear weapons, or operators who execute orders.[170] Differences in posture among nuclear weapon possessors mean that their NC3 varies considerably: for example, while China has dual-use land- and sea-based nuclear weapons,[171] the United Kingdom has only a sea-based nuclear deterrent, and its NC3 systems do not support any conventional operations.[172]

To understand how AI could affect the risk of a global nuclear war, it is important to distinguish between distinct escalation routes. Following a typology by Johnson,[173] we can distinguish intentional and unintentional escalation. Under (1) *intentional* escalation, one state has (or gains) a set of (AI + nuclear) strategic capabilities, as a result of which they knowingly take an escalatory action for strategic gain (e.g. they perceive they have a first-strike advantage, and launch a decapitation strike); this stands in contrast to various forms of (2) *unintentional* escalation— situations where "an actor crosses a threshold that it considers benign, but the other side considers significant".[174]

Specifically, unintentional escalation can be further subdivided into (2a) *inadvertent* escalation (mistaken usage on the basis of incorrect information); (2b) *catalytic* escalation (nuclear war between actors A and B, triggered by the malicious actions of a third party C against either party's NC3 systems); or (2c) *accidental* escalation (nuclear escalation without a deliberate and properly informed launch decision, triggered by a combination of human and machine interaction failures, as well as background organisational factors).[175]

Additionally, AI can be used in, around, and against NC3 in a number of ways, all of which can contribute to different combinations of escalation risk (and thereby GCR). We will therefore review some uses of military AI, and how these could increase the risk of one or more escalation routes being triggered.

Autonomised decision-making

The first risk involves integrating AI directly into NC3 nuclear decision-making.[176] This could involve giving systems the ability to authorise launches, and/or to allow AI systems to compose lists of targets or attack patterns following a launch order, in ways that might not be subject to human supervision.

It should be immediately noted that few states currently appear interested in the outright automation of nuclear command and control in any serious way.[177] While commentators within the US defence establishment have called for the US to create its own AI-supported nuclear 'Dead Hand',[178] senior defence officials have explicitly claimed they draw the line at such automation, ensuring there will always be a human in the loop of nuclear decision-making.[179] Likewise, Chinese programs on military AI currently do not appear focused on automated nuclear launch.[180]

Indeed, in addition to a lack of interest, there may be outstanding technical limits and constraints posed by existing AI progress. For instance, it has been argued that current machine-learning systems do not lend themselves well to integration in nuclear targeting, given the difficulty of collating sufficient (and sufficiently reliable) training datasets of imagery of nuclear targets (e.g. mobile launch vehicles), which some have argued will provide 'enduring obstacles' to implementation.[181] If that is the case, highly anticipated applications may remain beyond current AI capabilities.

Nonetheless, even if no state is known to have directly done so today, and some technical barriers remain for some time, this avenue cannot be ruled out and should be cautiously observed. If configurations of

AI decision-making with nuclear forces were developed, this could introduce considerable new risks of false alarms, or of *accidental* escalation—especially given the history of cascading 'normal accidents' that have affected nuclear forces.[182]

Human decision-making under pressure

More broadly, the inclusion of AI technology in NC3 may increase the pace of conflicts, reducing the time frame in which decisions can occur and increasing the potential likelihood for inadvertent or accidental escalation.[183] As the perception of an adversary's capabilities are equally as important in deterrence efforts as their actual capabilities, a military's understanding of what (their or their adversaries') military AI systems are in fact able to accomplish may also spur miscalculation and inadvertent escalation.[184] Therefore, AI systems might not need to be deployed to create a destabilising nuclear scenario, as long as they are perceived as creating additional pressures that can lead to miscalculation, or rushed and ill-informed actions.[185]

AI in systems peripheral to NC3

Furthermore, AI does not need to be directly integrated into NC3 itself in order to affect the risks of nuclear war. As noted by Avin and Amadae, while there has been extensive attention on first-order effects of introducing technologies into nuclear command-and-control and weapon-delivery systems, there are also higher-order effects which "stem from the introduction of such technologies into more peripheral systems, with an indirect (but no less real) effect on nuclear risk".[186] For instance, even if militaries believe that AI is not usable for direct nuclear targeting or command, AI systems can still bring about cascading effects through their integration into systems that peripherally impact the safe and secure functioning of NC3; these might include electrical grids, computer systems providing access to relevant intelligence, or weapon platforms associated with the transportation, delivery, or safekeeping of nuclear warheads.

AI as threat to the information environment and accurate intelligence

A fourth avenue of risk is regarding AI's effects on the broader information environment surrounding, framing, and informing nuclear decision-making. In recent years, researchers have begun to explore the ways in which novel AI tools can enable disinformation,[187] and how this may affect societies' epistemic security[188] in ways that make it harder to agree on truth and take coordinated actions that could be crucial for societies to mitigate GCRs (whether this includes coordinated de-escalation around nuclear risks, or other coordination to mitigate other GCRs). For instance, Favaro has mapped how a range of technologies, including AI, might serve as Weapons of Mass Distortion.[189] She distinguishes four clusters of technological effects on the information environment—those that "distort", "compress", "thwart", or "illuminate". A more contested or unclear information environment would also open up new attack surfaces that could be exploited by third-party actors to trigger catalytic escalation amongst its adversaries.

AI as cyber threat to NC3 integrity

Whereas some AI uses within NC3 might be dangerous because of the vulnerabilities they create (as failure points, human decision compressors, or attack surfaces), another channel could involve the use of AI as a *tool* for attacking NC3 systems (regardless of whether they involve AI). This could involve the use of AI-enabled cyber capabilities to attack and disrupt NC3.[190] Experts are increasingly concerned that NC3 is vulnerable to cyberattacks, and that the resulting escalation or unauthorised launch could potentially trigger a GCR scenario.[191] AI technology has been shown to be capable of facilitating increasingly powerful and sophisticated cyberattacks, with increased precision, scope, and scale.[192] Although there is no evidence of states systematically deploying AI-enabled cyber-offensive weapons to date, the convergence of AI and cyber-offensive tools could exacerbate the vulnerabilities of NC3.[193] This could lead to deliberate escalation of offensive cyber-security strategies.[194]

Cyber attacks also can be hard to detect and attribute (quickly);[195] therefore they may be misconstrued, leading to unintentional or catalytic escalation. For example, an offensive operation targeting dual-use conventional assets could be interpreted as an attack on NC3.[196] It is also broadly agreed that AI acts as a force multiplier for cyber-offensive capabilities.[197] However, it is less clear whether AI will strengthen cyber defence to the same degree as it might strengthen offensive capabilities. The precise effect on the offence-defence balance may be critical to the overall picture.[198] Stronger offensive capabilities could further increase the risk of pre-emptive cyber attacks and subsequently intentional escalation, which would be especially dangerous in the context of nuclear weapon systems.

Broader impacts of AI on nuclear strategic stability

Moreover, the broader deployment of military AI in many other areas could indirectly lead to the disruption of nuclear strategic stability, which could increase the risk of potential intentional or inadvertent escalation.

AI technology could be used to improve a state's capabilities in locating and monitoring an adversary's nuclear second-strike capabilities. For example, better and cheaper autonomous naval drones could track nuclear-armed submarines. This, in turn, could increase the state's perception of likely success in destroying said capabilities before the state's adversary is able to utilise them, and therefore may make a pre-emptive nuclear strike a more attractive strategy than before.[199] Other risks could come from the integration of AI in novel autonomous platforms that are able to operate and loiter in sensitive areas for longer.[200] Even if they were only deployed in order to monitor rival nuclear forces, their pre-positioned presence close to those nuclear assets might prove destabilising, by convincing a defender that they are being deployed to 'scout out' or engage nuclear weapons in advance of a first strike. In these ways, autonomous systems could increase the risks of intentional escalation (when they give a genuine first-strike advantage to one state, or are perceived to do so by another), inadvertent escalation (when errors in their information streams lead to a misinformed decision to launch), or accidental escalation risks, starting the chain of escalation towards a nuclear GCR. Zwetsloot and Dafoe concur that this increased perception of insecurity in nuclear systems could lead to states feeling pressured during times of unrest to engage in pre-emptive escalations.[201]

Finally, in an effort to gain a real or perceived nuclear strategic advantage against their adversaries, while engaging in an AI race, states may place less value on AI safety concerns and more on technological development.[202] This could result in what Danzig has called a "technology roulette"[203] dynamic, with increased risk of prematurely adopting unsafe AI technology in ways that could have profound impacts on the safety or stability of states' nuclear systems.

Contributing factors to AI-nuclear risks

It is important to keep in mind that the risks generated jointly by AI and nuclear weapons are a function of several factors. Firstly, nuclear force posture differs by country, with some forces being more aggressively postured, in ways that enable swifter or immediate use. Additionally, depending on NC3 system design and the degree of force modernisation, AI will interact differently with NC3's component parts—and even dangerously, with brittle legacy systems. Third, the relative robustness or vulnerability of NC3 systems to cyberattacks, for example, will impact systems' resilience to malicious attacks. Along those lines, states' perception of their own vulnerability (as well as the aggressiveness of attackers) will impact stability. This is especially true given that, within complex systems and even through the use of extensive red teaming, it is impossible to identify all system flaws. Fourth, governments' willingness to prematurely deploy AI, either within NC3 and surrounding systems or to augment offensive options for targeting NC3, will be a determinant of catastrophic risk. Fifth, open dialogue, arms control, and risk reduction measures can reduce the potential for nuclear escalation, and a lack of such dialogue can be detrimental. Lastly, luck and normal accidents will inevitably play a role—a fact which highlights unpredictable outcomes amid increased complexity.

Questions for the GCR community

The above discussion has covered a wide range of themes and risk vectors to explore whether—or in what ways—military AI technology is a GCR. Given this, what are the lessons and insights? What policies will be needed to mitigate the potential global catastrophic risks from military AI technology, especially at the intersection with nuclear risk?

Finally, going forward as a field, what are the new lines of research that are needed?

There are lessons specific for the different communities, future questions they should take on, and outlines for an integrated research agenda into military technology, actors, and GCRs that will need further urgent exploration. This chapter has highlighted the urgent need for greater conversation between the different communities engaged on GCRs; on the ethics, safety, and implications of AI; and on nuclear weapons and their risks. We require cross-pollination between these fields, as well as contributions from people with robust expertise in AI and nuclear policy.

In the first place, scholars in defence should reckon with safety and reliability risks around military AI in particular (especially insofar as it poses a GCR), including topics such as robustness, explainability, or susceptibility to adversarial input ('spoofing'). To mitigate these risks, there is value in working with defence industry stakeholders to draw red lines, and to clarify procurement processes.[204]

For nuclear thinkers, there should be greater understanding of the complexities and risks of introducing AI technologies in nuclear weapons. Practically, it will be critical to study how the changing risks of nuclear war—as mediated by AI and machine learning—will impact not just GCR risk, but also the established taboo on nuclear weapons use. How will these changing risks impact governments' calculus about maintaining nuclear arsenals? Are there grounds for optimism about whether or how the 'nuclear taboo' might be elaborated or even extended to a nuclear-AI taboo?

Finally, for experts in both the military and AI fields, more attention needs to be dedicated to investigating the complex and quickly evolving environment that is military AI—especially risks arising at the intersection between nuclear weapons and AI. As made clear in this chapter, concerns around this are not as clear-cut as one might believe upon first glance. Instead, there are a number of possible risk vectors arising from the use of AI throughout the wider landscape, all of which could lead to different forms of nuclear escalation.

In addition, while our analysis in this chapter has made it clear that, at present, there is a small risk of LAWS becoming GCRs, this may not always be the case. It would be useful not only to continue to monitor the development of LAWS to assess if the likelihood of them leading to global catastrophic events alters, but also to find out how they may interact with other potential GCRs. For example, what might be the possibility of using LAWS to deliver WMDs, and what kind of risk impact could the combination of the two feasibly have? This is another potentially worthwhile avenue for future research.

It is clear that the question 'Is military AI a GCR?' is not only complicated to address, but also a moving target owing to the rapidly evolving technology and risk landscape. To be clear: our preliminary analysis in this chapter has suggested that not all military AI applications qualify as GCRs; however, it also highlights that there are distinct pathways of concern. This is especially the case where emerging military AI technologies intersect with the existing arsenals and command infrastructures of established GCR-level technologies—most notably nuclear weapons. All in all, we invite scholars and practitioners from across the defence studies, GCR, and AI fields (and beyond) to take up the aforementioned challenges, ensuring that this next chapter in global technological risk is not the final one.

Acknowledgements

The authors thank the editors, and in particular SJ Beard and Clarissa Rios Rojas, for their feedback and guidance. For additional and particularly detailed comments on earlier drafts of this chapter, we thank Haydn Belfield and Eva Siegmaim. Matthijs Maas also thanks Seth Baum and Uliana Certan (Global Catastrophic Risk Institute) for conversations and parallel work that clarified some of the arguments and shape of this debate.

Notes and References

1   Beard, S.J. and R. Bronson, 'The story so far: how humanity avoided existential catastrophe', in this volume.

2   Picker, C.B., 'A view from 40,000 feet: International law and the invisible hand of technology', *Cardozo Law Rev., 23* (2001), pp.151–219; Allenby, B., 'Are new technologies undermining the laws of war?', *Bull. At. Sci., 70* (2014), pp.21–31; Deudney, D., 'Turbo change: Accelerating technological

disruption, planetary geopolitics, and architectonic metaphors', *Int. Stud. Rev., 20* (2018), pp.223–31.

3   Boulanin, V. and M. Verbruggen, *Mapping the Development of Autonomy in Weapon Systems, 147* (2017). https://www.sipri.org/sites/default/ files/2017-11/siprireport_mapping_the_development_of_autonomy_in_ weapon_systems_1117_1.pdf. Crootof, R., 'The killer robots are here: Legal and policy implications', *CARDOZO LAW Rev., 36* (2015), p.80; Haner, J. and D. Garcia, 'The artificial Intelligence arms race: Trends and world leaders in autonomous weapons development', *Glob. Policy, 10* (2019), pp.331–37.

4   De Spiegeleire, S., M.M. Maas, and T. Sweijs, *Artificial Intelligence and the Future of Defense: Strategic Implications for Small- and Medium-Sized Force Providers*. The Hague Centre for Strategic Studies (2017).

5   Amodei, D. et al., *Concrete Problems in AI Safety* (2016). Lehman, J. et al., 'The surprising creativity of digital evolution: A collection of anecdotes from the evolutionary computation and artificial life research communities', *Artif. Life, 26* (2019); Arthur Holland, M., *Known Unknowns: Data Issues and Military Autonomous Systems*. (2021). https://www.unidir. org/known-unknowns

6   Belfield, H., A. Jayanti, and S. Avin, *Written Evidence to the UK Parliament Defence Committee's Inquiry on Defence Industrial Policy: Procurement and Prosperity* (2020). https://committees.parliament.uk/ writtenevidence/4785/default/

7   Horowitz, M.C. and L. Kahn, 'How Joe Biden can use confidence-building measures for military uses of AI', *Bull. At. Sci., 77* (2021), pp.33–35. Horowitz, M.C. and P. Scharre, *AI and International Stability: Risks and Confidence-Building Measures* (2021). https://www.cnas.org/publications/reports/ ai-and-international-stability-risks-and-confidence-building-measures

8   Yudkowsky, E., 'Artificial intelligence as a positive and negative factor in global risk', *Global Catastrophic Risks*. Oxford University Press (2008), pp.308–45; Bostrom, N., *Superintelligence: Paths, Dangers, Strategies*. Oxford University Press (2014); Ngo (2020); Russell (2019); Burden, Clarke, & Whittlestone (2022).

9   Goertzel, B., 'Artificial general intelligence: Concept, state of the art, and future prospects', *J. Artif. Gen. Intell,. 5* (2014), pp.1–48.

10   Grace, K., J. Salvatier, A. Dafoe, B. Zhang, and O. Evans, 'When will AI exceed human performance? Evidence from AI experts', *J. Artif. Intell. Res., 62* (2018), pp.729–54.

11   Gruetzemacher, R. and J. Whittlestone, 'The transformative potential of artificial intelligence', *Futures, 135* (2022), p.102884.

12   Russell, S., *Human Compatible: Artificial Intelligence and the Problem of Control.* Viking (2019); Burden, J., S. Clarke, and J, 'From Turing's speculations to an academic discipline: A history of AI existential safety', in this volume.

13   Future of Life Institute, 'AI safety myths', *Future of Life Institute* (2016). https://futureoflife.org/background/aimyths/

14   Cremer, C.Z., 'Deep limitations? Examining expert disagreement over deep learning', *Prog. Artif. Intell., 10* (2021), pp. 449–64. https://doi.org/10.1007/s13748-021-00239-1

15   Karnofsky, H., 'AI timelines: Where the arguments, and the 'experts,' stand', *Cold Takes* (2021). https://www.cold-takes.com/where-ai-forecasting-stands-today/

16   Hendrycks, D., N. Carlini, J. Schulman, and J. Steinhardt, 'Unsolved problems in ML safety', *ArXiv210913916 Cs* (2021); Amodei (2016).

17   Amodei, D. and J. Clark, 'Faulty reward functions in the wild', *OpenAI* (2016). https://openai.com/blog/faulty-reward-functions/; Krakovna, V. et al., 'Specification gaming: The flip side of AI ingenuity', *Deepmind* (2020). https://deepmind.com/blog/article/Specification-gaming-the-flip-side-of-AI-ingenuity; Turner, A.M., L. Smith, R. Shah, A. Critch, and P. Tadepalli, 'Optimal policies tend to seek power', *ArXiv191201683 Cs* (2021).

18   Cotra, A., 'Why AI alignment could be hard with modern deep learning', *Cold Takes* (2021). https://www.cold-takes.com/why-ai-alignment-could-be-hard-with-modern-deep-learning

19   Ngo, R., *AGI Safety From First Principles.* (2020).

20   Turchin, A., *Could Slaughterbots Wipe Out Humanity? Assessment of the Global Catastrophic Risk Posed by Autonomous Weapons* (2018); Turchin, A. and D. Denkenberger, 'Military AI as a convergent goal of self-improving AI', in R. Yampolskiy, *Artificial Intelligence Safety and Security.* CRC Press (2018); Vold, K. and D.R. Harris, 'How does artificial intelligence pose an existential risk?', in C. Veliz, *Oxford Handbook of Digital Ethics.* Oxford University Press (2021).

21   Levin, J.-C. and M.M. Maas, 'Roadmap to a roadmap: How could we tell when AGI is a 'Manhattan project' away?', 1st International Workshop on Evaluating Progress in Artificial Intelligence - EPAI 2020. (2020).

22   Grace, K., *Leó Szilárd and the Danger of Nuclear Weapons: A Case Study in Risk Mitigation* (2015). https://intelligence.org/files/SzilardNuclearWeapons.pdf

23   Maas, M.M., 'How viable is international arms control for military artificial intelligence? Three lessons from nuclear weapons', *Contemp. Secur. Policy, 40* (2019), pp.285–311; Zaidi, W. and A. Dafoe, *International Control of Powerful Technology: Lessons from the Baruch Plan* (2021). https://www.fhi.ox.ac.uk/wp-content/uploads/2021/03/International-Control-of-Powerful-Technology-Lessons-from-the-Baruch-Plan-Zaidi-Dafoe-2021.pdf

24   Leung, J., *Who Will Govern Artificial Intelligence? Learning From the History of Strategic Politics in Emerging Technologies.* University of Oxford (2019). Ding, J. and A. Dafoe, 'The logic of strategic assets: From oil to AI', *Secur. Stud.* (2021), pp.1–31. https://doi.org/10.1080/09636412.2021.1915583; Ding, J. and A. Dafoe, 'Engines of power: Electricity, AI, and general-purpose military transformations', *ArXiv210604338 Econ Q-Fin* (2021).

25   Beard & Bronson (2023).

26   Baum, S.D. and A.M. Barrett, 'Global catastrophes: The most extreme risks', in V. Bier, *Risks in Extreme Environments: Preparing, Avoiding, Mitigating, and Managing.* Routledge (2018), pp.174–84.

27   Bostrom, N. and M.M. Ćirković, 'Introduction', *Global Catastrophic Risks.* Oxford University Press (2011).

28   Weinberger, S. *The Imagineers of War: The Untold Story of DARPA, the Pentagon Agency That Changed the World.* Random House LLC (2017); Roland, A. and P. Shiman, *Strategic Computing: DARPA and the Quest for Machine Intelligence, 1983–1993.* MIT Press (2002).

29   Gordon, T.J. and O. Helmer, *Report on a Long-Range Forecasting Study* (1964). http://stat.haifa.ac.il/~gweiss/courses/OR-logistics/Rand.pdf

30   Defense Science Board Task Force, *Report of the Defense Science Board Task Force on Command and Control Systems Management, 49* (1978).

31   Roland & Shiman (2002).

32   Biddle, S., 'Victory misunderstood: What the Gulf War tells us about the future of conflict', *Int. Secur., 21* (1996), pp.139–79.

33   Cross, S.E. and E. Walker, 'DART: Applying knowledge based planning and scheduling to CRISIS action planning', in M. Zweben and M. Fox, *Intelligent Scheduling.* Morgan Kaufmann (1994), pp.711–29; Hedberg, S.R., 'DART: Revolutionizing logistics planning', *IEEE Intell. Syst., 17* (2002), pp.81–83.

34   Scharre, P., *Autonomous Weapons and Operational Risk* (2016). https://s3.amazonaws.com/files.cnas.org/documents/CNAS_Autonomous-weapons-operational-risk.pdf

35   Scharre, P., *Autonomous Weapons and Stability*. King's College (2020).

36   Scharre (2020).

37   Haner & Garcia (2019).

38   Research and Markets Ltd., *Artificial Intelligence in Military Market by Offering* (*Software, Hardware, Services*), *Technology* (*Machine Learning, Computer vision*), *Application, Installation Type, Platform, Region—Global Forecast to 2025* (2021). https://www.researchandmarkets.com/reports/5306656/artificial-intelligence-in-military-market-by

39   Haner & Garcia (2019).

40   Haner, J.K., *Dark Horses in the Lethal AI Arms Race* (2019). https://justinkhaner.com/aiarmsrace

41   Trajtenberg, M., *AI as the Next GPT: A Political-Economy Perspective* (2018). http://www.nber.org/papers/w24245 doi:10.3386/w24245; Leung (2019)

42   Maas, M.M., *Artificial Intelligence Governance Under Change: Foundations, Facets, Frameworks*. University of Copenhagen (2020); Drezner, D.W., 'Technological change and international relations', *Int. Relat.*, 33 (2019), pp.286–303.

43   Morgan, F.E. et al., *Military Applications of Artificial Intelligence: Ethical Concerns in an Uncertain World*, 224 (2020). https://www.rand.org/content/dam/rand/pubs/research_reports/RR3100/RR3139-1/RAND_RR3139-1.pdf

44   Allen, G. and T. Chan, *Artificial Intelligence and National Security* (2017). http://www.belfercenter.org/sites/default/files/files/publication/AI%20NatSec%20-%20final.pdf

45   Kania, E., 'AlphaGo and beyond: The Chinese military looks to future "intelligentized" warfare', *Lawfare* (2017). https://www.lawfareblog.com/alphago-and-beyond-chinese-military-looks-future-intelligentized-warfare

46   Ding & Dafoe (2021).

47   Nelson, A.J., *The Impact of Emerging Technologies on Arms Control Regimes* (2018).

48   Allen & Chan, (2017).

49   Horowitz, M.C., 'Do emerging military technologies matter for international politics?', *Annu. Rev. Polit. Sci.*, 23 (2020), pp.385–400.

50   Defense Science Board, *Defense Science Board Summer Study on Autonomy* (2016). https://www.hsdl.org/?abstract&did=794641

51 Soare, S.R., *Digital Divide? Transatlantic Defence Cooperation on Artificial Intelligence* (2020). https://www.iss.europa.eu/content/digital-divide-transatlantic-defence-cooperation-ai

52 Adamsky, D., *The Culture of Military Innovation: The Impact of Cultural Factors on the Revolution in Military Affairs in Russia, the US, and Israel.* Stanford University Press (2010).

53 Verbruggen, M., 'The role of civilian innovation in the development of lethal autonomous weapon systems', *Glob. Policy, 10* (2019), pp.338–42.

54 Soare (2020).

55 Gilli, A., *Preparing for "NATO-mation": The Atlantic Alliance Toward the Age of Artificial Intelligence* (2019). http://www.ndc.nato.int/news/news.php?icode=1270

56 Verbruggen, M., 'Drone swarms: Coming (sometime) to a war near you. Just not today', *Bulletin of the Atomic Scientists* (2021). https://thebulletin.org/2021/02/drone-swarms-coming-sometime-to-a-war-near-you-just-not-today/

57 Gilli, A. and M. Gilli, 'Why China has not caught up yet: military-technological superiority and the limits of imitation, reverse engineering, and cyber espionage', *Int. Secur., 43* (2019), pp.141–89.

58 Amodei, D. and D. Hernandez, 'AI and compute', *OpenAI Blog* (2018). https://openai.com/research/ai-and-compute

59 Ayoub, K. and K. Payne, 'Strategy in the age of artificial intelligence', *J. Strateg. Stud., 39* (2016), pp.793–819; Horowitz, M.C., 'Artificial intelligence, international competition, and the balance of power', *Texas National Security Review* (2018).

60 Dafoe, A., 'On technological determinism: A typology, scope conditions, and a mechanism', *Sci. Technol. Hum. Values, 40* (2015), pp.1047–076.

61 Maas (2019).

62 Bleek, P.C., *When Did (and Didn't) States Proliferate? Chronicling the Spread of Nuclear Weapons, 56* (2017). https://www.belfercenter.org/sites/default/files/files/publication/When%20Did%20%28and%20Didn%27t%29%20States%20Proliferate%3F_1.pdf; Meyer, S., S. Bidgood, and W.C. Potter, 'Death dust: The little-known story of US and Soviet pursuit of radiological weapons', *Int. Secur., 45* (2020), pp.51–94.

63 Rosert, E. and F. Sauer, 'How (not) to stop the killer robots: A comparative analysis of humanitarian disarmament campaign strategies', *Contemp. Secur. Policy, 0* (2020), pp.1–25. https://www.tandfonline.com/doi/full/10.1080/13523260.2020.1771508; Belfield, H., 'Activism by the AI community:

Analysing recent achievements and future prospects', *Proceedings of the AAAI/ACM Conference on AI, Ethics, and Society.* ACM (2020), pp.15–21. https://doi.org/10.1145/3375627.3375814

64 McDonald, J., *What If Military AI Is a Washout?* (2021). https://jackmcdonald.org/book/2021/06/what-if-military-ai-sucks/

65 McDonald (2021).

66 Garfinkel, B. and A. Dafoe, 'How does the offense-defense balance scale?', *J. Strateg. Stud.*, 42 (2019), pp.736–63; Lieber, K.A., 'Grasping the technological peace: the offense-defense balance and international security', *Int. Secur.*, 25 (2000), p.71.

67 Payne, K., *I, Warbot: The Dawn of Artificially Intelligent Conflict.* C Hurst & Co Publishers Ltd (2021).

68 Boulanin & Verbruggen (2017).

69 Blain, L., *South Korea's Autonomous Robot Gun Turrets: Deadly From Kilometers Away* (2010). http://newatlas.com/korea-dodamm-super-aegis-autonomos-robot-gun-turret/17198/; Velez-Green, A., 'The foreign policy essay: The South Korean sentry—a "killer robot" to prevent war', *Lawfare* (2015). https://www.lawfareblog.com/foreign-policy-essay-south-korean-sentry%E2%80%94-killer-robot-prevent-war

70 Israel Aerospace Industries, *Harpy Loitering Weapon* (2020). https://www.iai.co.il/p/harpy.

71 Future of Life Institute, '5 real-life technologies that prove autonomous weapons are already here', *Future of Life Institute* (2021). https://futureoflife.org/2021/11/22/5-real-life-technologies-that-prove-autonomous-weapons-are-already-here/

72 Tucker, P., 'SecDef: China is exporting killer robots to the Mideast', *Defense One* (2019). https://www.defenseone.com/technology/2019/11/secdef-china-exporting-killer-robots-mideast/161100/

73 Trevithick, J., 'Turkey now has swarming suicide drones it could export', *The Drive* (2020).

74 UN Panel of Experts on Libya, *Letter dated 8 March 2021 from the Panel of Experts on Libya established pursuant to resolution 1973* (2021). https://undocs.org/pdf?symbol=en/S/2021/229; Cramer, M., 'A.I. Drone may have acted on its own in attacking fighters, U.N. says', *The New York Times* (2021).

75 Kesteloo, H., 'Punisher drones are positively game-changing for Ukrainian military in fight against Russia', *DroneXL* (2022). https://dronexl.co/2022/03/03/punisher-drones-ukrainian-military/; Trabucco, L. and

K.J. Heller, 'Beyond the ban: Comparing the ability of 'killer robots' and human soldiers to comply with IHL', *Fletcher Forum World Aff. 46* (2022).

76 Scharre, P., *Robotics on the Battlefield, Part II: The Coming Swarm, 68* (2014). https://www.cnas.org/publications/reports/robotics-on-the-battlefield-part-ii-the-coming-swarm

77 Hambling, D., 'Israel's combat-proven drone swarm may be start of a new kind of warfare', *Forbes* (2021). https://www.forbes.com/sites/davidhambling/2021/07/21/israels-combat-proven-drone-swarm-is-more-than-just-a-drone-swarm/

78 Michel, A.H., 'The killer algorithms nobody's talking about', *Foreign Policy* (2020). https://foreignpolicy.com/2020/01/20/ai-autonomous-weapons-artificial-intelligence-the-killer-algorithms-nobodys-talking-about/

79 Bergman, R. and F. Fassihi, 'The scientist and the A.I.-assisted, remote-control killing machine', *The New York Times* (2021).

80 Knight, W., 'A dogfight renews concerns about AI's lethal potential', *Wired* (2020).

81 US Department of Defense, *Department of Defense Announces Successful Micro-Drone Demonstration*. US Department of Defense (2017). https://www.defense.gov/News/Releases/Release/Article/1044811/department-of-defense-announces-successful-micro-drone-demonstration/

82 Chavannes, E., K. Klonowska, and T. Sweijs, 'Governing autonomous weapon systems: Expanding the solution space, from scoping to applying', *HCSS Secur., 39* (2020); Rosert, & Sauer (2020).

83 Carpenter, C., *'Lost' Causes, Agenda Vetting in Global Issue Networks and the Shaping of Human Security*. Cornell University Press (2014). https://doi.org/10.7591/9780801470363

84 Liu, H.-Y., 'Categorization and legality of autonomous and remote weapons systems', *Int. Rev. Red Cross, 94* (2012), pp.627–52; Anderson, K., D. Reisner, and M. Waxman, 'Adapting the law of armed conflict to autonomous weapon systems', *Int. Law Stud., 90* (2014), p.27.

85 Human Rights Watch, *Shaking the Foundations: The Human Rights Implications of Killer Robots* (2014).

86 Rosert, E. and F. Sauer, 'Prohibiting autonomous weapons: Put human dignity first', *Glob. Policy, 10* (2019), pp.370–75; Rosert, & Sauer (2020).

87 Kallenborn, Z., 'Meet the future weapon of mass destruction, the drone swarm', *Bulletin of the Atomic Scientists* (2021). https://thebulletin.org/2021/04/meet-the-future-weapon-of-mass-destruction-the-drone-swarm/

88   Bahçecik, Ş.O., 'Civil society responds to the AWS: Growing activist networks and shifting frames, *Glob. Policy,* 10(3) (2019), pp. 365–69.

89   Future of Life Institute, *Slaughterbots* (2017). Future of Life Institute, *Slaughterbots—If human: kill( )* (2021).

90   Bahçecik (2019).

91   Turchin, A. and D. Denkenberger, 'Classification of global catastrophic risks connected with artificial intelligence', *AI Soc., 35* (2020), pp.147–63.

92   Kallenborn, Z. and P.C. Bleek, 'Swarming destruction: drone swarms and chemical, biological, radiological, and nuclear weapons', *Nonproliferation Rev., 25* (2018), pp.523–43.

93   Kunz, M. and S. Ó hÉigeartaigh, 'Artificial intelligence and robotization', in R. Geiss and N. Melzer, *Oxford Handbook on the International Law of Global Security.* Oxford University Press (2021).

94   Rogers, J., 'The dark side of our drone future', *Bulletin of the Atomic Scientists* (2019). https://thebulletin.org/2019/10/the-dark-side-of-our-drone-future/

95   Mani, L., A. Tzachor, and P. Cole, 'Global catastrophic risk from lower magnitude volcanic eruptions', *Nat. Commun., 12* (2021), p.4756.

96   Solodov, A., A. Williams, S.A. Hanaei, and B. Goddard, 'Analyzing the threat of unmanned aerial vehicles (UAV) to nuclear facilities', *Secur. J. Lond. 31* (2018), pp.305–24.

97   Tang, A. and L. Kemp, 'A fate worse than warming? Stratospheric aerosol injection and global catastrophic risk', *Front. Clim., 3* (2021), p.144; Baum, S.D., T.M. Maher, and J. Haqq-Misra, 'Double catastrophe: Intermittent stratospheric geoengineering induced by societal collapse', *Environ. Syst. Decis. 33* (2013), pp.168–80.

98   Future of Life Institute, *An Open Letter to the United Nations Convention on Certain Conventional Weapons* (2017). https://futureoflife.org/autonomous-weapons-open-letter-2017/

99   Russell, S., A. Aguirre, A. Conn, and M. Tegmark, 'Why you should fear "slaughterbots"—a response', *IEEE Spectr.* (2018).

100   Turchin, &. Denkenberger (2020).

101   Aguirre, A., 'Why those who care about catastrophic and existential risk should care about autonomous weapons', *EA Forum* (2020). https://forum.effectivealtruism.org/posts/oR9tLNRSAep293rr5/why-those-who-care-about-catastrophic-and-existential-risk-2

102   Turchin (2018).

103   Ibid.

104   Aguirre (2020).

105   Brookings,   *What   Nuclear   Weapons   Delivery   Systems Really   Cost*   (2016).   https://www.brookings.edu/ what-nuclear-weapons-delivery-systems-really-cost/

106   Blumberg, Y., 'Here's how much a nuclear weapon costs', *CNBC* (2017). https://www.cnbc.com/2017/08/08/heres-how-much-a-nuclear-weapon-costs.html

107   UN Secretary-General, *Chemical and Bacteriological (Biological) Weapons and the Effects of Their Possible Use* (1969). Koblentz, G.D., *Living Weapons: Biological Warfare and International Security*. Cornell University Press (2011).

108   Scharre (2014).

109   Baum, S.D., A.M. Barrett, U. Certan, and M.M. Maas, *Autonomous Weapons and the Long-Term Future* (2022).

110   Sabbagh, D., 'Killer drones: How many are there and who do they target?', *The Guardian* (2019).

111   Vailshery, L.S., 'Global   consumer   drone   shipments   2020–2030', *Statista*   (2021).   https://www.statista.com/statistics/1234658/ worldwide-consumer-drone-unit-shipments

112   Hambling, D., 'The U.S. Navy plans to foil massive 'super swarm' drone attacks by using the swarm's intelligence against itself', *Forbes* (2020).

113   Turchin (2018).

114   Kemp, L., 'Agents of doom: Who is creating the apocalypse and why', *BBC Future* (2021).

115   Kallenborn (2021).

116   Baum, Barrett, Certan, & Maas, (2022).

117   Perkovich, G., 'Will you listen? A dialogue on creating the conditions for nuclear disarmament', *Carnegie Endowment for International Peace* (2018). https://carnegieendowment.org/2018/11/02/will-you-listen-dialogue-on-creating-conditions-for-nuclear-disarmament-pub-77614

118   Lewis, J., 'Point and nuke: Remembering the era of portable atomic bombs', *Foreign Policy* (2018). https://foreignpolicy.com/2018/09/12/ point-and-nuke-davy-crockett-military-history-nuclear-weapons/

119   Galison, P L. and B. Bernstein, 'In any light: Scientists and the decision to build the superbomb, 1952–1954', *Hist. Stud. Phys. Biol.*

Sci., 19 (1989), pp.267–347; Wellerstein, A., 'The leak that brought the H-bomb debate out of the cold', *Restricted Data: The Nuclear Secrecy Blog* (2021). http://blog.nuclearsecrecy.com/2021/06/14/the-leak-that-brought-the-h-bomb-debate-out-of-the-cold/

120 Horgan, J., 'Bethe, Teller, Trinity and the end of Earth', *Scientific American Blog Network* (2015). https://blogs.scientificamerican.com/cross-check/bethe-teller-trinity-and-the-end-of-earth/; Ellsberg, D., *The Doomsday Machine: Confessions of a Nuclear War Planner*. Bloomsbury USA (2017).

121 Scarry, E., *Thermonuclear Monarchy: Choosing Between Democracy and Doom*. W. W. Norton & Company (2016).

122 BBC, 'Hiroshima and Nagasaki: 75th anniversary of atomic bombings', *BBC News* (2020).

123 PBS News Hour, 'Types of nuclear bombs', *PBS NewsHour* (2005). https://www.pbs.org/newshour/nation/military-jan-june05-bombs_05-02

124 Toon, O.B. et al, 'Rapidly expanding nuclear arsenals in Pakistan and India portend regional and global catastrophe', *Sci. Adv., 5* (2019).

125 Rosenberg, D.A. and W.B. Moore, "Smoking radiating ruin at the end of two hours': Documents on American plans for nuclear war with the Soviet Union, 1954–55', *Int. Secur., 6* (1981), pp.3–38.

126 Rosenberg, D., 'Constraining overkill: Contending approaches to nuclear strategy, 1955–1965', *Naval History and Heritage Command* (1994).

127 Ellsberg (2017).

128 Badash, L., *A Nuclear Winter's Tale: Science and Politics in the 1980s*. MIT Press (2009). Sagan, C., 'Nuclear war and climatic catastrophe: Some policy implications', *Foreign Aff. 62* (1983), pp.257–92.

129 US Secretary of Defense, 'Nuclear winter: The view from the US Defense Department', *Survival, 27* (1985), pp.130–34.

130 Badash (2009).

131 Tannenwald, N., 'The nuclear taboo: The United States and the normative basis of nuclear non-use', *Int. Organ., 53* (1999), pp.433–68.

132 Sauer, F., *Atomic Anxiety: Deterrence, Taboo and the Non-Use of US Nuclear Weapons*. Springer (2015).

133 Robock, A. and O.B. Toon, 'Local nuclear war, global suffering', *Sci. Am., 302* (2010), pp.74–81.

134 Helfand, I., *Nuclear Famine: Two Billion People At Risk? Global Impacts of Limited Nuclear War on Agriculture, Food Supplies, and Human Nutrition*

(2013). https://www.psr.org/wp-content/uploads/2018/04/two-billion-at-risk.pdf

135 Coupe, J., C.G. Bardeen, A. Robock, and O.B. Toon, 'Nuclear winter responses to nuclear war between the United States and Russia in the whole atmosphere community climate model version 4 and the Goddard Institute for Space Studies Model', *Geophys. Res. Atmospheres, 124* (2019), pp.8522–543.

136 Reisner, J. et al., 'Climate impact of a regional nuclear weapons exchange: An improved assessment based on detailed source calculations', *J. Geophys. Res. Atmospheres, 123* (2018), pp.2752–772.

137 Frankel, M., J. Scouras, and G. Ullrich, *The Uncertain Consequences of Nuclear Weapons Use* (2015). https://apps.dtic.mil/sti/citations/ADA618999

138 Scouras, J., 'Nuclear war as a global catastrophic risk', *J. Benefit-Cost Anal., 10* (2019), pp.274–95.

139 Gavin, F.J., 'We need to talk: The past, present, and future of US nuclear weapons policy', *War on the Rocks* (2017). https://warontherocks. com/2017/01/we-need-to-talk-the-past-present-and-future-of-u-s-nuclear-weapons-policy/

140 Rodriguez, L., *How Likely Is a Nuclear Exchange Between the US and Russia?* (2019). https://rethinkpriorities.org/publications/how-likely-is-a-nuclear-exchange-between-the-us-and-russia; Baum, S., R. de Neufville, and A. Barrett, 'A model for the probability of nuclear war', *Glob. Catastrophic Risk Inst. Work. Pap.* (2018). https://doi.org/10.2139/ssrn.3137081; Baum, S., 'Reflections on the risk analysis of nuclear war', in B.J. Garrick, *Proceedings of the Workshop on Quantifying Global Catastrophic Risks*. Garrick Institute for the Risk Sciences (2018), pp.19–50.

141 Schlosser, E., *Command and Control: Nuclear Weapons, the Damascus Accident, and the Illusion of Safety*. Penguin Books (2014); Sagan, S.D., *The Limits of Safety: Organizations, Accidents, and Nuclear Weapons*. Princeton University Press (1993). https://doi.org/10.1515/9780691213064

142 Sagan, S.D., 'Learning from normal accidents', *Organ. Environ., 17* (2004), pp.15–19.

143 Maas (2019).

144 Maas, M.M., 'Regulating for "normal AI accidents": Operational lessons for the responsible governance of artificial intelligence deployment', *Proceedings of the 2018 AAAI/ACM Conference on AI, Ethics, and Society*. Association for Computing Machinery (2018), pp.223–28. https://doi. org/10.1145/3278721.3278766

145   Rodriguez, L., 'What is the likelihood that civilizational collapse would directly lead to human extinction (within decades)?', *Effective Altruism Forum* (2020). https://forum.effectivealtruism.org/posts/GsjmufaebreiaivF7/what-is-the-likelihood-that-civilizational-collapse-would; Wiblin, R., *Luisa Rodriguez on Why Global Catastrophes Seem Unlikely to Kill Us All.* 80,000 Hours Podcast (2021).

146   Belfield, H., 'Collapse, recovery and existential risk', in P. Callahan, M. Centeno, P. Larcey, and T. Patterson, *The End of the World as We Know It.* Routledge Press (2022).

147   Schubert, S., L. Caviola, and N.S. Faber, 'The psychology of existential risk: Moral judgments about human extinction', *Sci. Rep., 9* (2019), p.15100.

148   Kohler, S., *Cooperative Security and the Nunn-Lugar Act. 4* (1989).

149   Wunderlich, C., H. Müller, and U. Jakob, *WMD Compliance and Enforcement in a Changing Global Context* (2020). https://www.unidir.org/publication/wmd-compliance-and-enforcement-changing-global-context

150   Reif, K. and S. Bugos, 'US, Russia extend new START for five years', *Arms Control Association* (2021). https://www.armscontrol.org/act/2021-03/news/us-russia-extend-new-start-five-years

151   Kühn, U., 'Why arms control is (almost) dead', *Carnegie Europe* (2020). https://carnegieeurope.eu/strategiceurope/81209

152   Wan, W., *Nuclear Escalation Strategies and Perceptions: The United States, the Russian Federation, and China* (2021). https://unidir.org/escalation; https://doi.org/10.37559/WMD/21/NRR/02

153   Lucero-Matteucci, K.T., 'Signs of life in nuclear diplomacy: A look beyond the doom and gloom', *Georget. J. Int. Aff* (2019).

154   Kirstensen, H.M., 'US deploys new low-yield nuclear submarine warhead', *Federation Of American Scientists* (2020). https://fas.org/blogs/security/2020/01/w76-2deployed/

155   Fink, A.L. and O. Oliker, 'Russia's nuclear weapons in a multipolar world: guarantors of sovereignty, great power status & more', *Daedalus, 149* (2020), pp.37–55.

156   Piotrowski, M.A., *Russia's Status-6 Nuclear Submarine Drone (Poseidon)* (2018) https://pism.pl/publications/Russia_s_Status_6_Nuclear_Submarine_Drone__Poseidon_

157   Vaddi, P., 'Bringing Russia's new nuclear weapons into new START', *Carnegie Endowment for International Peace* (2019). https://carnegieendowment.org/2019/08/13/bringing-russia-s-new-nuclear-weapons-into-new-start-pub-79672

158   Edmonds, J. et al., *Artificial Intelligence and Autonomy in Russia* 258 (2021). https://www.cna.org/CNA_files/centers/CNA/sppp/rsp/russia-ai/Russia-Artificial-Intelligence-Autonomy-Putin-Military.pdf

159   Kristensen, H.M. and M. Korda, 'Chinese nuclear weapons, 2021', *Bull. At. Sci.*, 77 (2021), pp.318–36.

160   Kristensen, H.M. and M. Korda, 'China's nuclear missile silo expansion: from minimum deterrence to medium deterrence', *Bulletin of the Atomic Scientists* (2021). https://thebulletin.org/2021/09/chinas-nuclear-missile-silo-expansion-from-minimum-deterrence-to-medium-deterrence/

161   Wright, T., 'Is China gliding toward a FOBS capability?', *IISS* (2021). https://www.iiss.org/blogs/analysis/2021/10/is-china-gliding-toward-a-fobs-capability. Acton, J.M., 'China's tests are no Sputnik moment', *Carnegie Endowment for International Peace* (2021). https://carnegieendowment.org/2021/10/21/china-s-tests-are-no-sputnik-moment-pub-85625

162   Mills, C., *Integrated Review 2021: Increasing the Cap on the UK's Nuclear Stockpile* (2021).

163   Acton, J.M. *Is It a Nuke?: Pre-Launch Ambiguity and Inadvertent Escalation* (2020). https://carnegieendowment.org/2020/04/09/is-it-nuke-pre-launch-ambiguity-and-inadvertent-escalation-pub-81446

164   Futter, A. and B. Zala, 'Strategic non-nuclear weapons and the onset of a Third Nuclear Age', *Eur. J. Int. Secur.*, 6 (2021), pp.257–77.

165   Trabucco, L. and M.M. Maas, 'Into the thick of it: Mapping the emerging landscape of military AI strategic partnerships', in AutoNorms / Center for War Studies (SDU) conference "The Algorithmic Turn in Security and Warfare" (2022); Stanley-Lockman, Z., *Military AI Cooperation Toolbox: Modernizing Defense Science and Technology Partnerships for the Digital Age* (2021). https://cset.georgetown.edu/wp-content/uploads/CSET-Military-AI-Cooperation-Toolbox.pdf; Bendett, S. and E.B. Kania, *A new Sino-Russian High-Tech Partnership: Authoritarian Innovation in an Era of Great-Power Rivalry*, 24 (2019). https://www.aspi.org.au/report/new-sino-russian-high-tech-partnership

166   Thompson, N. and I. Bremmer, 'The AI Cold War that threatens us all', *Wired* (2018).

167   Borning, A., 'Computer system reliability and nuclear war', *Commun. ACM*, 30 (1987), pp.112–31.

168   Raushenbakh, B.V., 'Computer war', in A.A. Gromyko and M. Hellman (eds), *Breakthrough: Emerging New Thinking: Soviet and Western scholars Issue a Challenge to Build a World Beyond War*. Walker (1988).

169   Hoffman, D., *The Dead Hand: The Untold Story of the Cold War Arms Race and Its Dangerous Legacy*. Anchor (2010).

170   Harvey, J.R., 'US nuclear command and control for the 21st century', *Nautilus Institute for Security and Sustainability* (2019). https://nautilus. org/napsnet/napsnet-special-reports/u-s-nuclear-command-and-control-for-the-21st-century/

171   Cunningham, F., 'Nuclear command, control, and communications systems of the People's Republic of China', *Nautilus Institute for Security and Sustainability* (2019). https://nautilus.org/napsnet/napsnet-special-reports/nuclear-command-control-and-communications-systems-of-the-peoples-republic-of-china/

172   Gower, J., *United Kingdom: Nuclear Weapon Command, Control, and Communications* (2019). https://securityandtechnology.org/wp-content/uploads/2020/07/gower_uk_nc3_report_IST.pdf

173   Johnson, J., 'Inadvertent escalation in the age of intelligence machines: A new model for nuclear risk in the digital age', *Eur. J. Int. Secur.* (2021a) pp.1–23.   https://doi.org/10.1017/eis.2021.23;   Johnson,   J.,   ''Catalytic nuclear war' in the age of artificial intelligence & autonomy: Emerging military technology and escalation risk between nuclear-armed states', *J. Strateg. Stud.*, (2021b), pp.1–41.

174   Johnson (2021a).

175   Johnson (2021b).

176   Geist, E. and A.J. Lohn, *How Might Artificial Intelligence Affect the Risk of Nuclear War?*, 28 (2018). https://www.rand.org/pubs/perspectives/PE296.html; Fitzpatrick, M., 'Artificial intelligence and nuclear command and control', *Survival*, 61 (2019), pp.81–92; Field, M., 'Strangelove redux: US experts propose having AI control nuclear weapons', *Bulletin of the Atomic Scientists* (2019). https://thebulletin.org/2019/08/strangelove-redux-us-experts-propose-having-ai-control-nuclear-weapons/; Johnson, J., 'Delegating strategic decision-making to machines: Dr. Strangelove Redux?', *J. Strateg. Stud.*, 45(3) (2022), pp.439–77.

177   Despite speculation that Russia's 'Dead Hand' system is still in use, there is no definitive evidence that this is or will continue to be the case.

178   Lowther, A. and C. McGiffin, 'America needs a "Dead Hand"', *War on the Rocks* (2019). https://warontherocks.com/2019/08/america-needs-a-dead-hand/

179   Freedberg, S.J., 'No AI for nuclear command & control: JAIC's Shanahan', *Breaking Defense* (2019). https://breakingdefense.sites.breakingmedia.com/2019/09/no-ai-for-nuclear-command-control-jaics-shanahan/

180 Fedasiuk, R., 'We spent a year investigating what the Chinese army is buying. Here's what we learned', *POLITICO* (2021). Fedasiuk, R., J. Melot, and B. Murphy, *Harnessed Lightning: How the Chinese Military is Adopting Artificial Intelligence* (2021). https://cset.georgetown.edu/publication/harnessed-lightning/

181 Loss, R. and J. Johnson, 'Will artificial intelligence imperil nuclear deterrence?', *War on the Rocks* (2019). https://warontherocks.com/2019/09/will-artificial-intelligence-imperil-nuclear-deterrence/

182 Maas (2019). Schlosser (2014). Sagan, (1993).

183 Johnson, J.S., 'Artificial intelligence: A threat to strategic stability', *Strateg. Stud. Q.* (Spring 2020), pp.16–39. Payne, K., 'Artificial intelligence: A revolution in strategic affairs?', *Survival, 60* (2018), pp.7–32.

184 Johnson (2020).

185 Amadae, S.M. et al., *The Impact of Artificial Intelligence on Strategic Stability and Nuclear Risk Vol. 1.* SIPRI (2019).

186 Avin, S. and S.M. Amadae, 'Autonomy and machine learning at the interface of nuclear weapons, computers and people', in V. Boulanin (ed), *The Impact of Artificial Intelligence on Strategic Stability and Nuclear Risk.* Stockholm International Peace Research Institute (2019). https://doi.org/10.17863/CAM.44758

187 Citron, D. and R. Chesney, 'Deepfakes and the new disinformation war: The coming age of post-truth geopolitics', *Foreign Affairs, 98* (2019).

188 Epistemic security has been defined as the state which "ensures that a community's processes of knowledge production, acquisition, distribution, and coordination are robust to adversarial (or accidental) influence [such that] [e]pistemically secure environments foster efficient and well-informed group decision-making which helps decision-makers to better achieve their individual and collective goals". Seger, E. et al., *Tackling Threats to Informed Decisionmaking in Democratic Societies: Promoting Epistemic Security in a Technologically-Advanced World* (2020). https://www.turing.ac.uk/research/publications/tackling-threats-informed-decision-making-democratic-societies

189 Favaro, M., *Weapons of Mass Distortion: A New Approach to Emerging Technologies, Risk Reduction, and the Global Nuclear Order* (2021). https://www.kcl.ac.uk/csss/assets/weapons-of-mass-distortion.pdf

190 Johnson, J. and E. Krabill, 'AI, cyberspace, and nuclear weapons', *War on the Rocks* (2020). https://warontherocks.com/2020/01/ai-cyberspace-and-nuclear-weapons/

191   Sharikov, P., 'Artificial intelligence, cyberattack, and nuclear weapons—a dangerous combination', *Bull. At. Sci., 74* (2018), pp.368–73.

192   Schneier, B., *The Coming AI Hackers* (2021). https://www.schneier.com/wp-content/uploads/2021/04/The-Coming-AI-Hackers.pdf; Brundage, M. et al., *The Malicious Use of Artificial Intelligence: Forecasting, Prevention, and Mitigation* (2018). http://arxiv.org/abs/1802.07228

193   Futter, A., *Hacking the Bomb: Cyber Threats and Nuclear Weapons*. Georgetown University Press (2018).

194   Johnson and Krabill (2020).

195   Eilstrup-Sangiovanni, M., 'Why the world needs an international cyberwar convention', *Philos. Technol., 31* (2018), pp.379–407.

196   Johnson, J., 'The AI-cyber nexus: implications for military escalation, deterrence and strategic stability', *J. Cyber Policy* (2019).

197   Gartzke, E. and J.R. Lindsay, 'Weaving tangled webs: Offense, defense, and deception in cyberspace', *Secur. Stud., 24* (2015), pp.316–48.

198   Zwetsloot, R. and A. Dafoe, 'Thinking about risks from AI: Accidents, misuse and structure', *Lawfare* (2019). https://www.lawfareblog.com/thinking-about-risks-ai-accidents-misuse-and-structure

199   Geist, E. and A.J. Lohn, *How Might Artificial Intelligence Affect the Risk of Nuclear War?, 28* (2018). https://www.rand.org/pubs/perspectives/PE296.html . Fitzpatrick (2019).

200   Kallenborn, Z., 'AI risks to nuclear deterrence are real', *War on the Rocks* (2019). https://warontherocks.com/2019/10/ai-risks-to-nuclear-deterrence-are-real/

201   Zwetsloot and Dafoe, (2019).

202   Armstrong, S., N. Bostrom, and C. Shulman, 'Racing to the precipice: A model of artificial intelligence development', *AI Soc., 31* (2016), pp.201–06.

203   Danzig, R., *Technology Roulette: Managing Loss of Control as Many Militaries Pursue Technological Superiority, 40* (2018). https://www.cnas.org/publications/reports/technology-roulette

204   Belfield, Jayanti & Avin (2020).

Afterword

SJ Beard

This book was written as part of the 'Science of Global Risk' programme at the Centre for the Study of Existential Risk. The aim of this programme is to develop, implement, and refine a model systematic approach to addressing how global catastrophic and existential risk can best be identified, understood, managed, and mitigated. Many of the chapters it contains originated in sessions of an international conference hosted as part of this programme in 2020, which sought to survey the diversity of work already being undertaken in this field and position the centre's distinctive research in a constructive dialogue with a far wider community of researchers, decision-makers, and activists who were concerned about global risk.

The first five chapters of this volume developed arguments in relation to the study of global risk as an open and engaged field of academic study. Chapter 1 described how this study has long roots stretching back into the 20th century and beyond and has already made a number of significant contributions to making the world safer. Chapter 2 surveyed a range of methods that have been used to model the risks and causes of social and environmental collapse, and the directions in which these are currently being developed. Chapter 3 considered different approaches to the governance of risky scientific research and technological development, arguing for the importance of bottom-up— as well as more traditional top-down—approaches to this. Chapter 4 looked at how groups and individuals are contributing to the current level of global risk, and showed how the present reality of profound global injustice plays an important role in this causation. Finally, Chapter 5 looked at the increasingly important issue of diversity and inclusion,

  https://doi.org/10.11647/OBP.0336.11

and argued that within the field of global risk this is not only a pressing issue of justice and equity, but also of safety and resilience. Together, these chapters show how, even as it deals with unprecedented extreme future risks, our science can remain rooted in the real world and the realities of the here and now.

Building on these foundations, the remaining five chapters looked at a range of risk drivers (in 'Science of Global Risk' we often prefer to talk about individual risk drivers rather than individual risks, for the reasons I set out below). Chapter 6 looked at 'natural' risk drivers such as volcanoes and asteroids, and argued that even if these have anthropogenic causes, the current level of risk that we face is significantly determined by human-made vulnerabilities and exposures to such hazards. Chapter 7 considered more traditional anthropogenic environmental risk drivers, such as climate change, and argued that these undoubtedly contribute to the level of global risk, but that the traditional framing they have received in global risk research may be doing more harm than good with respect to our aim of understanding and addressing this. Chapter 8 provided a survey of recent developments in biotechnology with the potential to contribute to global risk, both positively and negatively, and argued that by enhancing existing science governance tools and mechanisms and introducing new risk management frameworks, these can be rendered far safer and more beneficial. Chapter 9 provided a contemporary history of thinking in the rapidly advancing field of AI safety, highlighting the shift away from safety concerns anchored only in the theoretical capabilities of AGI systems and towards thinking about the many challenges of aligning transformative AI with human society and human values. Finally, Chapter 10 considered the military use of AI, and argued that in recent years too much attention in this field may have been paid to the role of lethal autonomous weapons, and not enough to the connection of AI to nuclear weapons.

In their own way, each of these chapters shows us how this developing science is changing the way we understand and manage risks for the better by broadening the perspective of global risk researchers away from the most immediate hazards towards complex risk assessment, which also accounts for key vulnerabilities, exposures, and risk cascades, while still remaining relevant, and action guiding, to the most urgent problems facing humanity.

Together, then, these chapters highlight a field undergoing significant transformation and development. In previous work I have argued that this represents a natural result of previous developments in this crucial area of research.[1] While scholarship on global catastrophic and existential risk in the first decade of the 21st century was often marked by shared ethical and epistemological assumptions (such as commitments to utilitarianism, transhumanism, and Bayesian reasoning) that formed a coherent 'first wave' of research, a growing awareness of the scale of the challenges currently facing humanity—and a desire to harness additional resources to resolving these—led to a period of rapid expansion through the century's second decade. This saw the establishment of many new centres of research (including the Centre for the Study of Existential Risk itself) and the growth and development of existing centres through the generous support of committed funders. However, this in turn brought about a 'second wave' characterised by a far weaker set of assumptions and a growing desire to make research engaging for a wider audience, and to highlight the most urgent research and mitigation priorities. Yet, this second wave of research could never have been an end in itself, and as the field has continued to mature, its diversification and growth have brought in new research paradigms that may not only be based around different founding assumptions than those of previous waves of research, but also seek to articulate distinctive alternatives to the work that was already produced by them. This includes highlighting the importance of bottom-up as well as top-down governance mechanisms, global injustice as well as utilitarian efficiency, natural and environmental risk drivers as well as technological ones, and the importance of engaging with researchers who may not be personally committed to reducing global risks but whose work can nevertheless aid in this common endeavour.

Some key aspects of this emerging 'third wave' of research include a move from studying the aetiology of specific existential and global catastrophic risks (plural) to studying the interconnected drivers of existential and global catastrophic risk (singular); identifying the conditions and contexts within which risk is emerging and through which it can be managed; and working with experts from other disciplines, traditions, and cultures to achieve these aims. It is thus typified by the diversity of viewpoints on issues like how to classify risks, what the best methods for studying them are, and how to evaluate different possible outcomes. However, in exploring this greater diversity, scholars who contribute to this third wave have often coalesced around the complexity of risk as a phenomenon that emerges from systems characterised by non-linear changes and feedback loops. This marks a shift away from focusing on the direct impacts of existential hazards to considering humanity's vulnerabilities and exposure to indirect and cascading impacts as well.

These are also the themes that come up time and again in the preceding chapters, from arguing that AI risk needs to be understood via the interrelation of AI with human systems or that asteroids and volcanoes are far more dangerous than they might be because of the design of critical infrastructure, to appealing to the value of engaging with existing models for studying social and environmental collapse or the need to understand individual motivations through the lens of global injustice. However, more than this, these themes can also be seen in how these issues sit in dialogue with each other, drawing on and developing different aspects of science governance, international security, environmental breakdown, and other complex phenomena to produce a systemic approach to identifying, understanding, managing, and mitigating global risk. Above all, I would argue that the sheer disciplinary diversity present in not just the authors and editors who have contributed to this volume (ranging from technical AI experts, engineers, and life scientists, to complex system modellers and volcanologists, to economists, lawyers, and philosophers, to the director of the Bulletin of Atomic Scientists and NASA's Planetary Defense Officer) but even more so to the almost astronomical diversity of works cited by them, encompassing almost every field of human knowledge in one form or another.

Of course, my way of thinking about the history of the science of global risk is by no means universally shared, and others have articulated different understandings of the field and its development.[2] However, to take the long view of our own long-termism—and begin to see this field as something that has a history, and even a sociology, behind it, as well as to recognise that the field is undergoing processes of development and change in sometimes contradictory directions—is itself a new and important idea that can help us to understand the work that we do and how to improve it. And while I would not wish to foist such views on anyone, I sincerely hope that reading this book will have helped anyone interested in global risk to have improved not only their understanding of this risk, but also of how it is studied, how it can be reduced, and what role they might be able to play in achieving this goal.

Notes and References

1   Beard, S.J. and Phil Torres, *Ripples on the Great Sea of Life: A Brief History of Existential Risk Studies* (2020).

2   E.g. Moynihan, Thomas, *X-Risk: How Humanity Discovered Its Own Extinction*. MIT Press (2020); Cremer, Carla Zoe, and Luke Kemp, 'Democratising Risk: In Search of a Methodology to Study Existential Risk', *arXiv preprint arXiv:2201.11214* (2021).

Contributor Biographies

SJ Beard is an Academic Programme Manager and Senior Research Associate at the Centre for the Study of Existential Risk. They work across CSER's research projects, including foundational research on the ethics of human extinction; developing methods to study extreme, low probability, and unprecedented events; understanding and addressing the constraints that prevent decision-makers taking action to keep us safe; and building existential hope in the possibility of safe, joyous, and inclusive futures for human beings on planet earth.

They have a PhD in Philosophy and an MSc in Philosophy and Public Policy from the London School of Economics. As well as research, SJ has extensive experience across politics and policy-making, including as a researcher in the UK parliament, think tanks, and NGOs. They have taught moral and political philosophy and provide mentorship and supervision through Magnify Mentoring and the Effective Thesis Project.

Rachel Bronson is the President and CEO of the *Bulletin of the Atomic Scientists*. She oversees the publishing programmes, management of the Doomsday Clock, and a growing set of activities around nuclear risk, climate change, and disruptive technologies. Before joining the *Bulletin,* Bronson served as the vice president of studies at the Chicago Council on Global Affairs and taught "Global Energy" at the Kellogg School of Management. Prior to moving to Chicago, she worked at the Council on Foreign Relations, the Center for Strategic and International Studies, Harvard University's Belfer Center for Science and International Affairs, and Columbia University.

Rachel's writings have appeared in publications such as *Foreign Policy, Foreign Affairs, The National Interest, The New York Times, The Washington Post*, and *The Chicago Tribune*. She has appeared as a commentator on numerous radio and television outlets, including National Public Radio, CNN, Al Jazeera, the *Yomiuri Shimbun*, "PBS NewsHour," and "The Daily Show." She has also testified before the congressional Task Force on Anti-Terrorism and Proliferation Financing, Congress's Joint Economic Committee, and the 9/11 Commission. Her book, *Thicker than Oil: America's Uneasy Partnership with Saudi Arabia*, was published by Oxford University Press.

John Burden is a postdoc working at the Centre for the Study of Existential Risk and Leverhulme Centre for the Future of Intelligence. His work focuses on developing robust evaluation frameworks for AI systems in order to properly understand these systems' capabilities and limitations, as well as identifying links between an AI system's capability, generality, and the risks the system poses.

John has a background in Computer Science, having completed his PhD at the University of York, as well as holding a master's degree from Oriel College, Oxford.

Sam Clarke is the Strategy Manager at the Centre for the Governance of AI in Oxford. He researches actionable questions related to AI governance field-building strategy. He has a background in computer science and philosophy, and previously worked as an AI governance researcher at the University of Cambridge.

Nancy Connell is a Senior Scientist in the Board on Life Sciences at the US National Academies of Science, Engineering, and Medicine (NASEM). Trained in microbial genetics at Harvard, Dr Connell's work has focused on advances in life sciences and technology and their application to a number of developments in the areas of biosecurity, biosafety, biodefense and the responsible conduct of science. She has had a long-standing interest in the development of regulatory policies associated with biocontainment work and dual-use research of concern. Dr Connell is a past member of the Board on Life Sciences and currently serves on the Committee on International Security and Arms Control. She is a National Associate of NASEM, where she has served on more than 15 NASEM committees. Among other national and international committees, she served on the US National Science Advisory Board for Biosecurity. Dr Connell was Senior Scientist at the Johns Hopkins Center for Health Security and Professor in the Department of Environmental

Health and Engineering at the Johns Hopkins Bloomberg School of Public Health from 2018–2021. From 1992–2018, Dr Connell was an investigator in microbial genetics and drug discovery at Rutgers New Jersey Medical School (NJMS), finishing her long career there as Professor in the Division of Infectious Disease and Director of Research in the Department of Medicine.

Di Cooke is a Research Affiliate at the Centre for the Study of Existential Risk and a Tech Policy Fellow at the Center for Strategic and International Studies.

Douglas Erwin is a Senior Scientist and Curator at the National Museum of Natural History and an External Faculty member at the Santa Fe Institute. A paleontologist and evolutionary biologist, his research topics involve the end-Permian mass extinction and recovery, the early evolution of animals and the evolution of gene regulatory networks. He has just completed a book on evolutionary novelty and innovation.

Lindley Johnson graduated from the University of Kansas in 1980 with a BA in Astronomy and a commission from Air Force ROTC. He also has an MS degree in Engineering Management from the University of Southern California. He is now assigned to NASA Headquarters Science Mission Directorate, Planetary Science Division, as the Lead Program Executive for the Planetary Defense Coordination Office and the NASA Planetary Defense Officer, tasked with warning and response to any potential impact of Earth by an asteroid or comet. Prior to NASA he served twenty-three years of Air Force active duty, obtaining the rank of lieutenant colonel and numerous military awards and decorations while working on a variety of national security space systems.

After joining NASA in 2003, he was the Program Executive for NASA's Deep Impact mission to comet Tempel 1, launched in January 2005 to deliver an impact probe to the comet's surface on July 4, 2005, and explore the composition and interior structure of comets. He then served for eight years as the Lead Program Executive for the Discovery Program of mid-class Solar System exploration missions. NASA's Near-Earth Objects Observations programme has discovered over 19,000 near-Earth asteroids and comets since Lindley became its manager, over 87% of the total known. Lindley has received NASA's Exceptional Achievement Medal for his work on comet and asteroid missions.

Asteroid 5905 (1989 CJ1) is named "Johnson" to recognise Lindley's efforts in detecting near-Earth objects.

Natalie Jones is a Policy Advisor on Sustainable Energy Supply at the International Institute for Sustainable Development (IISD), where she conducts policy advocacy, aiming to influence governments and international institutions on phasing down oil and gas production in a just and equitable manner. Natalie is also an Affiliated Researcher at the Stockholm Environment Institute (SEI). Natalie was previously a Research Associate at the Centre for the Study of Existential Risk, where she worked at the intersection of global justice and global catastrophic risk, with a particular interest in climate change. Her projects included: elaborating the conceptual linkage between global justice and global catastrophic risk; assessing indigenous peoples' collective right to participate in global governance; and exploring how countries discuss fossil fuel production in their national communications under the Paris Agreement.

Prior to joining CSER, Natalie completed a PhD in international law at Trinity College, Cambridge and worked as a research assistant at the Lauterpacht Centre for International Law. She co-founded and was secretariat Co-Coordinator for the All-Party Parliamentary Group on Future Generations. Natalie holds an LLM in international law from the University of Cambridge, and an LLB(Hons) and BSc in physics from the University of Canterbury. Alongside her academic work, she writes for IISD's *Earth Negotiations Bulletin*, the de facto history of multilateral environmental negotiations.

Luke Kemp is a Research Affiliate with the Centre for the Study of Existential Risk (CSER) and Darwin College at the University of Cambridge. His research focuses on the deep history and future of catastrophic risks. He has advised the Australian Parliament on ratifying the 2015 Paris Agreement on climate change and has a decade of experience in international environmental negotiations. His work has been covered by media outlets such as the BBC, *The New York Times*, and *The New Yorker*. He holds both a doctorate in International Relations and a Bachelor of Interdisciplinary Studies with first class honours from the Australian National University. Luke is currently writing a book on societal collapse and transformation (*Goliath's Curse*) which will be published with Penguin in 2024.

Kelsey Lane Warmbrod is a Research Analyst specialising in biological and chemical weapons nonproliferation at Pacific Northwest National Laboratory, USA. Her work primarily focuses on improving national and global security by maximising the benefits of life science research while minimising risks to safety and security in an equitable manner. During the COVID-19 pandemic, Warmbrod was seconded to the World Health Organization to support their response to the pandemic. Warmbrod worked at the Johns Hopkins Center for Health Security, where she led projects on biological attribution, the bioeconomy, and the governance of life science research. Prior to Hopkins, she worked at Oak Ridge National Laboratory in the National Security Sciences Directorate, contributing to projects concerning the security of chemical, biological, radiological, and nuclear material. Lane is currently pursuing a PhD in public health genetics at the University of Washington.

Dr Kobi Leins (GAICD) is an Honorary Senior Fellow of King's College, London; Advisory Board Member of the Carnegie AI and Equality Initiative; Member of Standards Australia as a technical expert on the International Standards Organisation's work on AI Standards; Affiliate, ARC Centre of Excellence for Automated Decision-Making and Society; and former Non-Resident Fellow of the United Nations Institute for Disarmament Research.

Leins provides strategic advice on selection, implementation, and operation of technologies to drive business edge; creates systems for organisational and delegation of ownership for complex systems and data; and uses international benchmarking to analyse opportunities and risks in face of rapidly changing legal and governance landscapes and data literacy and public sentiment.

Leins has previously managed programs and teams in administrative law and justice, humanitarian law, human rights law, and disarmament with the UN and the International Committee of the Red Cross and worked in two different university faculties of Engineering and Computer Science.

Leins is the author of *New War Technologies and International Law: The Legal Limits to Weaponising Nanomaterials*, Cambridge University Press (2022). Further publications can be found at kobileins.com.

Kayla Lucero-Matteucci works jointly for Cambridge's Centre for the Study of Existential Risk and Leverhulme Centre on the Future of Intelligence, with primary interests in anthropogenic risks from climate change and artificial intelligence. She spent six years in the nuclear policy field, with prior experience as a Fulbright Scholar working with the UK Foreign and Commonwealth Office, as well as at the Carnegie Endowment for International Peace and Sandia National Laboratories. As a 2021 Marshall Scholar, she completed graduate studies at the University of Cambridge in Politics and International Studies and at the University of East Anglia in Climate Change and International Development.

Matthijs Maas is a Senior Research Fellow in Law and AI at the Legal Priorities Project and a Research Affiliate at the Centre for the Study of Existential Risk (CSER), University of Cambridge. His work focuses on mapping theories of change for the governance of advanced, transformative AI; different international institutional designs for AI, the effect of AI on international law, and arms control regimes for military uses of AI technology. Matthijs received his PhD in Law from the University of Copenhagen.

Lara Mani, PhD, is a Senior Research Associate at the Centre for the Study of Existential Risk, University of Cambridge, UK, where her research seeks to understand the efficacy of various communication methods and strategies for gaining traction for the mitigation and prevention of global catastrophic risks. Lara's work also focuses on volcanic risk and particularly on the global risks posed by large magnitude eruptions and their cascading impacts.

Martin Rees is the UK's Astronomer Royal and a Crossbencher in the House of Lords. He is based at Cambridge University where he is a Fellow (and former Master) of Trinity College. He is a former President of the Royal Society and a member of many foreign academies. His research interests include space exploration and cosmology. He is a co-founder of the Centre for the Study of Existential Risks at Cambridge

University (CSER), and has served on many bodies connected with education, space research, arms control, and international collaboration in science. In addition to his research publications he has written many general articles and ten books, including, most recently, 'On the Future: Prospects for Humanity', 'The End of Astronauts', and 'If Science is to Save Us'.

Catherine Richards has 15+ years of experience at the intersection of real assets, emerging technology, and sustainability. During her time at CSER (2020–2022), where she co-edited this book, Catherine's research developed our understanding of global risks, governance mechanisms and technical solutions in relation to complex critical infrastructure systems, largely focused on environmental risks, future foods biotechnology, digital twins, and artificial intelligence.

She is now working as a management consultant at a top tier firm. Previously, Catherine developed strategy for a climate tech start-up. She dabbled in novel materials and real estate constructions while completing her PhD(Eng) at Cambridge on energy transition, climate change and agri-food supply chain risk. Prior to that, she was an engineer at a top Fortune 500 company in the energy sector and government corporation in the water sector, the latter while completing her BEng(Civ) and BEng(Env) at University of Newcastle, Australia. Catherine has multiple publications in top academic journals, including the Nature portfolio; is a John Monash scholar; and was recognised in Forbes' 30 Under 30 for Industry Innovation.

Clarissa Rios Rojas is a science diplomat, a government science advisor and, currently, a Research Associate at the Centre for the Study of Existential Risk (University of Cambridge), where she works at the interface of science and policymaking. Clarissa researches the risks coming from emerging technologies and also builds science-policy interfaces that can provide scientific evidence and advice to different policy stakeholders (public sector, businesses and civil society).

Clarissa has worked closely with different international organisations building programmes for women's economic empowerment (UN Women), writing white papers on policy for economic transformation and frontier risks (WEF's Future Councils), collaborating on the production of reports on Foresight (G20, WHO), leading Science

Government Advice workshops (Global Young Academy/INGSA), and mentoring scientists in the Global South (UN's Biological Convention Program), among others. She is also an expert advisor for the OECD (on Global Catastrophic Risks), the UN Secretary-General's High-Level Advisory Board (on Effective Multilateralism), the UK parliament (bill on Future Generations), and the UNDRR (new scientific agenda for the Sendai Framework). Her website is: www.clarissarios.com/.

Sabin Roman is a Research Associate at the Centre for the Study of Existential Risk who works on the long-term modelling of societal evolution; having developed models for the historical dynamics of Easter Island, the Maya civilization, the Roman Empire, and Imperial China. He employs methods from dynamical systems theory, network science, stochastic processes, agent-based modelling, and machine learning. He has a background in mathematical physics, with a master's degree from the University of Edinburgh. He obtained a PhD in Complex Systems Simulation from the University of Southampton, where his research focused on the mathematical modelling of societal collapse.

Lalitha S. Sundaram is a Senior Research Associate at the Centre for the Study of Existential Risk who works in the area of bio-risk, with a particular emphasis on regulation and governance. She investigates risks—real or perceived—surrounding emerging biotechnologies such as synthetic biology and their convergence with artificial intelligence. Before joining CSER, Lalitha worked within the University of Cambridge and Edinburgh's Arsenic Biosensor Collaboration where she developed strategy to take this novel synthetic biology product from bench to field, focusing regulation and Responsible Research and Innovation (RRI).

Following this, she held a fellowship at King's College London investigating the opportunities and challenges facing emerging biotechnologies seeking to tackle global health challenges. Lalitha's PhD research, also at the University of Cambridge, used a combination of bioinformatic, next-generation sequencing and molecular biology tools to explore host-cell metabolic and microRNA changes following infection by the pathogenic parasite Toxoplasma gondii.

Sheri Wells-Jensen is the 2023 Baruch S. Blumberg NASA/Library of Congress Chair in Astrobiology, Exploration, and Scientific Innovation and an Associate Professor in the Department of English at Bowling Green State University. A linguist with research interests in phonetics, braille, language creation, and disability studies, her early work on the potential for non-physically mediated language acquisition (by AI or other non-human beings) led to an ongoing interest in ethical issues related to space exploration, as well as disability issues in space travel. Her current research centres on increasing access for people with disabilities in space including participation on the leadership board of Mission: AstroAccess, a project that promotes disability inclusion in space.

Sheri has presented at the Amazon Disability Month Presentation Series, the Potomac Institute for Policy Studies, the Institutions of Extraterrestrial Liberty Conference, the NASA Ames Research Center, and the Social and Conceptual Issues in Astrobiology conference. Her work has been published in the *Journal of the British Interplanetary Society*, *Futures*, *Scientific American*, the *METI International Blog*, and *Rejoinder*. She received a BA in psychology and sociology from Adrian College, an MA in Spanish and applied linguistics from Southern Illinois University, Carbondale, and a PhD in linguistics from State University of New York, University of Buffalo.

Jess Whittlestone is Head of AI Policy at the Centre for Long-Term Resilience. She was previously a Senior Research Fellow and Deputy Director of the AI: Futures and Responsibility Programme at the Leverhulme Centre for the Future of Intelligence and the Centre for the Study of Existential Risk, both at the University of Cambridge. She holds a PhD in Behavioural Science from the University of Warwick and a master's in Mathematics and Philosophy from University of Oxford.

Index

23–24, 122, 288. *See also* Doomsday
   Clock
Butler, Samuel 3, 19, 202
Campaign for Nuclear Disarmament
   6–7, 57
Carson, Rachel 9, 22, 114, 122
cascade failures vii, 133–136, 140, 149,
   153, 165, 221, 263, 288
cascading risk 134
catastrophe viii, xiii–xviii, xx, 2–3, 5–6,
   10, 12–13, 17–20, 22–23, 25, 32–33, 38,
   44, 49, 58–59, 73, 75, 79–84, 88, 91–93,
   103, 105–106, 114, 123, 126–127, 129,
   131–136, 138, 140, 144–145, 147, 150–
   155, 157, 159–160, 162, 164, 167–170,
   182, 201, 212, 215–216, 219, 221, 229,
   237–242, 246, 249–252, 254–256, 260,
   266, 268, 271, 276, 278–279, 285, 287
causal loop diagram (CLD) 35–37
Centre for the Study of Existential Risks
   (CSER) x, xii, xiv, 15–16, 113, 118,
   165, 285, 287
ChatGPT 190
Chelyabinsk impact event 132, 136
chemical weapons 189, 252
Chemical Weapons Convention (CWC)
   175, 177
Churchill, Winston 56
Cirkovic, Milan xxi, xxiii, 242, 271
climate change viii, xi–xii, xvi–xviii,
   2, 8–9, 11–12, 22–23, 30, 32, 46, 48,
   54, 79, 82–93, 95, 97–99, 105, 112,
   115, 126–129, 140, 147–159, 161–164,
   167–172, 176, 286
climate cooling 128
Climate World Risk Index 85
cliodynamics 44, 46, 54
Club of Rome 10, 22, 42, 159, 170
Cohen, Stanley 61, 97
Coherent Extrapolated Volition (CEV)
   204–205, 230
Cold War 5–6, 14–17, 242, 257–261,
   281–282
collapse xiii, xiv–xv, 1, 9, 16, 22, 27–28,
   30–36, 38–48, 50–54, 82, 101, 125,

134–135, 145, 147–149, 154–159, 165,
   167–169, 251, 257, 276, 280, 285, 288
collective action xvi, 70–71, 74
Collingridge Dilemma 70
comets 127, 130–131, 138, 143
complexity xvii, 16, 18, 27, 30–32, 35–36,
   38–46, 51, 64–65, 70, 83, 109, 123,
   127, 133, 149, 151–154, 168–169, 174,
   183, 185, 188, 194, 198, 208, 213, 217,
   224, 226, 235–236, 239, 245, 257, 260,
   266–267, 286, 288
Comprehensive AI Services (CAIS)
   213, 233
COVID-19 viii, ix, 17, 71, 90, 95, 98, 103,
   134, 171, 181–182, 188, 196, 199
Cuban Missile Crisis 8, 17, 21
Cuvier, Georges 123
cyber attacks viii, 249, 264–266
cyber defence 244, 265
cyber security 264
cyber warfare 237
DALL-E 190, 210
defense 136, 138, 145, 247, 256, 269,
   271–272, 274–275, 278, 281–282, 284,
   288
Defense Advanced Research Projects
   Agency (DARPA) 243, 248, 255, 271
degrowth 159
Diamond, Jared 30, 47, 50
diminishing returns 38–39, 51
disability xvi–xvii, 101–113, 116–117,
   119, 121
diversity viii, xiii, xvi–xvii, 46, 58, 61,
   64, 69–70, 73, 101, 107–108, 110–111,
   116, 119, 124–125, 167, 176, 179–180,
   184, 186, 194, 211, 237, 244–245, 285,
   287–288
DIY-bio 65–66, 77
DNA 60–62, 75–76, 174–175, 178–179,
   186, 188, 195–196
Doomsday Clock xiv, 1–2, 5, 11–12,
   14–16, 19–20, 55, 191. *See also Bulletin
   of the Atomic Scientists of Chicago (The
   Bulletin)*
Double Asteroid Redirection Test
   (DART) 137, 139, 243, 271

About the Team

Alessandra Tosi was the managing editor for this book.

Rosalyn Sword performed the copy-editing and proofreading.

Lucy Barnes indexed the book.

Jeevanjot Kaur Nagpal designed the cover. The cover was produced in InDesign using the Fontin font.

Melissa Purkiss typeset the book in InDesign.

Cameron Craig produced the paperback and hardback editions. The text font is Tex Gyre Pagella; the heading font is Californian FB.

Cameron produced the EPUB, AZW3, PDF, HTML, and XML editions — the conversion was made with open-source software such as pandoc (https://pandoc.org/), created by John MacFarlane, and other tools freely available on our GitHub page (https://github.com/OpenBookPublishers).

This book need not end here...

Share

All our books — including the one you have just read — are free to access online so that students, researchers and members of the public who can't afford a printed edition will have access to the same ideas. This title will be accessed online by hundreds of readers each month across the globe: why not share the link so that someone you know is one of them?

This book and additional content is available at:
https://doi.org/10.11647/OBP.0336

Donate

Open Book Publishers is an award-winning, scholar-led, not-for-profit press making knowledge freely available one book at a time. We don't charge authors to publish with us: instead, our work is supported by our library members and by donations from people who believe that research shouldn't be locked behind paywalls.

Why not join them in freeing knowledge by supporting us:
https://www.openbookpublishers.com/support-us

Follow @OpenBookPublish

Read more at the Open Book Publishers **BLOG**

You may also be interested in:

Transforming Conservation
A Practical Guide to Evidence and Decision Making
William J. Sutherland (ed.)

https://doi.org/10.11647/OBP.0321

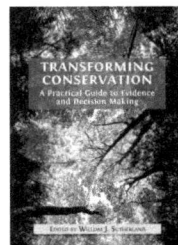

Negotiating Climate Change in Crisis
Steffen Böhm and Sian Sullivan (eds)

https://doi.org/10.11647/OBP.0265

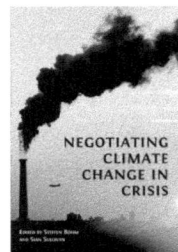

Earth 2020
An Insider's Guide to a Rapidly Changing Planet
Philippe Tortell (ed.)

https://doi.org/10.11647/OBP.0193

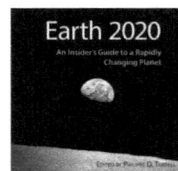

www.ingramcontent.com/pod-product-compliance
Lightning Source LLC
Chambersburg PA
CBHW070842300326
41935CB00039B/1348